Deafness in Mind

Working Psychologically with Deaf People across the Lifespan

Dedicated to my family: Dennis, Laelia, Rob, Fay and Steve Austen.
Sally

Dedicated to the memory of my father, which enables me to put life into perspective; and to my family, who support me in the belief that 'everything is possible'.
Susan

Deafness in Mind

Working Psychologically with Deaf People across the Lifespan

Edited by

SALLY AUSTEN

Consultant Clinical Psychologist, National Deaf Services,
Queen Elizabeth Psychiatric Hospital, Birmingham

and

SUSAN CROCKER

Clinical Psychologist, Nuffield Hearing and Speech Centre,
Royal National Throat Nose & Ear Hospital, London

W

WHURR PUBLISHERS
LONDON AND PHILADELPHIA

© 2004 Whurr Publishers Ltd
First published 2004
by Whurr Publishers Ltd
19b Compton Terrace
London N1 2UN England and
325 Chestnut Street, Philadelphia PA 19106 USA

Reprinted 2005

British Library Cataloguing in Publication Data

A catalogue record for this book
is available from the British Library.

10-digit ISBN 1 86156 404 X (P/B)
13-digit ISBN 978 1 86156 404 7 (P/B)

Typeset by Adrian McLaughlin, a@microguides.net
Printed and bound in the UK by Athenæum Press Ltd, Gateshead, Tyne & Wear.

Contents

Contributors

Twanette Acker has worked as a Paediatric Speech Therapist and Audiologist both in South Africa and England for the past 12 years. She is currently working in the Tygerberg Hospital/University of Stellenbosch Cochlear Implant Unit, Cape Town, South Africa.

Sally Austen is a Consultant Clinical Psychologist and has worked with d/Deaf people for over ten years. She is employed by Birmingham and Solihull Mental Health Trust and works at Denmark House, National Deaf Mental Health Service, Birmingham.

Joanna Atkinson is currently training as a Clinical Psychologist at Bristol University, and is employed by Taunton and Somerset NHS Trust. She previously worked for three years as a Research Psychologist in the Deaf Stroke Project team at City University, London.

Nigel Beail is a Clinical Psychologist working in Learning Disabilities in Barnsley and is also a part time clinical lecturer at Sheffield University.

Emma Coleman is an Advocacy Worker with Deaf people with mental health problems at Birmingham Citizen Advocacy, an independent voluntary organisation. Emma has previously worked as a Psychology Assistant within National Deaf Mental Health Service, Denmark House, Birmingham.

Andy Cornes is a Clinical Social Worker and Co-ordinator of the Psychological Health and Deafness Service at the Rivendell Adolescent Unit, Thomas Walker Hospital, under the Central Sydney Area Health Service.

Susan Crocker has worked as a paediatric Clinical Psychologist at the Nuffield Hearing and Speech Centre, Royal National Throat, Nose and Ear

Hospital for eight years. She is also Lead Clinical Psychologist at the Donald Winnicott Centre, Child Development Service for Hackney and the City of London.

Jim Cromwell is a Clinical Psychologist at National Deaf Services, London.

Bruce Davidson has worked as a Registered Mental Nurse in National Deaf Services, London for 7 years. For the past two years he has worked as a Clinical Case Manager for the Deaf Enhanced Support Team – an Assertive Outreach service for Deaf people with Severe Mental Illness.

Margaret du Feu is a Consultant Psychiatrist at Denmark House, National Deaf Mental Health Service, Birmingham and Solihull Mental Health Trust.

Lindsey Edwards is a paediatric Clinical Psychologist working at Great Ormond Street Hospital on the Cochlear Implant Programme, and also provides a Clinical Psychology service to the Ear Nose and Throat speciality within the Hospital.

Janet Fernando is Head of Psychotherapy for National Deaf Services, South West London and St George's Mental Health NHS Trust, London. She is a member of the Lincoln Clinic and Centre for Psychotherapy.

John Graham is a Consultant Otologist, and Director of the Cochlear Implant Programme at the Royal National Throat, Nose and Ear Hospital, London.

Alison Gray is a Consultant Psychiatrist with Denmark House, National Deaf Mental Health Service, Birmingham with an interest in rehabilitation, spirituality in psychiatry and mental health promotion. She is an honorary visiting fellow at the University of Leicester.

Mary Griggs completed a PhD in Deafness and Mental Health in 1998. Following several years at the Centre for Deaf Studies, University of Bristol, she is currently a trainee Clinical Psychologist in Bristol.

Sally Hind has worked as a Developmental Psychologist at the Institute of Hearing Research, Nottingham University for ten years.

Sylvia Kenneth worked at National Deaf Services, London, as a Health Care Assistant. Currently she is training to become a Registered Mental Nurse.

Nick Kitson was formerly Consultant Psychiatrist and Clinical Director, National Deaf Services, London. He is currently an adult general psychiatrist in Cornwall.

Cathy Lynch is an Audiological Scientist specialising in cochlear implantation. She has worked in several implant programmes including the Royal National Throat, Nose and Ear Hospital in London and currently the Emmeline Centre for Hearing Implants, Addenbrooke's Hospital, Cambridge.

Jane Marshall trained as a Speech and Language Therapist and is currently working as a Senior Lecturer in the Department of Language and Communication Science, City University, London.

Helen Miller is a Consultant Adult Psychiatrist at the National Deaf Services, London.

Jemina Napier is Research Fellow and Co-ordinator of the Auslan Interpreting Program in the Linguistics Department at Macquarie University, Australia. She is also an Adjunct Lecturer at Renwick College, University of Newcastle, and works freelance as an Auslan/ English interpreter.

Sue O'Rourke has worked in mental health and deafness for 15 years. She is Head of Clinical Psychology at Mayflower Hospitals, Manchester, which is a medium secure unit for Deaf people.

Emma Sands is a paediatric Clinical Psychologist at Guy's Hospital and at the Audiology Service, St. Thomas' Hospital, London.

Elizabeth Stone Charlson was for several years a Research Psychologist at the Department of Psychiatry, Center on Deafness at the University of California. Currently she is on the faculty of the Department of Child and Adolescent Development, San Francisco State University.

Alice Thacker trained as a Speech and Language Therapist and is currently a Senior Lecturer in the Department of Mental Health, St George's Hospital Medical School, London.

Bencie Woll is a linguist. She co-founded the Centre for Deaf Studies at Bristol University and has been Professor of Sign Language and Deaf Studies in the Department of Language and Communication Science, City University, London, since 1995.

Preface

Deafness in Mind has come about as the result of both my frustration at, and my enthusiasm for, the field of mental health and deafness.

When I returned to mental health and deafness after a period of working with hearing populations, I was frustrated at how little the published evidence base had grown in my absence and felt moved to begin to address the problem myself. I was also dismayed that little seemed to have been achieved in terms of preventing the development of mental health problems in deaf people:

- many deaf people are still reaching adulthood with issues of language deprivation, literacy problems, abuse, neglect and isolation that inevitably contribute to mental health problems;
- resources are still focused on treating the severely mentally ill rather than on primary mental healthcare provision or prevention;
- adult services still work in isolation from the child, family and education services, despite evidence that the majority of adult problems are rooted in childhood experience;
- the needs of deaf people with additional disabilities are still not sufficiently addressed;
- resources are still provided on the assumption that delivering services to deaf people can be achieved with the same time and money as treating hearing people.

However frustration fuels action and, with the encouragement of some amazing people throughout my career, my enthusiasm for my job as a clinical psychologist and for my speciality has thrived. I am glad to have the opportunity in this book to address these issues. I would like to take this opportunity to thank those whose influence on my career made the idea for this book possible: Sue O'Rourke, Nick Kitson, Chris Gilleard, Liz Charlson and Mary Plackett.

I am not generally short of ideas but they are ineffective by themselves. The difference between the idea and the reality of this book would not have been possible without the phenomenal intellect, pragmatism and humour of my co-editor Susan Crocker. We started the book as colleagues and finished it as dear friends; to her I give my greatest thanks. Her child and family clinical experience together with my adult experience informs a lifespan perspective on deafness that, while working together on this book, has enhanced the understanding of us both.

We are both extremely grateful to those that have contributed chapters of such a high standard to *Deafness in Mind*. We hope that you, the reader, are as enthused by reading this book, as we were in writing it.

Sally Austen

Introduction

Deafness in Mind is unique in its comprehensive application of psychological models to work with deaf people. Contributors to this book are mainly from the field of clinical psychology, although other aspects of psychology, psychiatry, medicine, speech and language therapy and audiology are represented.

This text applies evidence-based psychological practice to children, adults and older adults affected by deafness, by referencing peer reviewed research and current government developments.

In Part 1, 'Introducing deafness', opens with a description of some of the more controversial debates within the d/Deaf world and the reader is invited to consider subsequent chapters from each of these opposing standpoints. The medical, audiological and screening processes for deafness are outlined, and highlighting audiological and socio-political differences between people who are born Deaf and people who become deaf.

Throughout the book we use the terms deaf and deafness to represent all levels of hearing impairment from mild to profound. We have respected the standard way of identifying those who associate themselves with the Deaf community and who use a manual language by using a capital 'D' for the word Deaf. People who become deaf, who do not associate themselves with the Deaf community, and those who use predominantly oral skills are represented with a small 'd' when using the word deaf. Where no statement of identity or type of deafness is required, then the word deaf will have a small 'd'; where some importance is implied by the heterogeneous inclusion of all people of all types of deafness and identity then the label 'd/Deaf' is used. Where individual authors have used a different nomenclature they have included an explanation of this at the beginning of their chapter.

Deafness refers to an auditory phenomenon that tells us little about a person's psychological state or their identity. Even with the distinctions of

'Deaf' and 'deaf', many people do not fall neatly into these two categories, nor would they describe themselves in these ways. Furthermore, categorization is certain to evolve over time to encompass changes in society in general and changes specific to d/Deaf people. For example, the closure of Deaf schools and increase in mainstream education, technical advances such as cochlear implants and digital hearing aids, and increasingly early diagnosis of deafness as a result of neo-natal hearing screening, are all likely to blur the boundary between deaf and Deaf. Developments in medical science are resulting in fewer people being born deaf from causes such as ototoxicity or rubella. Other deaf people are surviving medical conditions, for example, prematurity and CMV, where previously they may have died. Changes in the demographics of the deaf population in the UK are also brought about by increased immigration of people from cultures where inoculations are less common, resulting in diseases where deafness may result, or from war torn countries where people are at risk of noise related hearing loss. Thus, this book attempts to unpack the needs of d/Deaf people regardless of culture, race, language, intellectual ability, life experience and so on.

In putting together the content for *Deafness in Mind*, we made the decision not to discuss culture, race and working with diversity separately, as we hope that each chapter deals with these aspects of clinical work within the wider structure and thinking within each topic area.

In Part 2, 'Psychological models applied to deafness', the proponents of different psychological models are challenged to apply their theory to deafness, with fascinating results. Although on the surface the systemic, psychodynamic, cognitive-behavioural and neuropsychological models may appear to contradict each other, an eclectic approach to the understanding of psychology and deafness can only benefit the d/Deaf client. Indeed, our understanding of the very definitions of mental illness used are challenged in the 'Deaf Wellness Explored' chapter, which provides a more sociological standpoint from which to consider the later chapters.

Anecdotally, the editors of *Deafness in Mind* had a sense that political correctness surrounding the d/Deaf world had resulted in deaf people's additional needs going unnoticed and therefore unresourced. It seemed that, as a back lash to the history of discrimination that deaf people experience, and in an overzealous attempt to promote deaf people as 'normal', the description of deaf people's needs have been restricted to their linguistic and cultural difference. In this book we have asked each contributor to be cognisant of the effects additional disabilities (physical, sensory, neuropsychological or developmental) have on a significant proportion of the deaf population. Here we look at the evidence, and consider ways of working that look at the whole person, in order to assess and work effectively alongside the d/Deaf client's wishes and with their informed consent.

In Part 3, 'Deafness and mental health', incidence findings and evidence-based practice form the backdrop for development and provision of both child and adult services. By including both child, parent and adult data, *Deafness in Mind* allows the reader to consider the transition through the ages and what effect, if any, the high levels of additional difficulties in children, particularly neuropsychological difficulties or language deprivation, have on the incidence and presentation of mental health problems in d/Deaf adults. By extrapolating from what is known about hearing people, the impact of psychosocial experiences on the prevalence of certain experiences, specifically schizophrenia and substance use disorders, are considered.

Also, the role of the psychologist in cochlear implantation and the role of the sign language interpreter in psychological therapies are both discussed and the need for inter-disciplinary working highlighted in both.

Finally, in Part 4, 'New developments in psychology and deafness', this book brings forth new developments in the field of mental health from a psychological perspective. Contributors whose work has focused on specific aspects of mental health and deafness share their ideas. Many of the chapters have formed part of PhD work and all are of an extremely high academic standard. Given that our clients' only commonality is their deafness, it is necessary that we consider the links between Psychology and other specialities. Thus, the links exemplified here with forensic services, training, neuropsychology, adult mental health and psychosomatic medicine are welcomed.

In writing any book, there are invariably areas that cannot be covered due to size restrictions. Here we are aware that those people who are deafened, have a progressive hearing loss or have a mild to severe hearing impairment are less well represented than adults and children whose deafness is profound. Also certain topic areas, such as education and mental health services for deaf children are not covered in this book. This is not an oversight, rather we hope that from the way the book is presented, readers will be able to infer and make links from the material to other age groups or clinical areas. Thus, the book is designed to be read as a whole. To avoid too much repetition, authors have been encouraged not to elaborate on points that are covered in more depth in other chapters.

Although the field of mental health and deafness is relatively small, there is a disproportionate lack of evidence-based written material available nationally and internationally. There seem to be two main reasons for this. Firstly, research in the field is extremely difficult, with few measures, tests or questionnaires having been validated for use with deaf people. Measures can lose validity and reliability when translated into sign language or are invalidated by being presented in written form, as the median reading age of the Deaf adult is less than 9 years. Furthermore, there are only a small number of professionals working with d/Deaf people each of whom has to prioritize the shorter term clinical needs of their clients over the longer term research needs.

The second reason for the dearth in evidence-based material is that professionals often consider that they only have something to offer if they have a set of skills specific to deafness. The premise of this book is that to work with specific client groups as a psychologist, a clinician needs to have an underlying framework for thinking, which can then be applied practically. This text moves away from the idea that clinicians require a whole new set of skills in order to work with deaf people. We all work in a range of settings, with differing client groups and across the life span. By applying robust scientific practice in the form of psychological models, all clinicians can apply their skills in the area of deafness. Likewise the needs of the deaf individual and the family can be understood in the specific context of the client group. Knowledge of sign language and of deaf culture is, of course, beneficial but it would be wrong to equate the understanding of mental health and deafness with the ability to sign only.

We have been pleased to have the opportunity to add to the psychological understanding of mental health and deafness evidence base, and we are extremely proud of the standard of the chapters that have been contributed by our colleagues and peers. We hope that 'Deafness in Mind' encourages the reader in their work with their d/Deaf clients and that its scientific rigour sets a benchmark for the application of psychological theory to future publications.

Susan Crocker
Sally Austen

PART 1
INTRODUCING DEAFNESS

CHAPTER 1

Controversy in deafness: *Animal Farm* meets *Brave New World*

SALLY AUSTEN AND EMMA COLEMAN

Introduction

Within the field of deafness and psychology there is much that is referred to as 'politics'. In this context 'politics' refers to areas of controversy that appear to be emotively rather than scientifically debated. This strong emotion has, in part, been fuelled by d/Deaf people's historical sense of oppression by hearing people and this will be described in two parts: broadly pre-twentieth century and post-twentieth century. It is not possible to do justice to the complexity of each debate. Thus, the aim of this chapter is briefly to identify the areas of controversy to (a) inform readers of the issues that have current import and (b) assist them to consider the subsequent chapters and other d/D literature objectively. Where possible, quotations and case examples from those directly affected by each situation have been documented.

Medical model versus Deaf culture

Wherever there is political disharmony you will usually find a dichotomy, the medical and cultural models of deafness being no exception. In attempting to convey the information simply it is inevitable that one perpetuates dichotomous descriptions. We would urge the reader to consider the multitude of positions that exist between any of the extremes described in this chapter. Throughout this chapter we will differentiate between the two broad groupings of deaf people by the lower or upper case letter 'D': lower case 'd' to refer to those people who regard their deafness as a disability and capital 'D' for those who see their deafness as a cultural choice.

Medical model

The 'medical model' holds that deafness is a disability that should be corrected where possible. In its pure form this model supports the use of assistive devices such as hearing aids and cochlear implants, oral education and integration into mainstream (hearing) society.

People who have had, and then lost, hearing are likely to regard themselves as having a disability and to regard being hearing as preferable to being deaf. They may need to grieve the loss of their hearing and of associated abilities. They are likely to refer to themselves as hearing impaired, hard of hearing or deafened. This group is likely to have lost hearing postlingually.

Cultural model

Alternatively, members of the 'Deaf community' would regard deafness as a normal human variant or a lifestyle choice and may react defensively to suggestions that they are disabled. They tend to be prelingually or congenitally Deaf and use native sign languages. They regard themselves as a linguistic and cultural minority, whose problem is not lack of hearing so much as the attitude of the hearing majority, most of whom do not sign.

Referring to themselves as Deaf with a capital letter 'D' they tend to be part of the Deaf community. Although there are occasional attempts to eradicate the distinction between Deaf, deaf and deafened, such that all are included in the same grouping, there is often strong exclusivity in the Deaf community. For those included, the Deaf community is thought to provide a sense of belonging, social support, and an ease of communication, which might not be available from their own families where language barriers are common (90% of deaf people have hearing parents).

Within the Deaf community it would be less common to find people who thought that being hearing was superior to being Deaf. Carver (1995) states his opinion that there are 'rich alternatives to being hearing' and that deaf children can expect to lead fulfilling lives without having to depend largely on their sense of hearing.

Baker and Padden (in Siple:1978) describe the Deaf community as

> . . . individuals who share a common language, common experiences and values and a common way of interaction with each other and with hearing people. The most basic factor determining who is a member of the deaf community seems to be what is called 'attitudinal deafness'. This occurs when a person identifies him/herself as a member of the deaf community and other members accept that person as part of the community.

Are Deaf people disabled?

Using the old World Health Organization (WHO) (1980) categories it might seem that the Deaf argument – that they are not disabled – is somewhat flawed. Although it is true that it may be society's attitudes and lack of sign language prowess that 'handicaps' them, this does not mean that they are not disabled by their lack of hearing. If the whole world signed, they would still be disabled by the inability to hear environmental sounds such as oncoming traffic and fire alarms. The Deaf view may, however, be that disability is a relative term, varying with the accessibility of new technology such as flashing doorbells and online interpreting services that reduce both handicap and disability (although not impairment). Proponents of the cultural model would point to the description of the population of Martha's Vineyard USA between the seventeenth and nineteenth centuries (Croce, 1985). The islanders had an unusually high proportion of genetic deafness and Croce describes a situation where deafness was considered virtually normal and where 'everyone here spoke sign language'. The newer WHO definitions (2002) of impairment, activity and participation were presumably developed to address just such contentions, but have not yet been widely used. In these definitions, activity (or limitation of activity) is assessed while allowing for the use of assistive devices. Thus, those with maximally functional hearing aids, interpreter or technological assistance may not be limited in their activity.

> I find the Deaf obsession with distancing themselves from disability an insult to people who have disabilities. Personally, I would say that deaf people are disabled and that there is nothing wrong with being disabled. (Hearing female health professional)

Hodges and Balkany (in Cotton and Myer, 1999) highlight the paradox of people who claim not to be disabled but who claim state disability allowances. Although their argument makes semantic sense, this view may suggest paternalism, i.e. willingly offering help to only those who agree to accept the majority's labels. However, the claim to the label of linguistic minority may be questioned as those from other countries who have not yet learned the majority language do not claim disability benefits. Furthermore, the true linguistic minorities have the capacity to learn the majority (spoken) language whereas Deaf people may not.

A further paradox is that, whereas limited English skills are true of the majority of Deaf people, a significant minority are not profoundly deaf, could function with spoken English as their first language, but choose not to. Most states support the provision of appropriate minority language services where the person is unable to communicate in the majority language. However, we would guess that few would be willing to go to the expense of offering such services where the person was perfectly fluent in the majority language and was merely expressing a language preference for cultural reasons.

Hodges and Balkany (1999) quote the California Department of Rehabilitation (Harris, Anderson and Novak, 1995) study that associates deafness with the lowest education levels, the lowest family income and the highest unemployment, as evidence that deafness is a disability. The Deaf community would probably regard the same data as evidence of the poor access for Deaf people to the education system and their rejection by the hearing majority: a fault they would see as perpetuated by the medical model that promotes the, in their opinion, unsuccessful oralist education.

> Some Deaf people believe they are not disabled but still collect disability benefits. This is not hypercritical but highlights the flaws within the system. I view DLA (Disability Living Allowance) as 'shut up money'. In a truly inclusive society everyone with any contact with Deaf people, including our doctors, would be able to sign or anticipate our need for an interpreter. Why should we have to do our own admin. and pay other people wages because the state has failed to provide us with the full access we are entitled to? DLA is accepted on a 'shut up and don't complain' basis: viewed by some as 'compensation' for the injustices we endure on a daily basis. (Deaf female)

Few writers challenge the dichotomies present in the study of deafness: possibly because of ignorance, possibly for fear of appearing politically incorrect. Refreshingly compromising, Peters (2000) describes deafness as 'a serious but addressable disability which as far as we can tell, uniquely among disabilities, results in a true culture, one unified primarily by its complete and independent language system . . .'

The oral/manual debate

It is hard to imagine a longer running or more emotionally fuelled debate in the history of education, than that of the oral/manual debate in the education of Deaf children. A simple disagreement, some think education of Deaf children should be conducted via speech, lip-reading and residual hearing; some think it should be conducted via sign language. Although the content of the debate is simple, the reasons for its existence are complex.

History of the 'oppression' of Deaf people: part I

In order to work psychologically with d/Deaf people it is important to have an understanding of the cultural, historical, political and sociological perspectives affecting their lives. Just as to begin to understand the conflict between warring factions in Ireland one must go back to Oliver Cromwell, in the Deaf world one must go back to Hitler, Alexander Graham Bell, the 1880 Milan Conference on Education and way beyond.

In 1880, the Milan Conference for the education of deaf people effectively banned the use of sign language in schools. In many parts of Europe, including the UK, this ruling still affects the implementation of the curriculum. There are still many schools where children are punished for signing and many people, particularly those who are older, still experience a sense of shame or stigma for using sign language. Alexander Graham Bell's infamy concerns his reference to the deaf as 'a defective variety of the human race' and his work to develop the first hearing aids. To the deaf he is a liberator; to the Deaf he is an oppressor. Bell's work and attitude fuelled the oral movement and encouraged a belief that, with enough dedication, all deaf children could learn to function entirely orally and could integrate into hearing society.

Many Deaf people regard the 'obsession' with hearing as being the cause of an unhappy and ineffectual education, sacrificed to the aims of speech and hearing therapy. Throughout history, education and health policy has been influenced by the belief that signing to children will prevent them from acquiring oral skills. However, a significant proportion of professionals now believe that signing improves general language skills, which in turn improves the acquisition of English skills. There is now a growing trend for teaching sign language to hearing babies to improve their communication. It does seem ironic that hearing babies have access to sign whereas deaf babies do not.

> The Milan 1880 Conference was one of the worst things ever to happen to Deaf people. It amounts to linguistic and educational experimentation, and thus is abuse. Milan still affects us now – we only need to look at today's standards of so-called Deaf 'education' to see that the decision made in 1880 was WRONG. (Deaf female)

On the other hand, supporters of oralism would say that being part of a hearing world is inevitable, that signing will not help with this and that children should receive as much oral/aural habilitation as possible if they are to integrate successfully into mainstream society. They believe that signing should be used as a last resort and that with early diagnosis and effective aiding, most children can learn strategies to cope in a mainstream environment. They may see signing as an indicator of having failed in the 'superior' oral system.

In 2003, British Sign Language was recognized as an official language by the UK government. Bilingual schooling is therefore becoming more acceptable, but advocates of signing or oralism often struggle to compromise and research still tends to focus on each end of the pendulum.

Mainstream versus specialist schools

The arguments concerning integration versus congregation are much the same in deafness as in other fields. The argument for integration says that d/Deaf children deserve the same education as hearing children, that extra provision should be provided in mainstream schools to make this possible and being 'the same' as hearing peers will enhance self-esteem. The argument for specialist schooling points to the different language needs of d/Deaf children and says that integration can be a very isolating experience: whether the child communicates orally or signs, there will never be enough resources to make children feel truly involved and they will have very few people with whom they can communicate fully. The two sides agree on the need for a peer group to enhance self-esteem but proponents of specialist schools consider one's 'true' peers to be other d/Deaf children and that integrated schooling only serves to negatively highlight the child's differences.

Within education, research seems to influence policy less than does rhetoric. The median reading age of profoundly prelingually deaf school leavers is low, at less than 9 years (Conrad, 1979). Advocates of specialist schooling or mainstream integrated schooling each blame the other for the poor results. Similarly, each blames the relatively low self-esteem, unemployment and increased mental health problems on the other.

Parents' choices

Advice to parents of newly diagnosed d/Deaf children has been at best mixed and confusing and at worst charismatically directive. In the past, many parents were told not to sign to their children and some believe this has resulted in language deprivation for thousands of d/Deaf people. The provider of the information holds power and influence that they may not consciously misuse. The aim, for example, of the neo-natal hearing screening described in a later chapter is to provide d/Deaf children with resources to develop their language skills from early on in life, in whichever mode of language and schooling that the parents choose. However, at a time when the child is being screened for medical difficulties, possibly in a hospital that provides cochlear implants, within a health service that employs few Deaf people, it may be difficult for hearing parents to see their child's deafness as anything other than a disability. Despite attempts to counsel the parents about the other options, it may be that choice is skewed and that an oral route is determined from the moment of diagnosis.

It also seems that parents are often provided with choices based on only one theory at a time and are not shown the bigger picture. For example, late diagnosis of deafness can lead to language delay so the neonatal screening programme looks to address this. However, like so many attempts to redress past errors, the pendulum swings to the other extreme and aims to diagnose in the first few days of life. Although the option for parents to improve their child's language opportunities is positive, to some extent the historical position of speech at any cost has been replaced with a language at any cost mission statement. The consequence of such early diagnosis on parental mood, bonding, acceptance of the child and family dynamics are not yet known, so the parents cannot consider this information while deciding whether and when to have their child screened.

The 'postcode lottery' of service provision further restricts parental choice: integrated or specialist, oral or signing will depend on where you live, the philosophy of the education service near you and the services to which you are entitled.

Hodges and Balkany (in Cotton and Myer, 1999) describe how some Deaf people would argue that hearing parents of deaf children do not have the right skills and experience to make decisions for their children and that the Deaf community should be given this role. The argument would follow that since 90% of deaf children are born to hearing parents, that these children belong more to the Deaf community than they do to the parents, and thus the Deaf community should make the decisions on such issues as schooling, language and cochlear implantation. However, the ethics, medical and legal worlds state that, whether the parents are deaf, Deaf or hearing, only they have the right to make such decisions. There are times when all sides (the deaf, Deaf and hearing) seem to regard the others as incompetent to make decisions on behalf of d/Deaf children. An increase in the number of d/Deaf professionals may help bridge some of the gaps between the Deaf and hearing worlds.

Deafness and genetics

People say we are playing God. But if we don't play God, who will?' (Watson, 2003)

There are at least 400 types of hereditary deafness that account for 50% to 60% of moderate to profound prelingual deafness (Arnos, 2002). While those who see deafness as a disability are working hard to make use of the human genome project to eradicate deafness, those who are concerned for the demise of the Deaf community are considering its use in maintaining prelingual deafness. Each side of the debate is shocked by what it sees as the inhumanity of the other's position: Deaf people believing that

hearing people wish them personally exterminated; hearing people thinking that afflicting deafness on others is barbaric.

History of the 'oppression' of Deaf people: part II

Hitler is, of course, the most famous proponent of eugenics, but he was
not the first by any means. By the time Hitler came to power in 1930s
Germany, the Americans, in particular, had been practising eugenics for
some time. It is the beliefs and actions of such groups that fuel much of
the suspicion and defensiveness of today's Deaf community. Eugenics
describes the attempt to manipulate the gene pool to maximize the func-
tionality of future generations. This term has become associated with
oppression, particularly as a result of forcible sterilization, which was
widely used in the USA in the 1930s; both sterilization and extermination
being used by Nazi Germany during the 1930s and 1940s (Schou, 1934;
Wiethold, 1934; Boestroem, 1935). Throughout history, deaf people have
been advised or forced not to mate (or even to meet) in order to prevent
the creation of a deaf baby.

The end of the twentieth and the beginning of the twenty-first centuries
saw the human genome project map the genetic make-up of humans so
that it is now possible to pinpoint some of the genes that lead to hereditary deafness. This opens up two possible routes for genetic selectivity:
abortion of the foetus or selection of embryos prior to in-vitro implantation. Watson (2003) is very clear that he hopes the human genome project
will serve to eradicate any state of being that burdens the rest of society.
Deafness, seen as a disability or seen in tandem with its oft-times associated disabilities or relatively poor socio-economic functioning, could fall
into this category. At its most sophisticated, the aim of genetic engineering
would be to have the people who would otherwise be deaf to be hearing;
the less sophisticated would be for them not to exist at all.

> Biotechnology poses an enormous challenge to the Deaf community.
> Decisions about the use and regulation of genetic technologies relating to
> deafness do not just affect future generations of Deaf people, they say some-
> thing about the value we place on Deaf people's lives today. Such decisions
> will determine the kind of society we live in – a society that seeks relent-
> lessly to assimilate minorities, or a society that celebrates difference and
> diversity. (British Deaf Association, Genetics Policy Statement)

Watson emphasizes his difference to the Nazi regime in that he regards
eugenics as the choice of the parents and not the state. He may not have
considered that some Deaf parents, given the opportunity, may use
eugenics for the procreation of Deaf children. Some Deaf people would
very much like to have Deaf children with whom they will share their

culture and language. Genetic counsellors are obliged to provide an objective service, providing information but not influencing the parents' choices. They may soon be in a situation where they are required to support Deaf parents in excluding hearing embryos or aborting hearing foetuses – aborting babies on the grounds only that they are entirely healthy (Arnos, 2002). Despite Watson's assertion that eugenics should be a choice offered to parents, it seems likely that the state will become involved in such significant decisions, particularly in countries such as Britain where the state would be financing much of it (foetus selection as part of IVF, selective abortion, sperm or egg donation and so on).

Caplan (1995) predicted that this would be an issue but few took it seriously until 2002 when a Deaf lesbian couple made international headlines for deliberately choosing a five-generation Deaf man as the sperm donor for their second baby to ensure it was born Deaf (Savulescu, 2002). Although their first 'designer' Deaf baby (fathered by the same man) had gone unnoticed by the press, this conception raised discussion of the ethics of selecting in or selecting out deafness, and selection generally, in virtually every living room in the western world.

Cochlear implant

Few medical interventions are associated with such controversy as the cochlear implant. Welcomed to restore hearing to the deafened, and relatively unhelpful for adults who were prelingually deafened, the implantation of born deaf children has fuelled fierce objection from factions of the Deaf community, and equally fierce defence from the audiological professions.

Deaf extremists see cochlear implants as a combination of eugenics to eradicate deafness and the Deaf community, and the harmful obsession with oralism that reduces people to an audiological measurement. Demonstrators opposed to implants, particularly of young children, have picketed numerous cochlear implant conferences. Demonstrators outside the Seventh International Cochlear Implant conference quoted the deaths through meningitis of implantees as evidence of the 'murderous tendencies' of the cochlear implant surgeons (Anon, 2002). (Summerfield and Graham (2003) presented research at the British Cochlear Implant Group in April 2003 refuting the direct link between cochlear implants and meningitis related deaths.) Some Deaf people who are against implants liken the attempt to correct deafness through surgery as similar to attempting to 'correct' an Afro-Caribbean person's blackness through surgery. Peters (2000), although supportive of Deaf culture, thought this argument irritating, illogical and unhelpful.

Those enlisting a more academic opposition to cochlear implants say that there is not enough evidence that they are useful or that they are not physically or psychologically harmful (Pollard, 1993; Lane and Bahan, 1998; Peters, 2000; Moores, 2002). It is pointed out that the research quoting the success of implantation is mostly funded by cochlear implant companies who often only include their most successful users in their research samples and leave out non-users (those who had an implant but stopped using it). They point out that if the cochlear implant companies are to survive financially they need to implant Deaf children. There is suspicion that the neonatal hearing screening programmes fit conveniently with the implant company's need to implant increasingly younger children and babies. However, there are many who are confident that evidence does show implants to be useful and safe (Knutson, 1988; NIH, 1995; Hodges and Balkany, 1999).

Balkany and Hodges (1995) say that activists are misleading the Deaf community with misinformation and inflammatory, illogical rhetoric using terms such as 'genocide' and 'child abuse'. They quote the low reading age of the average Deaf school leaver as evidence that a small elite is able to control the interpretation and distribution of complex information to many Deaf people. (However, it should be added that misinformation can also be provided by both d/Deaf and hearing people in support of cochlear implants.)

The opposition's attempts to be conciliatory often state that implantation should be postponed until children are old enough to give consent themselves. The small number of Deaf people employed in the audiological field means that few Deaf people are aware that the window of opportunity for children to develop speech and hearing is restricted to the first few years of life. Likewise, few Deaf people would know that after meningitis, ossification of the cochlea can occur, such that delay may render implantation impossible.

> The Deaf community views the use of surgery which prevents a child from developing within the [Deaf] cultural minority to be a form of genocide prohibited by the United Nations Treaty on Genocide. Cochlear implants of young healthy deaf children is a form of communication, emotional, and mental abuse. (Canadian Association of the Deaf, press release, 25 January 1994)

Both sides of the debate accuse the other of exploiting vulnerable parents of deaf children, the Deaf community to ensure its survival and the medical profession and implant manufactures in search of power or profit.

The continuation of the Deaf community

Davis (in Graham and Martin, 2001) says that because of increasing survival, the number of hearing-impaired people is likely to rise by 20% in the next 20 years. Despite this, extremists of the Deaf community see all oralism, mainstreaming, cochlear implants and genetic engineering as potential threats to their existence, leading to the eradication of deafness, sign language or both. The end of the Deaf community was also predicted with the advent of radio aids but it never happened (Laurenzi, 1995). Some agree that there will be fewer deaf people, particularly as many will have cochlear implants and that as such, the Deaf community will shrink. Others point to the attitudinal membership requirements of the Deaf community and hypothesize that more hearing, partially deaf people and implant users (who will still be deaf) will be welcomed as a means of maintaining numbers.

Peters (2000) reports that some Deaf activists argue that cochlear-implanted children will be ostracized by the Deaf community, but that he regards this as 'nothing other than cultural terrorism'. Although there is anecdotal evidence that people with implants have been ostracized, there is also evidence that the community is beginning to assimilate beliefs that one can be both implanted and Deaf (Hodge, Barman and Walker, 2002). Laurenzi (1993) reminds us that cochlear implants are not a 'cure' for deafness and blames the media for fuelling this myth by sensationalizing stories of its benefit.

Many cochlear implant teams are now supporting the use of sign language for their implantees (although in some cases, it may be seen only as a temporary aid to spoken language and not as a persistent language of equal worth). There is a growing lobby that says that children will attain better spoken and aural language skills if they have good general language skills (Heiling, 1995). This lobby reasons that in the absence of – or during the post-implant wait for – meaningful sound recognition, that sign is a useful way of developing general language skill. However, there are still teams that work on the premise that an oral only approach increases performance after cochlear implant.

Victim-perpetrator

As with many political dichotomies, the group that considers itself to be oppressed often replicates the behaviours of the group it considers oppressive. In therapy this is referred to as the 'victim-perpetrator split'. Thus, a common response to the reality or the sense that sign language is being oppressed is to ban the use of speech. Those Deaf parents, such as the Deaf lesbians mentioned earlier, ensured genetically that their child was Deaf, but some Deaf parents also decide that their child should be linguistic and culturally Deaf. In such scenarios children are given neither cochlear implants nor hearing aids and parents protest that the child can choose for themselves to use such devices when old enough to consent. Without early oral/aural input however, this child will not truly be able to choose between speech and sign, as the option to develop any useful speech will have gone. Thus, in extreme cases, we see the desire to maintain sign language in the family resulting in not only the banning of other languages, but the parents making it biologically impossible for the child to use speech. Whereas understandably the Deaf community express disgust that schools used to make children sit on their hands to prevent signing, the irreversibility of this biological language enforcement is tantamount to cutting out a Deaf child's tongue so that they cannot learn to speak. Bertling's 1994 autobiography pulls no punches in his assertion that his oral skills and residual hearing were sacrificed in the name of Deaf culture.

Cultural terrorism

What Peters (2000) referred to as 'cultural terrorism' is also responsible for an extremely strong tendency to 'out grouping'. This refers to how a group will exclude people in an attempt to have a strong sense of identity in its 'in group'. As a result a lot of deaf people are 'fence deaf': they sit between the Deaf and deafened worlds with no community to support them. Profoundly prelingually deaf people who communicate orally, those who have good speech or who are highly intelligent, and those with additional disabilities may be excluded or ostracized. In some situations those who have hearing parents will be excluded, in favour of the 'proper', genetically Deaf. The historical sense of being excluded by hearing society is replicated in the Deaf community's exclusion of those they consider 'others'. Where some deaf people can experience the stress of having to 'pass' in a hearing world (Breakwell, 1986), some may also experience stress in having to 'pass' in the Deaf world.

Homogeneity

Consideration of the desire to ensure the continuation of the Deaf community reminds us that Deaf people are not a homogenous group. Some Deaf people come from families where deafness is the norm, many generations of relatives having been Deaf. Maintaining something that is 'normal' makes semantic sense. It may be that, for the purposes of both debate and research, a distinction should be made between those who have genetic deafness and are from a Deaf family, those who have genetic deafness and are from a hearing family and those who have deafness that is acquired either prelingually or postlingually.

The Deaf community does not appear to encourage the continuation of the Deaf community through adventitious deafness. For example, there is no movement to ban inoculations for rubella or encourage children to listen to extremely loud music. Thus, it may be more useful in future studies to focus in on which aspects of deafness within Deaf culture are really valued and which are being lumped together incorrectly in the rhetoric of politic debate. It may be that the Deaf lesbians, who were happy with the birth of their genetically deaf baby, may have had a different reaction to having a hearing baby who was then deafened prelingually through rubella or postlingually through meningitis.

Culture

It seems to be an accepted fact that a shared language has an important role in passing on culture. However, the continuation of the culture is not dependent on the exclusion of all but one language. Minority languages and cultures, such as Welsh in Great Britain and French in Canada, are maintained without restricting access to the majority language. This is achieved by respecting both languages, emphasizing the positive aspects of the minority language and ensuring regular access to both.

Interestingly, Aoki and Feldman (1991) showed statistically that for the survival of sign language (and presumably therefore the Deaf community) it is essential that hearing people pass on sign language. They show that the majority of deafness is caused by the recessive as opposed to the dominant genes and that a likely scenario is that a deaf generation will be followed by a hearing generation. If this hearing generation does not pass on sign to the subsequent deaf generations then the language will be lost from that family. Ironically, the 'enemy' of the activists, the hearing people, may be the very people who ensure the survival of the Deaf community.

Politics versus science in mental health and deafness

As with most opposed factions, the Deaf world and the audiology world share little common ground. Relatively few Deaf people are employed in the field of audiology, and audiological professionals are rarely invited to give their views to the Deaf community. Thus, the debates are often fuelled by ignorance and fear on both sides: 'd/Deaf politics' gets the better of 'd/Deaf science'.

However, the world of mental health and deafness seems to have embraced Deaf culture in a way that medicine has not, and that education has, though only recently. Unfortunately however, 'embracing' an issue is very different from being cognisant of that issue, and an over concern with political correctness can lead to subjectivity and therefore to poor science.

The chair of the World Federation of the Deaf (WFD), a political body, was given a platform for a keynote speech at the Sixth Conference of the European Society of Mental Health and Deafness (ESMHD), a scientific body in May 2003. The chair of the WFD reported that 'no deaf group in the world is fighting for better hearing' and went on to link all good experiences that Deaf people have had to the use of sign language and all bad experiences – including terrorism – to oralism. Such bold and untested statements are common in minority groups that have fairly recently started to assert themselves. However, it cannot be so usual to have eminent research and clinical scientists in the audience, applauding such rhetoric.

> In a reversal of the perceived oppressive/hostile or simply ignorant/uncaring attitude of hearing society, there are some hearing individuals, either professionals or lay members of the public, who embrace the Deaf 'cause' with semi-religious fervour.

> I have observed hearing adults who've found they have a flair for sign language, latch on to Deaf people and try to immerse themselves in the Deaf Community – it's as if they're drunk on deafness. (Hearing female professional)

Additional difficulties

At a clinical level the idea that all bad comes from oralism and all good from sign language leads to a belief that all a Deaf person's difficulties and the solutions to these are associated with communication mode. This can result in the Deaf person's additional disabilities being missed or untreated. There is no benefit for the patient if the culture of 'they are just deaf' of 80 years ago (when Deaf people were commonly considered stupid and were afforded no resources) moves to a culture of 'they are just Deaf' (meaning that all this person needs is sign language) as they will still not be afforded extra resources. The authors have seen patients whose learning disabilities, social deprivation, physical health problems and mental health problems have gone undiagnosed and untreated as a result of political correctness among professionals.

Fear of labelling

Starting work in Deaf mental health services, the first sign that the first (hearing) author was taught was 'bad attitude'. It seems that the fear of being accused of having a 'bad attitude' to deafness is similar to the fear of being labelled as 'racist'. Although it is crucial that we all work towards equality across diversity, it is also important to note that the Deaf people who have the power to hand out the damning labels to hearing people are also the people who have been previously discriminated against by hearing professionals. It would therefore not be unexpected for a Deaf person to unconsciously 'project' or attribute discriminatory beliefs, thoughts or feeling onto the hearing person.

The fear of being labelled seems to paralyse the hearing professionals' capacity to be objective, or to follow up concerns in the same way that they would if working with hearing people. At the ESMHD conference mentioned earlier, the representative made a statement on the ESMHD's position on cochlear implantation, saying that 'the European Society of Mental Health and Deafness neither rejects nor supports cochlear implantation': a statement of avoidance rather than scientific rigour or leadership. In a field where the cochlear implant has been associated with every outcome from miracles to child abuse and murder, the representative scientific body really should have an opinion. However, the fear of ridicule or attack seems to prevent scientific hypothesis and investigation.

> I think that some of the behaviours considered to be elements of Deaf culture are actually symptomatic of brain damage associated with the cause of deafness. But I couldn't research that: I'd get lynched. (Hearing male mental health professional at the aforementioned ESMHD conference)

Scientific rigour and the 'impostor complex'

Perhaps part of the motivation behind our lack of scientific rigour is that we are concerned that that same rigour may be used to assess our own practice. The 'impostor complex' refers to the sense that many of us have at times that we are not good enough and that our inadequacies will be found out. Specific to mental health and deafness we may be concerned that we have too few Deaf professionals, that our hearing staff's signing is not good enough and that we are often functioning from a position of little training and even less evidence-based practice. As a result of such concerns an atmosphere of collusion results. Unchallenged by Deaf people who have little access to our work or by our hearing colleagues (who are in awe of our ability to sign and relieved that they don't have to take responsibility for the Deaf people in their catchment-area), we are also able to, if not required to, refrain from challenging each other in order to maintain the status quo.

In the UK, a Department of Health (DoH) consultation document called the 'Sign of the times' (Department of Health, 2002) identifies that mental health services for sign language users often exist only as the result of the dedication of a few key individuals in specific geographical areas and is calling for co-ordinated and improved services. However, as the bulk of those consulted are the same few key individuals who are responsible for the existing services, new ideas may be limited. Whether this opportunity can be fully grasped will depend on whether, as scientists, we can *appraise* the various political views where others have *taken* the political view.

Conclusion

Whether hearing or d/Deaf oneself, in order to work effectively in the field of mental health and deafness, one must have an understanding of the social, political, economic and historical issues affecting d/Deaf people. Professionally our responsibility is to understand and implement strategies that maximize the mental wellbeing of d/Deaf people. There are a number of stormy debates raging. Emotive reasoning and sensationalist reporting makes the gathering of evidence-based information difficult and some professionals are reticent to assert science over politics. This is harmful to the clients whom we seek to serve.

Human nature seems bent on dichotomous reasoning, and extrapolated extremes are chosen to illustrate and justify debate. We have to some extent been guilty of this in this chapter. However, while some debates continue to swing from one extreme to the other, some have negotiated common middle ground.

In the second half of the twentieth century other battlegrounds of oppression and identity demonstrated that progress is possible, if not perhaps inevitable. Racial and ethnic groups have fought oppression but at the same time have themselves become more welcoming of diversity. Similarly the women's movement, starting with a somewhat uniformed fanaticism, has promoted a greater equality for women, and has gone on to embrace the opinions and support of a range of women and men. Equality of all people regardless of race, gender or ability is becoming a more commonly accepted goal.

Examples of oppression and language seem also to be taking a predestined route to co-existence. Languages such as Welsh or Guernsey Patois were discouraged in the early part of the twentieth century as they were seen to represent parochialism and were replaced with majority languages that represented progress. But progress was achieved at the expense of the sense of culture, history and identity that the minority languages enshrined and their resurgence, promoted by the state and by the individual, is being seen in many corners of the First World.

In the field of mental health and deafness we are likewise making progress to achieve common ground. British Sign Language has officially been recognized as a language (as has Cornish) and we have seen the qualification of the first deaf clinical psychologist in the UK. Previously oral schools are now allowing signing. People with cochlear implants and those with good oral skills are being welcomed into the Deaf community and d/Deaf youngsters have expectations of education to degree level and beyond. Ear, nose and throat surgeons are seeking the advice of Deaf colleagues and d/Deaf people are accessing more information about audiological issues. Hearing babies are being taught sign and the importance of language skills and psychosocial factors are being considered alongside the issues of speech and hearing.

Maximizing mental health is a journey, not a destination. Sometimes we seem to go backwards and sometimes we seem to stay in the same place or go round in circles. Hard as it is to remember in the face of such controversy as has been discussed here, debate is crucial to growth.

References

Anon (2002) The Dying Children: A 14-Year Coverup. Flyer handed out at the Sixth International Cochlear Implant Conference, Manchester, UK.

Aoki K, Feldman MW (1991) Recessive hereditary deafness, assortative mating and persistence of a sign language. Theoretical Population Biology 39: 385–72.

Arnos KS (2002) Ethical issues in genetic counselling and testing for deafness. In Gutman V (ed.) Ethics in Mental Health and Deafness. Washington: Galludet University Press, pp. 149–61.

Balkany TJ, Hodges AV (1995) Misleading the Deaf community about cochlear implantation in children. Annals of Otology, Rhinology and Laryngology 166: 148–9.

Baker C, Padden C (1978) Focusing on the non-manual components of ASL. In Siple P (ed.) Understanding Language Through Sign Language Research. New York: Academic Press.

Bertling T (1994) A Child Sacrificed to the Deaf Culture. Wilsonville OR: Kodiak Media Group.

Boestroem A (1935) Important decisions in the administration of justice in the court and higher court of eugenics. Fortschritte der Neurologie und Psychiatrie 7: 271–84.

Breakwell GM (1986) Coping With Threatened Identities. London: Methuen.

Caplan A (1995) Moral Matters: Ethical Issues in Medicine and the Life Sciences. Chichester: Wiley.

Carver R (1995) Cochlear Implants in Prelingual Deaf Children: a Deaf Perspective in Cochlear Implant and Bilingualism. Kimpton, Herts: Laser Publications.

Conrad R (1979) The Deaf School Child. London: Harper Row.

Croce NE (1985) Everyone Here Spoke Sign Language: Hereditary Deafness on Martha's Vineyard. London: Harvard University Press.

Davis A (2001) The prevalence of deafness and hearing impairment. In Graham J, Martin M (eds) Ballantyne's Deafness Sixth Edition. London: Whurr, pp. 10–25.

Department of Health (2002) A Sign of the Times – Modernizing Mental Health Services for People who are Deaf. www.doh.gov.uk/mentalhealth/signofthetimes

Harris JP, Anderson JP, Novak R (1995) An outcome study of cochlear implants in deaf patients. Archives of Otolaryngology, Head and Neck Surgery 121: 398–404.

Heiling K (1995) The Development of Deaf Children: Academic Achievement Levels and Social Processes. International Studies on Sign Language and Communication of the Deaf. Stockholm: Hamling Signum Press.

Hodge M, Barman P, Walker G (2002) Cochlear Implant Panel Discussion. Deafway II. Washington DC: Galludet University.

Hodges AV, Balkany TJ (1999) Controversies in cochlear implantation: ethical issues. In Cotton RT, Myer CM (eds) Practical Pediatric Otolaryngology. Philadelphia PA: Lippincott-Raven, pp. 315–27.

Knutson JF (1988) Psychological variables in the use of cochlear implants: predicting success and measuring change. Presented at NIH Consensus Development Conference May 2-4 Washington, USA.

Lane H, Bahan B (1998) Ethics of cochlear implantation in young children: a review and reply from a Deaf-World perspective. Otolaryngolgy, Head and Neck Surgery 119(4): 297–313.

Laurenzi C (1993) The bionic ear and the mythology of paediatric implants. British Journal of Audiology 27: 1–5.

Laurenzi C (1995) Cochlear implants and the British Deaf community. Journal of Audiological Medicine 4(2): ii–iii.

Moores DF (2002) Actions have consequences – cochlear implants: an update. American Annals of the Deaf 147(4): 3–4.

National Institute of Health (1995) Cochlear implants in adults and children. National Institute of Health Consensus Statements 13(2): 1–30.

Peters (2000) Our decision on a cochlear implant. American Annals of the Deaf 145(3): 263–7.

Pollard R (1993) Psychological risks in childhood cochlear implantation. Times Union (Rochester, New York). www.weizmann.ac.il/deaf-info/psych-risk.html

Savulescu J (2002) Deaf lesbians, 'designer disability', and the future of medicine. British Medical Journal 325: 771–3.

Schou HI (1934) Sterilization of the mentally ill and abnormal in Germany. Ugeskrift-foer-Laeger 96: 1125–6.

Summerfield Q, Graham JM (2003) Update on Meningitis Survey. Presentation to the British Cochlear Implant Group, Academic Meeting. Belfast, 4 April 2003.

Watson J (2003) DNA (television documentary). Channel 4 (UK), 30 March 2003.

Wiethold F (1934) The law on the prevention of hereditarily abnormal offspring. Kriminalistische-Monatschefte 8: 27–32.

World Health Organization (1980) International Classification of Impairments, Disabilities and Handicaps. Resolution WHA 29.35 of the Twenty-Ninth World Health Assembly, May 1976. Geneva, Switzerland: WHO.

World Health Organization (2002) Towards a Common Language for Functioning, Disability and Health: ICF. Geneva: World Health Organization.

CHAPTER 2

Newborn hearing screening: the screening debate

SALLY HIND

Introduction

The potential value of newborn hearing screening for the infant with permanent childhood hearing impairment (PCHI) has been a polemical issue since the techniques for neonatal screening and assessment became available. In the latter part of the twentieth century universal newborn hearing screening was introduced in specific states in the US, yielding data to enable systematic assessment of the impact of early identification on developmental outcomes. Data from the state of Colorado suggest a significant impact on the child's language development when PCHI is identified, and an appropriate intervention programme introduced prior to 6 months of life (Yoshinaga-Itano et al., 1998).

Although in a minority, there are professionals who consider that neonatal hearing screening is neither necessary nor desirable, and there are others, probably the majority, who believe wider psychological issues of early identification need addressing alongside technological and medical advances. This chapter will endeavour to present the arguments for and against implementing a newborn hearing screening programme. The author, a developmental psychologist, is the Information Coordinator for the Newborn Hearing Screening Programme (NHSP) in England. She believes the arguments in favour of introducing a sensitively designed neonatal hearing screening programme outweigh those against, and hence may stand accused of a biased presentation.

Criteria for national screens

Firstly, it is sensible to consider if a low incidence, non-life threatening condition with no systematic cure, warrants the introduction of a neonatal screening programme. This is especially pertinent given that a

21

universal infant hearing screen, the Infant Distraction Test (IDT), is already in place in the UK. However, there are serious problems with the IDT screen. It cannot be used with neonates; has poorer sensitivity and specificity; and is less cost-effective than the new screening techniques (Stevens et al., 1998).

The National Screening Committee in the UK has extended the original criteria for the practice of population screening originally proposed by the World Health Organization (Wilson and Jungner, 1968) to cover evidence-based effectiveness and concern about any adverse effects. All criteria need to be satisfied for a national screen to be implemented. Permanent childhood hearing impairment now meets all criteria.

An important criterion is acceptability by the target population. With neonatal screening, this must extend beyond the target population to include parents. Do parents want their baby's hearing screened at birth? Large scale surveys by Watkin et al. (1995) and Hind and Davis (2000) show the majority of parents of children with PCHI report they would prefer to know about a hearing impairment at or around birth. Hence, there is justification for introducing a newborn hearing screen programme (NHSP). The majority of professionals working with children who have PCHI also promote its introduction.

The author's conviction of the need for a nationally implemented NHSP grew primarily from experience with families of children with PCHI who reported having to 'fight' to get their children referred. These parents, typically the mothers, were commonly accused of being 'neurotic' by the primary care professionals they consulted. Data from the MRC Institute of Hearing Research's Trent Outcomes Study 'show a depressing picture of unnecessary and long delays' between parental suspicion of hearing impairment and diagnosis (Bamford et al., 2000). Reluctance to refer inevitably results in delayed diagnosis. The median age at diagnosis before the introduction of the NHSP in England was 20 months, across severity, rising to 35 months for a moderate hearing impairment.

How early should the screen be conducted?

From a clinical and family-friendly perspective, there is a relatively short window of opportunity for optimum screening of infants' hearing using available techniques. These require the baby to be settled, and preferably asleep, to expedite accurate outcome. As the child becomes more environmentally aware, screening becomes increasingly difficult to conduct. The earlier the child is referred for a hearing assessment, the more likely diagnosis can occur without recourse to sedation or anaesthetic. From a child- and family-friendly perspective this is desirable as, though very slight, sedation can carry risks. Hence it is preferable to conduct a full audiological assessment within a maximum of 4 weeks following a positive screen. Offering the hearing screen within a few days of life ensures sufficient opportunity, where necessary, for follow-up within the stipulated timeframe, and makes only limited demands on most families as clear responses are obtained at this stage for most babies.

There could be deleterious factors associated with a neonatal screen, however, which are considered by some to make the introduction of a NHSP unacceptable. The following section deals with some of the psychological processes associated with neonatal hearing screening and discusses objections to introducing a national programme.

The role of psychology in the screening process

Which psychological factors may affect the value of a newborn hearing screen and the parent's decision to have their baby's hearing screened? The potential positive impact of early diagnosis on the child's cognitive and language development is a major value (Yoshinaga-Itano et al., 1998). However, there may be psychological disadvantages to neonatal hearing screening and these are the main objections raised against introduction (see, for example, Bess and Paradise, 1994). The immediacy of a positive outcome (whether true or false) may affect parents in various ways. This section will deal with ways in which neonatal hearing screening could affect the parents and child adversely or positively.

Potential for stress or anxiety

Parents may become stressed or anxious by a positive outcome when the mother is still recovering from the physical and psychological effects of childbirth. De Uzcategui and Yoshinaga-Itano (1997) conducted a postal questionnaire survey of families in Colorado whose babies were referred for hearing tests. The response rate, typical for a postal survey, was low (34%). Hence it is necessary to be cautious when interpreting findings. Only 14% of the respondents reported a negative reaction to the programme, and 7% of them had children with confirmed hearing impairment. De Uzcategui and Yoshinaga-Itano concluded the majority of families do not experience lasting negative impact from newborn hearing screening. Generally parents reported that the process had a positive impact on their childcare, making them more aware of speech, language and hearing development. Identified weaknesses in the programme, which may have contributed to the negative reactions included (a) the way information and results were delivered; (b) the staff's ability to comfort parents, and help them to feel less angry, shocked or depressed; and

(c) understanding the needs of families whose first language is not English. They recommended increased training for those involved in the screening and testing process to provide a more sensitive programme.

Pipp-Siegel, Sedey and Yohsinaga-Itano (2001) studied parental stress of 184 mothers of children with PCHI. They found no significant association between age of identification and maternal stress, suggesting that any associated stress need not last long. Parents of children with PCHI had similar stress levels to a normative sample on the Parenting Stress Index (Abidin, 1995). Other studies (for example, Barringer and Mauk, 1997) found most parents were not greatly stressed by their experiences. Again the majority reported that the benefits of early detection outweighed any unnecessary stress experienced. One month following the hearing screen, Stuart, Moretz and Yang (2000) compared stress levels of mothers whose babies had clear responses with those of mothers whose babies had not. There was no significant difference in stress levels between the two groups. A study by Weichbold, Welzl-Mueller and Mussbacher (2001) asked 90 new mothers if newborn hearing screening should be performed despite the possibility parents become worried by false-positive results. The majority (84%) were in favour of screening.

Watkin et al. (1998) administered the State Trait Anxiety Inventory to two groups of mothers in a London hospital: one whose babies had received a positive hearing screen outcome in the first few days of life, and a control group whose babies had not had the screen. They found no significant difference in the anxiety state of the mothers.

Other studies exploring the impact of neonatal screens on parental concern or anxiety suggest various implicating factors, for instance number of assessments (see, for example, Vohr, Letourneau and McDermott, 2001; Owen, Webb and Evans, 2001), low parent education level, or being informed of outcome via telephone (see, for example, Tluczek et al., 1992). Owen et al. found the mean parental anxiety score (range 0–5) rose from 0.86 at first screen to 3.45 by audiology testing, but the screen was still well received by parents. Vohr, Letourneau and McDermott (2001) found similar effects, and identified socioeconomically disadvantaged mothers to be at greater risk. They propose a screening programme should aim to minimize false-positive rates, and to educate mothers about the screening process. Tluczek et al. (1992) found that parents who were informed of the follow-up test results for cystic fibrosis by telephone were more likely to have misunderstood the outcome and to have continued concerns with false positives.

Information from all these studies should be taken seriously when implementing a newborn hearing screen. The screen should be offered and, to facilitate informed choice, sufficient information should be provided in an accessible form – ideally, independent of level of parent's education. The protocol should limit the number of screening events, and results of any screen or hearing assessment must be given in person, using professional translators where necessary, with appropriate counselling and advice immediately available.

Therefore, from the available evidence, it would seem unlikely that neonatal screening is associated with long-term effects of stress or anxiety. The NHSP Evaluation Team will check this systematically in the short term. The Implementation Team will check it in the longer term. However, if anxiety arises in the short term, it could impinge on the parent–child relationship (see, for example, Avant, 1981). The next section will explore this issue.

Parent–infant relationship

Unless prewarned of a potential or real problem, most pregnant women and their partners expect to have a 'perfect' baby. Hearing impairment does not generally present overtly. Hence parents are initially misled into thinking there is nothing threatening the developmental potential of their baby. Anecdotally, some professionals argue for parents enjoying a few weeks in ignorance to enable them to develop a firm bond with their baby so they are in a stronger position psychologically to accept the condition when the diagnosis is made.

Some view the early days and weeks of life as important because this is when a life-enhancing parent–child bond is being formed (see, for example, Bowlby, 1988). One of the anomalies of a proposed critical period for attachment is highlighted by Trevathan (1987) with the acknowledgement that close attachment and a motivation to nurture can develop in adoptive mothers. Despite decades of study, there is no unequivocal evidence of the need for bonding to occur for healthy child development, but it is inadvisable to be complacent. It is possible a mother may reject her baby, at least in the short term, if a positive screen occurs, be it true or false. This needs to be considered when thinking of introducing any neonatal screen.

As stated earlier, the majority of parents of children with PCHI would prefer to learn of their child's hearing impairment at or around birth (Bamford et al., 2000). Hind and Davis (2000) conducted in-depth interviews with 100 of the responding families to explore the reasons for this response. Four main explanations were identified:

- the issue has to be faced at some point; the sooner it is accepted the better;
- knowing early permits dealing with the grieving process when the child is less likely to be affected;

- no unnecessary 'time is lost' in the child's development through ignorance, and
- there is more time to consider communication options, and learn
  about hearing impairment before important early developmental milestones are reached.

Hence, to all intents and purposes, it would seem appropriate to promote
newborn hearing screening. However with very early screening – before
48 hours of age – there is a greater possibility of false-positives. For false-
positive screens, the parent–infant relationship and interaction patterns
may be unnecessarily affected, which some report may have long-term
adverse effects for the child (for example, Cadman et al., 1984). A study
by al-Jader et al (1990) checking parental attitudes towards neonatal
screening for cystic fibrosis, report about 14% of parents acknowledge
temporary rejection of their babies during the follow-up period when
there was uncertainty, or following the procedures for diagnosis. It is
probable that some mothers who fear their child may be extremely ill and
could die at an early age may initially feel afraid to commit themselves
emotionally, but there is no unequivocal evidence that this happens.
Parsons et al. (2002) found neonatal screening for the life-threatening
condition, Duchenne Muscular Dystrophy, showed no evidence of long-
term disruption to the mother–baby relationship.

Hearing impairment is a very different condition to those mentioned
above as it neither creates illness nor limits life expectancy, and known
habiliative interventions exist. A Swedish study by Hergils and Hergils
(2000) on impact of neonatal hearing screening, concluded most of the
87 parents they questioned whose baby had been screened were reas-
sured by the newborn screen, and the risk of disturbing the parent–child
relationship seemed small.

Yoshinaga-Itano (2002) discusses the value of focusing on parental counselling and social-emotional factors as part of the habiliative programme for
parents of infants with PCHI. Such provision may facilitate more positive
parent–child interaction, which has been shown to be associated with
greater expressive language gain for the child (see, for example, Pressman
et al., 1999). The Department for Education and Skills (DfES), Department
of Health (DoH), and the voluntary sector are working together in England
to produce effective intervention programmes for babies identified through
the NHSP and their families, as part of the Early Support Pilot Programme.
This initiative aims to serve all types of disability in early infancy, and has
been awarded a substantial amount of government funding for the development, monitoring and evaluation of early intervention.

The intervention will be family- and child-centred and thereby potentially sensitive to specific needs of parents and will introduce

intervention aimed at ameliorating the impact on family function generally. It is possible some parents could experience undue stress or anxiety if screeners cannot obtain clear responses and the child is referred for full audiological assessment, even if there is no hearing impairment. A neonatal programme will need processes designed to reduce this potential impact.

Minimizing negative impact

Appropriate accessible information may help to engender informed choice and reduce anxiety. Evidence from research with cancer patients (for example, Hinds, Streater and Mood, 1995) suggests information is valued positively. In the large scale survey by Hind and Davis (2000) parents reported dissatisfaction with information when:

- it was non-existent;
- it was too complex; or
- good information existed but was not given unless requested.

Helping parents to cope with a positive outcome at the screen will involve ensuring they are adequately informed of the very low chance of a PCHI being associated with no clear responses, and the reassurance that appropriate and sensitive help will be available if there should be a PCHI. It is important not to understate the risk of PCHI. A small number of children who do not show clear responses at the screen will have a PCHI, yet to be confirmed.

Arguably the two potentially negative aspects of a NHSP discussed in this section could be largely overcome provided the screening programme is sensitive to parental needs. The next section will deal with the potential for an early diagnosis of PCHI to impact positively on the parents.

Grief resolution

The vast majority of children with PCHI are born to hearing parents. Hence when a diagnosis is confirmed the parents usually experience some degree of distress, which can be considerable. Most parents, receiving a diagnosis of a serious or chronic condition in their child, will initially be in a state of crisis or 'grief'.

Siegel (2000) conducted a pilot study with 16 families from the Colorado programme. The parents were asked questions from Pianta and Marvin's (1993) Reaction to Diagnosis Intervention (RDI) which aims to explore issues associated with grief resolution (GR). Judging by their responses to the RDI, 10 of the families had and six had not resolved their grief. The numbers were too small to conduct robust inferential statistics but the trend was in the direction of earlier diagnosis relating to better GR. The average age at diagnosis for the resolved group was 8.1 months as opposed to 16 months for the unresolved group. Furthermore, the children of families who had resolved their grief had expressive language skills 6 months in advance of the children from families who had not.

The present author and her team from the MRC Institute of Hearing Research assessed GR in 49 families of children with PCHI. Considering the Siegel study indications, it was predicted age at suspicion of PCHI, and identification and first fitting of hearing aids would be related to GR. The larger sample size permitted partial correlations, controlling for severity, age, presence and severity of other disability, and interval between diagnosis and interview. No association between age at diagnosis and first fitting of hearing aids was found with GR. However, there was a significant relationship between greater unresolved grief and child's age at parental first suspicion of hearing impairment. This association with less resolved grief was interpreted as mainly due to continuing feelings of guilt and sadness at the time 'lost' in their child's development, and anger with professionals for the associated delay.

There was a significant relationship between speech intelligibility and GR – the parents of children who had better speech intelligibility had better GR, and a significant relationship between speech intelligibility and age at first fitting of hearing aids – the earlier the hearing aids were fitted the better the speech intelligibility. These relationships suggest early identification is better for the child, and family in the longer term.

Overall it seems unlikely that introducing a NHSP will cause undue anxiety, stress or interfere with the parent–child relationship, provided a sensitively delivered programme which fully informs and supports the parents at all stages is implemented.

The NHSP began its initial roll-out across England in late 2001. All England, and most of the UK, with be participating by April 2005. From this point in the chapter, the assumption will be made that a NHSP is acceptable and desirable, and the following sections will deal with other practical and psychological factors requiring consideration to ensure delivery of an excellent programme.

Requirements of screens in the modernized NHS

Hind and Davis (2000) report an association between parental dissatisfaction with hearing services and poorer quality of family life irrespective of age at identification. Hence they promote the need for appropriate and family-friendly services. Dissatisfaction with services related to information and support provided at diagnosis, first fitting of hearing aids and present day provision. Improvements to services will need to include provision of more useful information, and a more supportive family-friendly service generally, including an all-year service from education – not just support within school term times. This is important as the teacher of the deaf is generally the key contact for the family, and will most likely continue to be so even for children aged 0 years to 3 years.

Information

The UK National Screening Committee has directed a need for change in the way screening programmes are introduced in the health services, notably in the domain of information provision. They recommend that full information should be provided, including information about risks and benefits, to ensure informed choice. There is no unequivocal evidence in the literature that such provision provides an effective mechanism for decision making, or informed choice, though women value the information provided for antenatal testing (Rowe et al., 2002). These researchers, like others (such as O'Cathain et al., 2002; Stapleton, Kirkham and Tomas, 2002), identify an important potential barrier to effectiveness – the process of information distribution. If there is no clear strategy for distribution and no accompanying explanation at point of distribution, the value of most informative materials may be minimal.

The NHSP has developed high quality information materials in various media, and a stipulated dissemination protocol. All material is highly accessible and family-friendly, and this has been confirmed by an independent quality assurance review (Tyler and Evans, 2002). The next section will expand on the concept of family-friendly services.

Family-friendly hearing services – meeting the needs of children and families

The NHS Plan highlights the need for all practices to be patient-/parent-centred/friendly. The National Screening Committee set, as a prerequisite to their recommending the introduction of a NHSP in England, the need to demonstrate the screening process would be 'family friendly'.

Research conducted by the NDCS and this author before the introduction of the NHSP show some hearing services in England, though most likely unintentionally, do not always provide a family-friendly service. For example, diagnosis is not always dealt with adequately. As most parents of children with PCHI are hearing, with little or no experience of hearing impairment, it is accepted that most will not welcome the initial diagnosis;

although for those who have had to 'fight' for the assessment there can be a sense of relief. Some clinics use the ENT consultant as the messenger. This is due to the belief, that as the families will have more dealings with audiology than ENT, it is better if they do not start off in a negative relationship with Audiology. This is clearly well meant but identifies a lack of understanding or training in how to deal with these situations. If disclosure is conducted in a sensitive and supportive way the parents will not necessarily 'hate the messenger'. Some interviewed parents who received the diagnosis from a skilled informer spoke highly of the interaction, kindness and consideration shown and the help provided.

Insensitive treatment sometimes occurs when families have a second child with a hearing impairment. Many clinics take the stance that the parents are 'expert' with dealing with hearing impairment so need little or no support. In reality, many of these parents are devastated to learn they have another child with PCHI and report they would have appreciated more support, and understanding.

Some clinics appear insensitive to the needs of parents who are themselves deaf. There are two main difficulties:

• no or very limited interpretation available for users of British Sign Language; and
• ignorance about the expectations of deaf parents.

Further or renewed training in giving diagnoses and communicating generally with all (deaf or hearing) parents may be required to ensure the quality of service is maintained across services in England.

Parents also report they would prefer better liaison between the different agencies working with their child. A major aim of the NHSP is to ensure seamless well coordinated multi-agency working through the development of children's hearing services working groups which are currently either in place or being set up across England. It is envisaged such groups will promote innovative seamless practice such as shared assessment.

Although targeted neonatal hearing screening has been in place for many years, a significant number of children with congenital PCHI have no risk factors. Hence, delivering a universal screen may lead to an initial peak in early referrals to hearing services. The next section assesses the potential challenges and methods of dealing with impact on hearing services.

Impact on hearing services

The introduction of a NHSP could affect at least three potential levels of services: capacity and form of services; the partnerships required for the screen and follow-up; and the leadership needed at different levels of the programme. Inadequacies in any of these levels could have a negative impact.

In some areas, there may be a shortage of appropriately trained staff, but as this is a low incidence condition and the screen has relatively high specificity, this should not be a major problem. There may be a short-term dearth of those experienced at working with very young children, but targeted neonatal hearing screening has been widespread for several years so there is developing expertise across disciplines. More recently the DoH and the DfES have introduced initiatives to combat this potential problem.

A training programme has been introduced for the NHSP, including audiological assessment. Workshops on areas of growing concern, for example, auditory neuropathy have been organized. A systematic upgrading of pediatric audiology is occurring through the Modernising Children's Hearing Services programme (initiated by the Department of Health and due to be fully implemented by 2005), which includes training and the introduction of leading-edge technology (equipment and hearing aids). It is estimated that another 100 paediatric audiologists will be needed by the time the NHSP is fully implemented. There is no certainty this additional number of specialists is available in England.

The anticipated impact on paediatric cochlear implant services is earlier consultation with a greater demand for earlier implantation. Programmes are preparing for this, and some are lowering the age of implantation to meet demand. The increase in caseload is expected to be manageable, but there may be a need for further staff recruitment in the short term. Although expertise in working with young children is already well developed in existing national paediatric cochlear implant teams, there is a recognised need to develop practice to meet the needs of the much younger infants and their families.

Teachers of the deaf, who often act as the key contacts for families, are typically contracted to work to education term time, and with children over 2 years of age. The DfES has agreed that a year-round service will be appropriate following the introduction of the NHSP to ensure a fully family-friendly service and have produced best practice guidelines for working with under 3 year olds. It is anticipated the reduction in over-referral from the Infant Distraction Test will eventually compensate to some extent for the increase in early referrals to audiology, and in the longer term, the initial increase in workload for education will be ameliorated by a reduction in requirements, at the child, family and school level, as the child develops (Davis et al., 1997).

There is also an acknowledged shortage of speech language therapists and child psychologists, and again a need in some areas for training to work effectively with very young infants. The Early Support Pilot Programmes are developing guidelines and information sources to help with service development and linking to other initiatives, e.g. in the North West Region of England a 'virtual' Early Excellence Centre is being developed which enables the sharing of expertise across Authority boundaries, joint training across disciplines, joint service development across individual services and regional groups. In the short term it is unlikely that all children's and family's needs in all areas of the country will be met appropriately.

The partnerships required to implement the NHSP, and to ensure seamless multi-agency working for the children and their families present another challenge to services. To date, several screening sites report that planning for the introduction of the NHSP has provided a catalyst for better joint working, which should complement other government initiatives aimed at improving delivery of services for children and their families – for example, the Children's Trust Pathfinders (Department for Education and Skills, 2003a).

Implementing the NHSP requires the transformation of culture, ways of working, attitudes and of systems in local NHS organizations. It is critical that leaders at all levels are willing to embrace change, and have the authority to promote the programme.

There will be some impact at the primary care level, mainly health visitors (HV). The role of the HV, in terms of hearing screening, will change. They will have responsibility for surveillance and general support for – and provision of – information on hospital programmes. This new role will be equally important. In areas where HVs conduct the screen, changes are in terms of the method and timing of the hearing screen as well as responsibility for surveillance and information provision.

An evaluation of the introduction of the NHSP will check the benefits, effects, costs and practical implications of the implementation, and provide evidence of impact on services. It will be possible to comment more specifically when the NHSP Evaluation Team reports are published. Currently in all services involved, the general opinion is that the NHSP provides an impetus for massive improvements in services for hearing impaired children and their families. The NHSP is to benefit from a direct link to the new NHS numbers for babies software system, which generates an NHS number for babies within seconds of their details being entered. The introduction of the NHSP complements the systematic introduction of other antenatal and child health programmes which is taking place across the nation, and promotes the values of the Children's National Service Framework (Department of Health, 2002).

Conclusion

Permanent childhood hearing impairment (PCHI) has the potential to impact negatively on developing children and their families, especially when the family has no history of hearing impairment. Evidence suggests very early identification and intervention may positively affect a child's language and cognitive skills. This chapter has attempted to present arguments for and against the introduction of a NHSP. The author believes early identification, following a newborn hearing screen, provides the best potential for the child and family.

However, it is equally important that a family-friendly, efficacious and supportive service is in place to ensure the potential for positive outcomes for true cases is realised. To this end, parents should be well informed at all stages of the screen or assessment, and the number of screens and assessments leading to diagnosis should be limited, without compromising outcome. A named key contact should be identified and introduced to the family at or soon after diagnosis to fit the needs of the family, and professionals working with the family should provide a coherent seamless service.

Although there is a potential for a true or false positive outcome to impact on the child–parent relationship initially, there is no unequivocal evidence this occurs, or that the effect lasts long term. The majority of parents of both hearing and hearing-impaired children, including those from the Deaf culture, are in favour of newborn hearing screening. For hearing families, identifying a PCHI very early in life permits time in which to come to terms with, and learn more about the condition and communication methods, before the child reaches important developmental milestones. Children will not have to fail to develop before suspicions are raised. Such early identification should also help to reduce some of the parental feelings of guilt and anger associated with late diagnosis. Possibly most importantly of all, the children will be given the opportunity to receive appropriate input from babyhood and thus improve their chances of reaching closer to their full potential. For those who have the newborn hearing screen there should be no more cases of mentally able children being misdiagnosed with learning difficulties.

The Department for Education and Skills (2003b) reports that the NHSP

> makes it possible for families to take very early action on behalf of their child and to intervene before language and communication deficit has become established. Where children have no other learning difficulty or disability, this brings a fundamental shift in emphasis away from remediation of a problem which has already developed, towards facilitation of development within the pattern and time frame expected for other children.

Provided the resources are made available by the DoH and DfES to implement recommendations, the vast majority of babies who are born deaf
will have the opportunity to have their condition recognised, understood
and an appropriate habiliative programme introduced during their very
early formative life.

Mothers whose babies have been screened by the NHSP say they value
the screening programme (Tyler and Evans, 2002) and see it as an example of a 'modern' NHS.

References

Abidin RR (1995) Parenting Stress Index. 3 edn. Odessa FL: Psychological
    Assessment Resources.
al-Jader LN, Goodchild MC, Ryley HC, Harper PS (1990) Attitudes of parents of
    cystic fibrosis children towards neonatal screening and antenatal diagnosis.
    Clinical Genetics 38(6): 460–5.
Avant KC (1981) Anxiety as a potential factor affecting maternal attachment.
    Journal of Obstetric, Gynecological and Neonatal Nursing 10: 416–19.
Bamford J, Davis A, Hind S, McCracken W, Reeve K (2000) Evidence on very early
    service delivery: what parents want and don't always get. In Proceedings of the
    International Conference, A Sound Foundation Through Early Amplification,
    October 1998. Chicago, IL, pp. 151–7.
Barringer DG, Mauk GW (1997) Survey of parents' perceptions regarding hospi-
    tal-based newborn hearing screening. Audiology Today 9: 18–19.
Bess F, Paradise JL (1994) Universal screening for infant hearing impairment: not
    simple, not risk-free, not necessarily beneficial, and not presently justified.
    Pediatrics 98: 330–4.
Bowlby JM (1988) A Secure Base: Clinical Applications of Attachment Theory.
    London: Routledge.
Cadman D, Chambers L, Feldman W, Sackett D (1984) Assessing the effectiveness
    of community screening programs. Journal of American Medical Association
    251(12): 1580–5.
Davis A, Bamford J, Wilson I, Ramkalawan T, Forshaw M, Wright S (1997) A criti-
    cal review of the role of neonatal hearing screening in the detection of con-
    genital hearing impairment. Health Technology Assessment 1(10): 59.
Department for Education and Skills (2003a) Children's Trust Pathfinders. 10 July.
    Press Notice 2003/0143. London: DfES.
Department for Education and Skills (2003b) Developing Early
    Intervention/Support Services for Deaf Children and their Families. London:
    DfES.
Department of Health (2002) National service framework for children template for
    the children's NSF. London: Department of Health. See http://www.doh.gov.uk/
    nsf/children/template.pdf.
De Uzcategui CA, Yoshinaga-Itano C (1997) Parents' reactions to newborn hear-
    ing screening. Audiology Today 24: 27.

Hergils L, Hergils A (2000) Universal neonatal hearing screening – parental attitudes and concern. British Journal of Audiology 34(6): 321–7.

Hind S, Davis A (2000) Outcomes for children with permanent hearing impairment. In Proceedings of the International Conference, A Sound Foundation through Early Amplification. October 1998. Chicago IL, pp199–212.

Hinds C, Streater A, Mood D (1995) Functions and preferred methods of receiving information related to radiotherapy – perceptions of patients with cancer. Cancer Nursing 18(5): 374–84.

O'Cathain A, Walters SJ, Nicholl JP, Thomas KJ, Kirkham M (2002) Use of evidence based leaflets to promote informed choice in maternity care: randomised controlled trial in everyday practice. British Medical Journal 324(7338): 643.

Owen M, Webb M, Evans K (2001) Community based universal neonatal hearing screening by health visitors using otoacoustic emissions. Archives of Disease in Childhood Fetal and Neonatal Edition May; 84(3): F157–62

Parsons EP, Clarke AJ, Hood K, Lycett E, Bradley DM (2002) Newborn screening for Duchenne muscular dystrophy: a psychosocial study. Archives of Disease in Childhood Fetal and Neonatal Edition. 86(2): F91–5.

Pianta R C, Marvin RS (1993) Manual for Classification of the Reaction to Diagnosis Interview. Unpublished manuscript. Charlottesville VA: University of Virginia.

Pipp-Siegel S, Sedey A, Yohsinaga-Itano C (2001) Predictors of parental stress in mothers of young children with hearing loss. Journal of Deaf Studies and Deaf Education 7: 1–17.

Pressman L, Pipp-Siegel S, Yoshinaga-Itano C, Deas A (1999) The relation of sensitivity to child expressive language gain in deaf and hard-of-hearing children whose caregivers are hearing. Journal of Deaf Studies and Deaf Education 4: 294–304.

Rowe RE, Garcia J, MacFarlane AJ, Davidson LL (2002) Health Expectancy 5 (1): 63–83.

Siegel S (2000) Resolution of Grief of Parents with Young Children with Hearing Loss. Unpublished manuscript. Boulder CO: University of Colorado.

Stapleton H, Kirkham M, Tomas G (2002) Qualitative study of evidence based leaflets in maternity care. British Medical Journal 324(7338): 639–43.

Stevens JC, Hall DM, Davis A, Davies CM, Dixon S (1998) The costs of early hearing screening in England and Wales. Archives of Disease in Childhood. 78(1): 14–9.

Stuart A, Moretz M and Yang EY (2000) An investigation of maternal stress after neonatal hearing screening. American Journal of Audiology 9(2): 135–41.

Tluczek A, Mischler EH, Farrell PM, Fost N, Peterson NM, Carey P, Bruns WT, McCarthy C (1992) Parent's knowledge of neonatal screening and response to false-positive cystic fibrosis testing. Journal of Developmental Behavior Pediatrics 13(3): 181–6.

Trevathan WE (1987) Human Birth: An Evolutionary Perspective. Hawthorne NY: Aldine de Gruyter.

Tyler S, Evans M (2002) Results of a Review of the Information Materials associated with the Newborn Hearing Screening Programme. Report commissioned by NSHP Implementation Team. Nottingham: MRC Institute of Hearing Research.

Vohr BR, Letourneau KS, McDermott C (2001) Maternal worry about neonatal hearing screening. Journal of Perinatology 21(1): 15–20.

Watkin PM, Beckman A, Baldwin M (1995) The views of parents of hearing impaired children on the need for neonatal hearing screening. British Journal of Audiology 29(5): 259–62.

Watkin PM, Baldwin M, Dixon R, Beckman A (1998) Maternal anxiety and attitudes to universal neonatal hearing screening. British Journal of Audiology 32(1): 27–37.

Weichbold V, Welzl-Mueller K, Mussbacher E (2001) The impact of information on maternal attitudes towards universal neonatal hearing screening. British Journal of Audiology 35(1): 59–66.

Wilson JMG, Jungner YG (1968) Principles and practice of screening for disease. Public Health Paper Number 34. Geneva: WHO, 1968.

Yoshinaga-Itano C, Sedey AL, Coulter DK, Mehl A (1998) Language of early- and later-identified children with hearing loss. Pediatrics 102(5): 1161–71.

Yoshinaga-Itano (2002) The social-emotional ramifications of universal newborn hearing screening, early identification and intervention of children who are deaf or hard of hearing. In Proceedings of the International Conference: A Sound Foundation through Early Amplification. October 2001. Chicago IL, pp. 221–31.

CHAPTER 3

Medical and physiological aspects of deafness

JOHN GRAHAM

Introduction

This chapter will deal with congenital deafness in children and acquired deafness in children and adults. I will begin by defining and describing some common terms. Throughout the chapter, when a new technical term is introduced, it is printed in bold text, to make it easier for the reader to refer back to it or to look it up. The rest of the chapter will describe the structure and function of the ear and hearing system. Types and causes of deafness will be described, and some treatments mentioned. Finally there is a brief discussion of the term 'medical model of deafness'.

Definitions

- *Loudness.* This is measured in units called **decibels,** which are shown on the vertical axis of an audiogram chart (see Figure 4.1, p. 55).
- *Frequency.* This is the **pitch** of a sound. It is measured in units called Hertz (Hz). A thousand Hz. are called a kilohertz, abbreviated as kHz. Frequencies range from deep, bass sounds, like that produced by a fog horn, to high pitched, treble sounds like that of a scream.
- *Deafness.* The word 'deafness' in this chapter will be used to refer to any form of hearing that is not within the normal range. 'Normal range' includes people with pure tone audiometric thresholds of between 0 dB and 20 dB. Technically, '0 dB Hearing Level' is a level of sound that can only just be heard by an 'otologically normal' person, aged between 18 and 30, who is 'in a normal state of health, free from all signs or symptoms of ear disease and wax, and with no history of undue exposure to noise'. This definition is part of the International Standards Organization's description of the ability of an individual to hear (ISO 389-1, 1998)
- *Hearing Loss.* This is used interchangeably with the word 'deafness' in this chapter.

- *Audiometry.* This means measuring hearing. The commonest form of audiometry involves placing headphones over the person's ears and finding the quietest pure tone at each frequency that the person can just hear. There are other forms of audiometry, such as testing the ability to hear and understand words or sentences, with or without lip-reading, measuring the hearing of children, either by using a child's natural curiosity in which the child turns his or her head to see where the sound is coming from (behavioural testing), or by conditioning a slightly older child to play a game, such as performing a simple task whenever the child hears a sound. In addition, there are forms of audiometry based on measurement of the electrical activity of the nerve of hearing or more central pathways of hearing in the brain (electric response audiometry: ERA) or detecting the activity of the outer hair cells in the cochlea (oto-acoustic emissions: OAE).

When professionals talk about deafness or hearing loss, they usually qualify it by the descriptions 'mild' 'moderate' 'severe' and 'profound'. An audiogram is a chart that shows a person's levels of hearing at different pitches (frequencies). Figure 4.1 in Chapter 4 shows the usual audiogram chart, with degrees of severity of deafness. In this chapter, Figure 3.1 shows an audiogram chart with, superimposed on it, the approximate pitch (frequency) and loudness (intensity) of speech sounds and common environmental sounds. Figure 3.2 shows an audiogram chart with the distribution of speech sounds only. The loudness and pitch of the sounds of conversational speech are broadly distributed in an area known by audiologists as the 'speech banana', because of its shape.

Normally, the lowest frequency measured is 125 Hz, one octave below the musical note middle C. Hearing is usually measured at octave intervals, doubling the frequency with each step, up to 8 kHz. The normal way of performing an audiogram is for the subject to sit with headphones over both ears, unable to see the tester. The tester chooses a frequency and, by pressing a button, causes a pulse of sound to come from one or other headphone. This sound, or tone, should last about a second, at the selected frequency and with a degree of loudness judged to be rather more than the subject's actual threshold of hearing. The tones are then presented more and more quietly until the subject stops responding, and are then increased just to the level at which the person responds again. This level of loudness, in dB, is normally taken as the person's threshold of hearing for that tone.

The normal ear and system of hearing

Figure 3.3 shows a diagram of the ear. The **pinna,** the easily visible outer part of the ear, has the function of slightly altering, or 'filtering' the

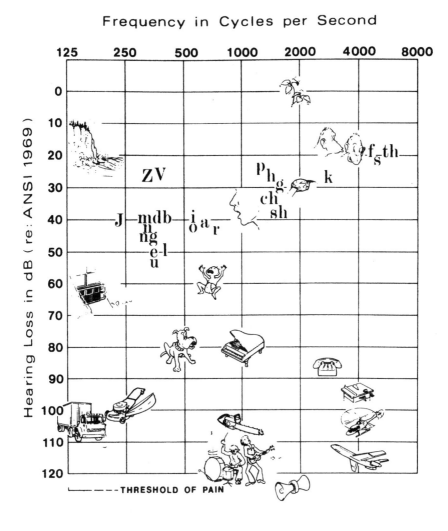

Figure 3.1 Audiogram chart showing pitch and loudness of some environmental and speech sounds. From McCormick B (2003) Paediatric Audiology 0–5 years. London: Whurr. Reproduced with permission.

sounds reaching the entrance to the external ear canal. The pinna does this because of its irregular shape.

This means that the quality of a sound reaching someone's ear from, for example, in front of them is different from the same sound arriving from behind them. In this way the pinna helps us know from which direction sounds are coming.

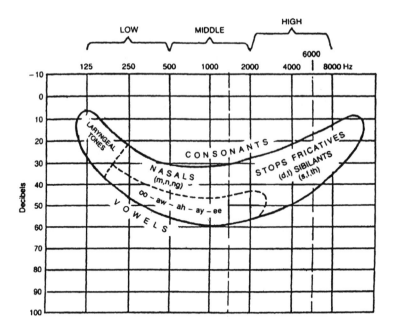

Figure 3.2 Audiogram chart showing the main pitch and loudness of different speech sounds. This diagram is sometimes called the 'speech banana'. From Graham JM, Martin M (eds) (2001) Ballantyne's Deafness. London: Whurr. Reproduced with permission.

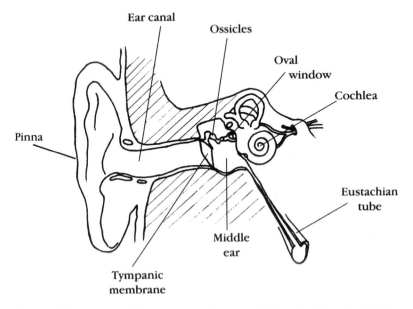

Figure 3.3 Anatomy of the ear. From Graham JM, Martin M (eds) (2001) Ballantyne's Deafness. London: Whurr. Reproduced with permission.

The **external ear canal** forms a tube that allows the sound to reach the tympanic membrane. The cartilage of the external ear surrounds the outer part of this tube, and the inner part of the tube is a hole in the outer bone of the skull. The skin that lines the outer part of the tube has glands in it that secrete wax, and also may have hairs growing from it.

The **tympanic membrane**, or 'eardrum', is a thin, more or less circular disc that closes off the inner end of the external ear canal and separates the outer ear from the middle ear. The membrane is thin and light, so is relatively easily made to vibrate when sound waves reach it . The handle of the first of the tiny bones, or ossicles (Figure 3.4), the **malleus**, is sandwiched between the outer and inner layers of the tympanic membrane. The outer layer of the membrane is a special kind of **skin**, the inner layer consists of what is known as **mucosa**, the moist surface that also lines the inside of our noses and throats, and the Eustachian tube connecting the back of the nose to the middle ear. These inner and outer layers sandwich the middle layer, which is made of tough fibres, which make the tympanic membrane hold its shape. As you can see in Figure 3.4, the malleus handle tents the tympanic membrane inward a little, helping it to catch the sounds that reach it through the external ear.

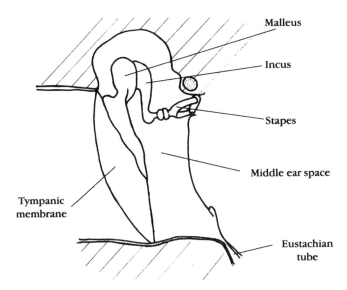

Figure 3.4 Diagram of the middle ear and ossicles. From Graham JM, Martin M (eds) (2001) Ballantyne's Deafness. London: Whurr. Reproduced with permission.

The **middle ear** (Figure 3.4) is a box in the bone of the skull. It contains air, constantly supplied from the back of the nose through the Eustachian tube. The middle ear has an upward extension called the attic, and a backward extension leading to the air cells of the mastoid, behind the ear. Supported by various ligaments and also attached to each other are the three **ossicles**. When sound reaches the tympanic membrane it causes the membrane to vibrate; as the malleus is held between the two layers of the membrane it also vibrates; the two other ossicles, the incus and stapes are therefore also made to vibrate. The stapes is set into an oval-shaped window into the cochlea, so the function of the middle ear is to pass the vibrations, or sound waves, from the tympanic membrane to the inner ear.

The inner ear in humans is like a snail shell wound around itself two-and-a-half times (Figure 3.5).

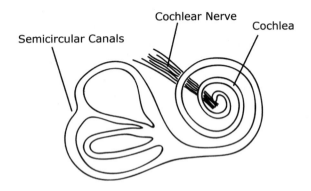

Figure 3.5 Diagram of the cochlea and semicircular canals.

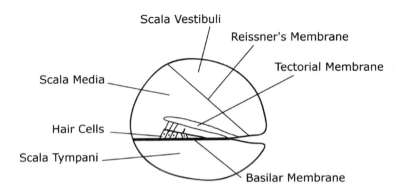

Figure 3.6 Cross-section of part of the cochlea, showing the fluid compartments and hair cells.

It is called the **cochlea**. Figure 3.6 shows what the cochlea looks like if it is cut vertically in half. It is like a spiral tunnel or a hollow snail shell. Cutting across the tunnel, you can see that it is divided into three compartments. The upper and lower compartments, the **scala vestibuli** and the **scala tympani** are full of a fluid called **perilymph,** which is the same as the **cerebrospinal fluid** that surrounds our brain. The perilymph communicates with the cerebrospinal fluid, which is why, in meningitis, when the cerebrospinal fluid is infected by bacteria, these bacteria also invade the cochlea, causing deafness. The middle channel, sandwiched between the scala tympani and the scala vestibuli, is the **scala media** which is full of a different liquid called **endolymph;** suspended in this are the **hair cells.** When the fluids inside the cochlea are vibrated by the movements of the stapes, these hair cells are displaced backwards and forwards and drop a chemical onto the endings of the nerves which lie just underneath them. The arrival of this chemical triggers electrical impulses, which pass along the **auditory nerves** that connect the cochlea to the brain, allowing us to hear.

Types of deafness

Conductive deafness

This is a hearing loss produced by a blockage or abnormality in the **external** ear, or an abnormality in the **middle** ear such as a perforation in the tympanic membrane, fluid in the middle ear, chronic infection in the middle ear or stiffening of the ossicles. When this happens, the sounds reaching the cochlea are quieter than they should be, so the patient has a degree of deafness. The cochlea itself may or may not be functioning normally. The true level of hearing in the cochlea itself can be judged by delivering the tones through a vibrator onto the part of the skull behind the ear. By vibrating the skull in this way, the cochlea is stimulated and can hear the tone produced by vibrating the bone of the skull. In conductive deafness, therefore, the level of hearing produced by this method of 'bone conduction' is better than when the sound is delivered normally to the external ear by 'air conduction'.

Sensorineural deafness

This is a hearing loss produced by malfunction of the cochlea or the nerve of hearing or both. In the majority of cases of sensorineural deafness, it is the cochlea that is at fault rather than the nerve, although when there is damage to the cochlea the nerves to which the signal from the cochlea is normally passed may suffer some secondary damage. Tumours can arise on the nerves of hearing or, usually, the nerve of balance, blocking the messages from the cochlea to the brain. 'Central' deafness has been described, following damage to the nerve pathways of hearing within the brain, but this form of deafness is extremely rare.

It is, of course, possible for someone to have both conductive and sensorineural deafness.

Progressive deafness

This is a form of hearing loss in which there is progressive worsening of the levels of hearing. Some degree of progressive deafness is a fairly normal event during the life of an individual, particularly after the age of 60. However, some forms of progressive hearing loss can appear at a much earlier age and become worse at a much faster rate.

Causes of deafness

Congenital deafness

Congenital deafness is deafness that is present at birth. Some forms of congenital deafness are programmed into the genetic profile of the developing foetus and therefore are inevitably present well before birth. However, the term 'congenital deafness' also includes hearing losses that are present at birth following earlier damage to the ears, from infections of the foetus during pregnancy.

The first type of hearing loss, that which is programmed into the developing foetus at conception, is called genetic. About 50% of all cases of congenital deafness are known to be of genetic origin in the UK, and of the remainder – 30% to 50% – are also likely to be genetic. This is a field in which much scientific progress has been made over the last few years. In the **human genome** or catalogue of our **genes,** there are many genes that control the development of hearing in the growing foetus. Abnormalities in these genes can result, therefore, in deafness.

Genetic abnormalities are traditionally divided into **dominant** and **recessive.** They can also be divided into those that cause deafness only and those in which as well as being deaf the child has other physical abnormalities.

Having a 'dominant' genetic abnormality means that if one parent has this dominant gene, then that parent will have the **phenotype** (the parent will actually have the disorder linked to the gene) and that, if the parent marries someone who does not have the same genetic condition, there is roughly a 50% chance of each of their children inheriting the abnormality. In some cases, the 'penetrance' of the gene is incomplete, so the 50% rule may end up being less than 50%.

Recessive genes are those where both parents have the same abnormal gene, but the gene is not one that causes them to have the abnormality, or phenotype, themselves. One recently discovered form of recessive gene is the 'Connexin 26' gene, which is responsible for about 20% of all genetic childhood deafness. Abnormal recessive genes are more common than dominant ones.

'Syndromal' genetic abnormalities, in which deafness is linked to other congenital abnormalities, are easier to recognize and are responsible for about 30% of cases of genetic deafness. Some forms of inherited deafness are linked to abnormalities of vision, abnormalities in the kidneys, or abnormalities in the skin, which makes those particular syndromes much easier to classify without specialised genetic testing.

Apart from genetic causes, a baby can be born with reduced or absent hearing because of infection suffered by the foetus while still in the womb. German measles used to be a common cause of hearing loss in the newborn. This is because the rubella virus, which causes German measles, causes damage to the cochlea if a mother catches the virus in the first three months of pregnancy

There are other viruses such as the cytomegalovirus (CMV) and the tox-oplasma virus and other infective organisms such as the syphilis organism that can cause damage to the inner ears of the developing foetus. In some cases, where a baby is born with a hearing loss caused by a virus, the con-tinued presence of the virus in the ear causes the hearing to deteriorate further in the first months or even years of the child's life.

There are also problems from which a baby may suffer at the time of birth that can cause damage to the cochlea. The main one at present is prematurity. Prematurely born children are more likely than other chil-dren to have a hearing loss, and this is probably related to the fact that in very small premature babies, the blood flow to the brain and inner ears is easily disrupted by short periods of lack of oxygen. Congenitally deaf chil-dren may also have malformations of the external ear and middle ear.

Prevalence

It has been estimated (Fortnum and Davis, 1997) that in the UK 1.12 chil-dren per thousand live births have a congenital permanent hearing loss of 40 dB or greater across the frequencies of 0.5, 1, 2 and 4 kHz and that this number increases to 1.33 in children who reach the age of 5 years, because of additional cases of acquired hearing loss. Profound congenital hearing loss is less common, with a figure of 0.24 per thousand live births.

Identification, or diagnosis, of cases of congenital deafness by screening tests

The identification of deafness in a baby can occur in several ways. In a child born into a family where there are already a number of people with congenital deafness or where a hereditary form of deafness has been identified in the family, that child should have a hearing test as soon as possible after birth. Children without a family history of deafness but for whom there are factors that are known to be associated with deafness are described by the paediatricians as being 'at risk' of deafness, and will have special hearing tests to measure their levels of hearing.

Some children do not come from families where there is known to be a history of hearing loss and do not have the factors described above. Among these children, the first suspicion that there might be a hearing loss may come from the child's own parents who notice that he or she does not respond to sounds or may respond to sound less than the family's older children did at a comparable age. The parents may then ask their family doctor to find out whether the child has normal hearing

In some children, hearing loss is not suspected but is detected during a screening exercise. In the UK, screening programmes were set up in the 1960s, following some pilot studies in the north of England. This **universal screening** of children's hearing currently takes place in children at the age of approximately 9 months using 'distraction tests' of hearing, and later at school entry, using audiometry. In 2003, however, pilot studies for screening all children at birth, 'neonatal screening', have been set up in the UK to test both the effectiveness of this screening in detecting hearing loss and also to make sure that the system of screening does not allow children to fall through the net and miss being tested. Once the pilot studies are complete and have been analysed, it is proposed to set up universal neonatal hearing screening throughout the UK. This *should* allow all cases of congenital deafness to be detected. There will, of course, be other children who are born with normal hearing but develop a hearing loss later: it is likely that some form of later screening test will be necessary. At present, many children with 'glue ear' or fluid in the middle ears would not have their deafness detected without the preschool and school screening programmes that are now in existence: it is likely that these types of screening will need to be maintained after universal neonatal screening has begun.

Acquired deafness

External ear

If people with normal hearing put their fingers in their ears, their hearing will be reduced. Hearing loss can occur when anything blocks the external ear canal in one or both ears, preventing sounds from reaching the tympanic membrane. The external ear can be blocked by wax, or by pus and debris filling up the external ear canal when there is an external ear infection (otitis externa). Otitis externa can be caused by bacteria or by a fungal infection, and most commonly occurs after swimming in water containing bacteria, but can also occur when eczema in the external ear canal acquires a secondary infection by bacteria. Treatment of wax is either by syringing, by careful removal with an instrument or, in some cases, by sucking the wax out of the ear canal while examining the ear with a microscope. In otitis externa, the debris has to be sucked or mopped out of the ear. The state of the external ear canal and tympanic membrane are then assessed. Medical treatment, in the form of antibiotics and antibiotic eardrops, is administered to eliminate the infection.

Middle ear

Otitis media with effusion (OME or 'glue ear') causes conductive deafness with a hearing loss of between 25 and 50 dB. It is much more common in children than in adults. Of children in the UK under the age of 5 years, up to 19% (Tos et al., 1986) may have it at any time. It seems to be most frequent at the age of 2 years and 6 months and at the age of 5, although it is not clear whether these are true peaks in the prevalence of glue ear or whether they coincide with times when children are more likely to have their hearing tested. There are a number of factors that may cause it to be present. A child may have had a middle-ear infection in which the ear fills up with fluid containing viruses or bacteria. This fluid may then fail to drain away down the Eustachian tube (Figure 3.3) and simply persist in the middle ear. Infections or allergy affecting the nose and sinuses may cause swelling of the lining of the Eustachian tube. This will prevent air from travelling up the Eustachian tube, from the back of the nose to the middle ear. The middle ear then fills with fluid. Treatment of OME may not be necessary since many cases resolve by themselves. If OME appears at an early age, and persists at the time when a child would normally be developing speech and language, it may have an effect on this development. It may also cause discomfort in children from repeated infections, and can cause poor balance. Often, the hearing changes from day to day or from week to week when OME persists. This can be confusing for a child.

Medical treatment consists of a short course of antibiotics, if there is an obvious infection in the nose, and treatment of allergy where this is present. When the OME does not get better, insertion of grommets into the middle ear under a short general anaesthetic may be advised. A grommet is a tiny plastic tube, which is placed in a small slit in the tympanic membrane, and allows air to enter the middle ear through the tympanic membrane so that the fluid can drain naturally down the Eustachian tube and the hearing improves.

If an adult develops OME, the doctor should be careful to check the space at the back of the nose to make sure that there is no swelling or disease there that could be blocking the Eustachian tube. Generally, OME clears up by itself in adults although occasionally grommets need to be inserted.

Chronic suppurative otitis media (CSOM) is a group of conditions in which chronic infection of the middle ear causes damage to the tympanic membrane with or without damage to the ossicles. There may be a hole, or 'perforation' in the tympanic membrane. This can let infection into the middle ear, causing a discharge of pus into the external ear canal. Perforations can usually be repaired by an operation called 'myringoplasty'. There is a worse form of CSOM, called 'cholesteatoma', in which a weakened part of the tympanic membrane does not perforate, but is pulled inwards, as a pocket, into the middle ear. Here it can destroy the ossicles, damage the facial nerve – causing paralysis of the face on that side – grow into the cochlea, causing permanent profound deafness, or even erode into the brain, causing meningitis or brain abscesses. Since cholesteatoma usually grows into the mastoid bone, behind the ear, an operation to remove cholesteatoma is called a 'mastoidectomy'. An operation to repair the damage to the ossicles, and so improve the hearing, is called 'ossiculoplasty'.

Traumatic middle ear damage. Damage to the tympanic membrane and ossicles can occur from trauma. This could be when an unfortunate person pokes a cotton bud or some other object too deeply into their ear, from a slap on the ear, from sudden decompression in the cabin of an aeroplane in flight, and, of course, from bomb blasts. The degree of damage from trauma ranges from a simple perforation of the tympanic membrane, which generally heals by itself if it does not become infected, to loss of the entire tympanic membrane with disruption of the ossicles and even damage to the cochlea. This severe degree of damage is more common in bomb blast injuries.

Otosclerosis is another condition that causes conductive hearing loss. It is a hereditary condition with 'dominant' inheritance, although occasionally cases appear in people in whom there is no other family history of deafness. In otosclerosis there is a localized hardening of the footplate of the stapes, which progressively reduces the movement of the stapes, causing progressive conductive deafness. Otosclerosis can affect one or both ears and usually appears for the first time in early adult life. The hearing can be restored by a delicate middle-ear operation called 'stapedectomy', in which the footplate of the stapes is removed, or a hole made in it, and a piston of plastic or metal is hooked onto the incus; the other end is placed through the stapes footplate, to make the cochlear fluid vibrate. Alternatively the patient may prefer to use a hearing aid.

In some cases of conductive deafness the patient is unable to wear a normal hearing aid with a plastic insert in the ear. In such people a **bone-anchored hearing aid** may be extremely helpful.

Inner ear and nerve of hearing (sensorineural deafness)

Presbyacusis is the commonest form of acquired sensorineural deafness in adults, the progressive loss of hearing that begins in most people after the age of 50 or 60. This is generally caused by the gradual death of the hair cells in the cochlea.

Noise-related hearing loss occurs when excessive levels of noise reach the ears either from prolonged exposure to high continuous noise levels, or from multiple episodes of exposure to sudden bursts of noise, such as gunfire, or from a single episode of blast, for example from a bomb. Recreational noise-induced deafness, from listening to amplified music for long periods of time, is also increasingly common; in this case each exposure to noise drags the hearing a little further downwards. Prevention is the best policy for this kind of hearing loss. Earplugs protect our ears against excessive noise: employers in the UK are obliged by law to provide ear protection, in the form of earplugs or ear defenders, to employees who may be exposed to excessive noise levels at work. Custom-made earplugs can be made by audiologists and are usually better fitting and more effective.

Menière's disease is a condition in which, for no currently known reason, the fluid in the endolymph compartment of the cochlea develops a high pressure. The signs of Menière's disease are fluctuation in the level of hearing in one or both ears, episodes of vertigo and tinnitus, which may also become worse when the hearing and balance are worse. It can be controlled by medical treatment and there are also operations that may help some people with this problem.

Many cases of hearing loss occur suddenly, in one, or occasionally both ears and for no detectable reason. If someone suffers a **sudden hearing loss,** whether this is in one or in both ears, it is sensible for such a person to be seen urgently in an ENT or audiology clinic. Many doctors will recommend that such a patient is admitted to a hospital bed for observation, daily audiometry, empirical treatment with corticosteroid and other drugs and for investigations to try to identify the cause of the deafness. It must be admitted that in most cases a cause is not found, but it seems likely that better ways of identifying the causes of sudden deafness will be discovered in the future.

Acoustic neuromas are benign (non-cancerous) tumours that usually arise on the **vestibular** nerves, the nerves of balance, rather than the neighbouring nerves of hearing, but the tumours press on the auditory nerve and cause deafness. These tumours are generally diagnosed by MRI scanning and often need to be removed, because if they continue to grow inside the skull they can be life threatening. Some acoustic neuromas may be treated by radiotherapy.

Balance

The cochlea shares the same fluid system of perilymph and endolymph with the semicircular canals (see Figure 3.5) in the same way that the front and rear brakes of a car are generally connected by pipes containing the same brake fluid. In many cases where hearing is damaged the patient's sense of balance may also be affected, producing either **vertigo** – a sense of movement of the patient or of the patient's surroundings – or loss of the ability to balance, especially when walking or standing. When vertigo begins suddenly and severely it can be accompanied by nausea and by vomiting. In this situation the patient feels very ill and is usually helped by medicines that suppress the part of the brain that deals with balance, 'vestibular sedatives', which are also used as sea-sickness remedies. These drugs are useful in the early stages of an attack of vertigo but prolonged use can be counterproductive. In most cases where the balance mechanism has been damaged, the brain will be able to compensate for the change in the signal pattern arriving in the nerves of balance from the two inner ears. Tests exist to measure the function of the organs of balance in the semicircular canals in the two ears separately. Physiotherapists are trained to help people with poor balance to regain some or all of their balance by helping the central compensation mentioned above to take place more quickly.

Hearing devices

People who develop sensorineural deafness are prescribed hearing aids. For people whose hearing loss is more profound cochlear implants form a useful and effective safety net.

'Different' and 'abnormal', and the concept of the 'medical model' of deafness

A term sometimes encountered is the **medical model** of deafness. This seems to have appeared as a corollary of the medical and educational management of people who are deaf. Most adults who lose hearing, and most hearing parents of deaf children, will turn to doctors for help. This is a normal expectation among the general population of any country, and certainly not something 'invented' by medical professionals. Applying the term 'medical model' to deafness seems as illogical as it would be to say that there is a 'medical model' for death, living, pneumonia, or any other natural state. Deafness, or absence of hearing, whether partial or total, is a state that is familiar, not simply to doctors, but to the general population of the world, 99% of whom are born with normal hearing. These people do not require medical degrees to know whether or not a person they meet has hearing or is deaf. Since only 0.1% of the adult UK population has a hearing loss in their better ear of 105 dB or more (Davis, 1989), only 0.2% a loss of 95 dB or more, and only 1.1% a loss of 65 dB or more, and since only about 0.18% of children are born with deafness severe enough for them to need hearing aids (Fortum and Davis, 1997), it is hardly surprising that the majority of the population will regard a deaf person as not having 'normal' hearing, or as having 'abnormal hearing'. This is simply a commonplace reality of life, rather than something cooked up by doctors to dupe non-professionals.

This is not, of course, to say someone with deafness should in any way be viewed as being an 'abnormal person', which would be both incorrect and insulting and the sort of attitude that professionals in the field of hearing, whether medically trained or not, spend much of their working lives trying to combat. Deafness is an abnormal, but natural state, and it is certainly not correct to use morally weighted words like 'right' and 'wrong' in relation to hearing. On the other hand it should be accepted that to be deaf is not viewed as a normal state by the 99% of the general population born with normal hearing, who therefore would be surprised to be asked to view such a well-known phenomenon as deafness as a 'model' invented in some way by doctors.

In dealing with an adult who loses hearing, or with a child born deaf, a doctor's duty is viewed by the population at large as to 'cure' or help the patient in any way possible, whether by surgery, medical treatment or the provision of hearing aids. Again this is a general expectation, not unique to doctors. The majority of normally hearing people would be surprised to receive the advice that a deaf person should be encouraged to enjoy their deafness as a 'normal' state. However, well-informed doctors and other professionals who work in the field of hearing, are aware of the existence of the 'deaf community', its culture and use of sign, and rightly respect it. Professionals and doctors in the field of hearing are thus more likely than the general population to be sympathetic to the views and needs of the deaf community, although they are just as likely to resist calls to abandon medical interventions such as the provision of cochlear implants for adults, or, when requested by their parents, for young children. They should, of course, also be aware of the balance between oralism and signing, and try to counsel deaf people and the parents of deaf children appropriately.

References

Davis AC (1989) The prevalence of hearing impairment and reported hearing disability among adults in Great Britain. International Journal of Epidemiology 18: 911–17.

Fortnum H and Davis AC (1997) Epidemiology of permanent childhood hearing impairment in Trent region, 1985–1993. British Journal of Audiology 31: 409–46.

ISO389-1 (1998) Reference zero for the standardization of audiological equipment, part 1. Reference equivalent threshold SPLs for pure tones and supra canal earphones. Geneva: International Standards Organization.

Tos M, Stangerup SE, Hvid G, Andreassen UK, Thomsen J (1986) Epidemiology and natural history of secretory ototis. In Sade J (ed.) Acute and Secretory Otitis. Amsterdam: Kugler, pp. 95–106.

CHAPTER 4

Tip-toeing through technology

Twanette Acker and Susan Crocker

Introduction

The main aim of this chapter is to give an overview of different hearing devices that are available. The focus will be on the types and functioning of current amplification technology and who might benefit from these. The psychological considerations for people, especially children, who are recommended to wear a hearing device will be discussed. Some practical aspects of device fitting will be linked with the child's experience of wearing a hearing aid or cochlear implant, as rehabilitation and technology can only be useful if a device is worn.

Thoughts about best practice for audiology teams will be discussed, along with practical tips to help children integrate a hearing device into their everyday lives. It may be useful to have an understanding of normal hearing and the different types of hearing loss before reading this chapter.

Treatment of hearing loss

There are three different ways to treat a hearing loss and all of these depend on the cause, type and degree of the loss:

- surgical treatment (usually indicated for outer and/or middle-ear abnormalities, disease or removal of growths/tumours in the middle ear or affecting the auditory nerve);
- medical treatment (usually indicated for outer or middle-ear disease);
- amplification/hearing devices (indicated for 'untreatable' conductive hearing loss and more commonly for sensorineural hearing loss).

Advantage of hearing devices and the importance of using these

There are several factors affecting the degree of handicap caused by a hearing loss. These include the age of onset, severity, site of lesion and family support (Davis and Hardick, 1986). For adults and older children, the acceptance of amplification is linked to the acceptance of the hearing loss, as wearing hearing aids can bring up anxieties related to their hearing impairment. Some individuals feel that by accepting the use of hearing aids they are betraying their lost hearing or rejecting their residual hearing (see Mueller and Grimes in Alpiner and McCarthy, 1987).

Oral communication makes us uniquely 'human' as we listen and think using speech and language. Hearing is an integral part of learning to use and maintain oral communication. A hearing loss does not only have an impact on the quality of communication (following conversation, speech, voice quality and control, language acquisition, and so forth), but also on psychosocial aspects of development in children (such as cognition, symbolic play, academic achievement, socio-emotional development, self-concept) and adults (Ling, 1976; Alpiner and McCarthy, 1987; Davis and Hardick, 1986; Northern and Downs, 2002).

The majority of children who are hearing impaired have some residual hearing. When properly aided, many children can detect most, if not all, of the speech spectrum. The use of an optimal amplification system could provide sufficient access to speech (and environmental) sounds for the child to be able to develop spoken language as a first language in a natural way through the auditory modality. As most deaf babies are from hearing families, the parental goal might be for the child to attend a mainstream school or at least use the home language. In order to benefit from the 'critical periods' of neurological linguistic development, the identification of the hearing loss, as well as use of technology to stimulate hearing, must occur as early as possible (Davis and Hardick, 1986; Northern and Downs, 2002). If hearing is not accessed during this critical language learning period (0–2 years), a child's ability to use acoustic input meaningfully will deteriorate due to physiological (deterioration of auditory pathways) and psychosocial (attention, practice and learning) factors (Webster, 1983).

The benefits from a hearing aid will be a function of how well the client can differentiate or learn to differentiate sounds. The success of this depends on the client and the ear, and not on the properly functioning hearing aid. Hearing aids function poorest in the situations in which the majority of hearing-impaired individuals need them most. Thus, realistic expectations are crucial to successful hearing aid use (Hodgson in Katz, 1985).

It is rarely the small child's aim to be able to hear. Thus, audiological intervention and rehabilitation will always involve the family, particularly the parents. It is generally the parents who hold the goals of improved hearing, and the motivation to undertake the interventions required to improve hearing for their child. As will be discussed in other chapters, grief, denial and other emotions associated with loss may get in the way of a family accepting a child's hearing loss (Tye-Murray, 1998). This in turn may result in the child not wearing the amplification as the family show ambiguity about the device, with the hearing aids making the invisible disability more visible. (Refer to the section on 'wearing the device').

Limitations of hearing aids/amplification

In most cases, wearing prescription glasses for common visual problems, will 'normalize' vision despite the fact that it is not a cure. Unfortunately, hearing aids (including cochlear implants) have more limitations. Not only are they not a cure for deafness but neither do they normalize hearing. With a conductive hearing loss there is usually little distortion in the amplified auditory signal. With a sensorineural hearing loss, distortion is expected due to damage sustained by sound receptors in the cochlear and nerve fibres involved in the transmission of sound to the higher auditory centres (Davis and Hardick, 1986). A hearing aid primarily makes sounds louder and not clearer (although louder sound will be more intelligible) and listening in noise and at a distance is always hard with a hearing aid (Crandell and Smaldino, in Tyler and Schum, 1995).

A parent must initially supply motivation to children to wear hearing aids. Consistent use of amplification is needed in young children to give them access to sound, to learn *to* listen and to learn *through* listening.

Factors affecting the outcomes of using amplification

The ultimate goal with amplification is probably a well-adjusted, well-integrated person who uses listening and speaking to successfully interact with others at home and school, in the community and in the wider world. To look at performance outcomes (the benefits or limitations) one must decide which aspects will be considered in terms of measuring success: language acquisition, integration into the deaf or hearing world, positive self-esteem and acceptance of deafness, speech intelligibility, academic performance or feeling 'in touch' with the world (even if it is only by detection of loud sounds).

Several factors have been identified that could have an affect on the performance outcomes of children fitted with amplification (Davis and Hardick, 1986; Tye-Murray, 1998; Chute and Nevins, 2002). These include:

- variables within the client in terms of:

  - hearing status (cause, type and degree of hearing loss, duration of deafness);
  - amplification (age at time of amplification, wear-time of the device, proper fitting and functioning of the device);

  - presence of other disabilities (including intellectual);
  - presence and sophistication of a formal language system;
  - visual motor skills;
  - attention;
  - expectations;
  - educational environment and mode of communication;
  - availability and quality of support services.

- family variables:
  - socioeconomic status;
  - acceptance of hearing loss;
  - family structure;
  - amount and quality of family support;
  - presence of a second language at home.

Selecting the appropriate amplification

Tye-Murray (1998) identified the main goals within the (re)habilitation process:

- alleviating the difficulties related to hearing loss;
- minimizing the consequences of the hearing loss (including the diagnoses, quantification of the hearing loss, provision of appropriate listening devices, communication strategies and counselling);
- teaching communication strategies;
- training listening and speech perception skills.

Probably the most critical element of aural (re)habilitation is selecting and fitting the most appropriate form of amplification for optimum presentation of the speech signal. The first consideration is usually a combination of medical history or details and the audiological findings. Other important factors include communication needs, communication environment, acceptance of hearing loss, motivation for change, body image, self-esteem and so on (Alpiner and McCarthy, 1987; Tye-Murray, 1998; Chute and Nevins, 2002).

The pure tone audiogram is the most convenient information to consider in deciding whether a client is a suitable candidate, and to decide on the most appropriate means of amplification (see Figure 4.1). An in-the-ear hearing aid may be considered for a patient with a mild to moderate sensorineural hearing loss, where a profound loss might be an indication towards considering cochlear implantation (see Table 4.1). The shape of loss and results of more specific assessment will give an indication of the 'fine tuning' of instruments to optimise hearing.

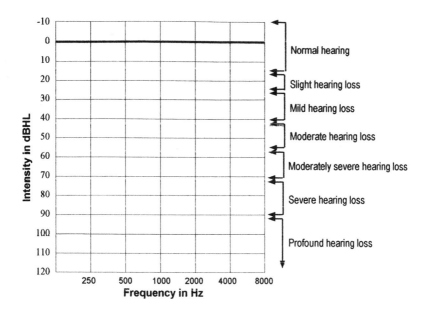

Figure 4.1 An audiogram indicating different degrees of hearing loss.

There are no universally agreed methods of hearing-aid selection, fitting and verification. Most are selected and fitted based on the adult client's acceptance after a brief trial period. Several prescription methods are available for children, adults and the older adult population (Pollack, 1975; Erber, 1993).

Other factors in selecting the style of the device are cost, user preference, lifestyle and physical status (Tye-Murray, 1998).

Table 4.1 Amplification devices

Type of amplification	Types available	Summary of selection criteria and contra-indications	Basic principles of functioning
Air conduction hearing aids	• Behind-the-ear • In-the-ear • In-the-canal • Body worn (external components only)	Mild, moderate or severe sensorineural hearing losses.	Acoustic

Table 4.1 Amplification devices (contd)

Type of amplification	Types available	Summary of selection criteria and contra-indications	Basic principles of functioning
Bone conduction hearing aids	• Eye glass aid • Body worn aid (external components only)	Conductive hearing loss when chronic external ear conditions precludes the use of an ear mould. Malformation of the earlobe or ear canal. For children who are too young to undergo surgery or adults awaiting surgery for a bone-anchored hearing aid. Dependant on the severity of the air-bone gap. Not permanent.	Vibro-tactile
Bone-anchored hearing aids	• Osseointegrated (internal and external components)	Conductive or mixed hearing loss when chronic external ear conditions precludes the use of an ear mould. Malformation of the earlobe or ear canal. Not dependant on the severity of the air-bone gap. Permanent.	Vibro-tactile
Cochlear implants	• Body worn • Behind the ear • Ongoing research on fully inplantable devices (internal and external components)	Bilateral severe to profound sensorineural hearing loss. No minimum or maximum age for referral. Restricted access to speech sounds with conventional hearing aids.	Electric

Available amplification technology

Air conduction hearing aids

Functioning

The hearing aid is an electronic instrument that amplifies sound in such a way that it can generally compensate for the disability of hard-of-hearing people (see Figure 4.2). Aids are not cures, however, and problems with aids have already been discussed. A hearing aid essentially consists of:

- Microphone – picks up the acoustic/sound signals from the environ-ment and converts it into electrical energy.
- Amplifier– amplifies the electrical signal in accordance with the settings based on the patient's hearing loss.
- Battery – power supply.
- User controls – influence the operation of the hearing instrument.
- Receiver – converts the electrical signal back into an acoustic signal. (From Davis and Hardick, 1986)

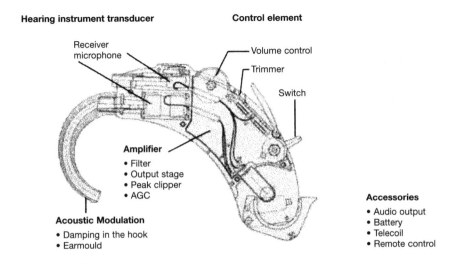

Figure 4.2 Basic components of a BTE hearing instrument (courtesy of Cochlear Europe).

Mueller and Hawkins (in Sandlin, 1995) identified three main considera-tions in hearing aid selection: directional microphones, binaural amplification and loudness discomfort level. The amount of gain and fre-quency responses can be adjusted and optimised by altering the ear mould, ear hook and internal settings of the hearing aid. Details of how to individualize hearing-aid settings to suit a patient's need is beyond the scope of this chapter.

Types available

Hearing aids are continuing to become smaller and smaller and we have moved from bodyworn, to behind-the-ear (BTE) to in-the-ear (ITE) hear-ing aids (see Figure 4.3). Although ITEs are cosmetically most acceptable, there are some problems preventing all clients being candidates. These include limitations in gain and output potential caused by the size of the aids. Some clients may also experience problems with dexterity and therefore with management. This very small hearing aid is often not powerful enough for sufficient amplification for people with severe to profound hearing losses. These aids are custom made for the shape and size of the client's ear canal and because this will change with normal growth, children are not considered to be suitable candidates.

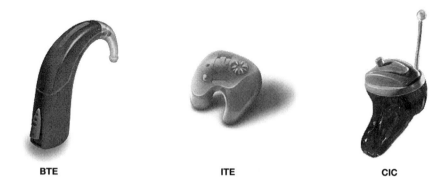

BTE   ITE   CIC

Figure 4.3 Examples of different types of hearing aids (courtesy of Phonak).

Candidacy

An air conduction hearing aid is usually considered for individuals with a permanent sensorineural hearing loss. The degree of loss will give an indication of options that can be considered. The shape of the loss will also play a part in what is expected of the hearing instrument in terms of frequency response and gain. When a hearing loss is unilateral, the presence of a normal ear often precludes the need for amplification on the side with a loss. However, the ideal goal in the rehabilitation process is to attempt to restore binaural hearing. Financial constraints sometimes make this impossible.

A conductive hearing loss would normally be corrected by medication or surgery but if this is not indicated for whatever reason, clients with a conductive hearing loss could also be considered.

Traditional bone-conduction hearing aids

Functioning

A bone vibrator is positioned on the mastoid (the bone behind the earlobe) and held in place by a headband and connected via a cord to a body worn device. The vibratory flat surface that rests on the mastoid transduces sound waves into vibro-tactile sensation, thereby stimulating the cochlear cells via the bone conduction (BC) auditory pathway (Northern and Downs, 2002). The BC receiver operates on the 'reaction' principle – that is, a magnetic driving system vibrates a mass inside an enclosed case. The vibrations of the mass are transmitted through the supporting spring to the case and then to the skin and bony structure of the head.

A BC hearing aid is not permanent and is usually used as an interim before surgery can take place to either resolve the loss or until the patient is fitted with a permanent bone-anchored hearing aid (see Figure 4.4).

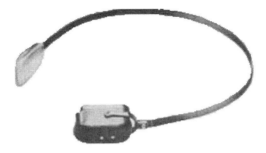

Figure 4.4 A traditional bone-conduction hearing aid (courtesy of Entific Medical Systems).

Types available

Two major forms are available, the body aid and the eyeglass aid. In the body aid, a bone receiver is substituted for the air receiver and held against the mastoid bone of the patient by a headband. In the eyeglass form, a bone receiver is mounted in the portion of the eyeglass temple behind the ear, with a vibratory pad facing towards the head.

Candidacy

The BC hearing aid is used with patients with a conductive hearing loss where surgery is not possible and in cases where the wearing of an ear mould is also not possible (e.g. due to chronic discharges of the middle ear or malformations of the earlobe and/or ear canal).

A BC receiver for a given electrical input produces a sensation level in a normal ear roughly 40 dB lower than does a comparable air-conductor receiver, so bone conduction hearing aids can generally be effective only when the air-bone gap exceeds about 35 dB.

Traditional BC devices also have several drawbacks being both cumbersome and obtrusive. Headaches caused by pressure on the skull, sore skin caused by abrasion and poor sound quality are well documented.

The need for BC type aids has become small because of the success of stapes surgery in deducing the air-bone gap.

Bone-anchored hearing aids (BAHA)

Functioning

Hearing by bone conducted sound is a natural way of hearing. When one listens to one's own voice one is listening to both airborne and bone-conducted sound and these seem to be of equal value. This is the reason why most people do not recognize their own voices on a recording – only the airborne component is recorded. With BAHA there is no occlusion of the ear canal to aggravate inflammation. As the system is based on osseointegration, using a fixture to attach the sound processor, there is no pressure from the transducer against the skin thus avoiding the headaches and soreness often associated with conventional bone conductors. BAHA is a predictable and safe solution (see Figure 4.5).

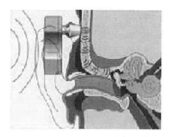 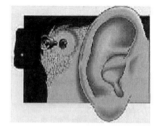

Figure 4.5 The bone-anchored hearing aid is fixed into the bone for sound to travel directly to the inner ear (courtesy of Entific Medical Systems).

A bone-anchored hearing aid consists of a sound processor attached to a small titanium implant, which is fixed in the bone behind the ear during a routine surgical procedure. The bone acts as a pathway for sound to travel to the inner ear without involving the outer ear and ear canal. The percutaneous transducer is attached to the fixture with a bayonet coupling. The air filled gap of the transducer is adjusted to an appropriate length and the resonance frequency and damping are chosen according to the amplification need for the specific hearing loss.

Types available

There are currently two models available:

- The BAHA Classic 300 (standard model) is indicated for a mild to moderate conductive hearing loss (the average bone conduction threshold should be 45 dB HL).

- The more powerful BAHA Cordelle II is indicated for patients with a moderate conductive loss (average bone conduction threshold up to 70 dB HL).

Candidacy

A BAHA is indicated for patients who have a conductive or mixed hearing loss and can still benefit from sound amplification. It works independently of the severity of the air bone gap.

The BAHA allows sound amplification and hearing by bypassing the outer and middle ear, so it is suitable for many people suffering from chronic draining of the ear, inflammation or infection of the ear canal. Another category of patients using conventional BAHA devices is those with congenital ear malformations with either missing or incomplete ear canals.

It is also appropriate for clients with bilateral conductive hearing loss due to disease of the middle ear bones who are not appropriate for surgical correction or unable to be aided by conventional hearing devices.

Cochlear implants (CI)

Functioning

A cochlear implant has several different parts, some of which are internal (cannot be seen) and some of which are external (worn outside the body) (see Figure 4.6).

Types available

There are currently three companies manufacturing cochlear implant systems in the world. The benefit outcomes for recipients using the different systems correlate well. All the different systems function on the same principles but have different features in terms of the implant and electrode array, speech processor functions and available speech coding strategies. Each one is a digitally programmable system, providing the audiologist with the ability to fine-tune each processor to an individual's hearing needs. The first speech processors were body worn and these are still often fitted to young children due to the fact that they are easier to wear (in a body-worn harness versus a processor behind a tiny 'floppy' ear) and to trouble shoot (see Figure 4.7). More and more recipients do choose the less visible, lighter and more convenient behind-the-ear (BTE) speech processor. The body-worn processors function on rechargeable batteries. A lot of research is carried out to improve the power consumption and cost involved in the batteries for the BTE.

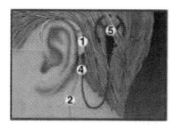
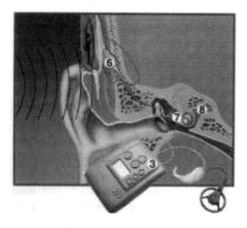

Figure 4.6 A cochlear implant.

1. Sounds are picked up by a microphone and turned into an electrical signal.
2. A thin cable carries the signal from the microphone to the speech processor.
3. The speech processor filters, analyses and digitises the sound into coded signals. The speech processor can be a body worn or ear level design.
4. The coded signals are sent from the speech processor to the transmitting coil.
5. The transmitting coil sends the coded signals across the skin by radio waves to the cochlear implant, which contains a receiver.
6. The implant delivers the pattern of small, safe electrical pulses to the array of electrodes in the cochlea.
7. These small pulses stimulate the remaining auditory nerve fibres in the cochlea.
8. The auditory nerve carries this information to the brain, where it is recognized as sound.

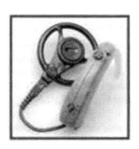
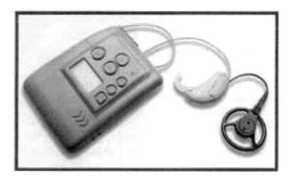

Figure 4.7 Esprit 24 behind the ear speech processor and Sprint body worn speech processor (courtesy of Cochlear Europe).

Candidacy

A CI could be considered in clients with a severe to profound sensorineural hearing loss with restricted access to speech when using
conventional hearing aids. The main aim is to provide access to the full

speech spectrum to aid the learning of spoken language or to 'restore' access to speech sounds for clients who are using spoken language, but have lost their hearing.

The criteria for children are:

- bilateral severe-to-profound sensorineural hearing loss;
- no minimum age for referral (the earlier the better);
- restricted or no useful benefit from hearing aids;
- child and parental motivation to use audition and speech.

The criteria for adults are:

- bilateral severe-to-profound sensorineural hearing loss;
- no upper age limit for referral;
- pre- or post-linguistic hearing loss with oral/aural communication skills;
- restricted or no useful benefit from hearing aids;
- motivation to use audition and speech.

Assistive listening devices (ALDs)

There are several options to use in conjunction with hearing instruments. A number will be discussed. The aim of assistive listening devices is to shorten the distance between output and input, so that amplification of distortion is reduced.

Induction coil (loop)

This is built into some hearing aids as well as the latest cochlear implant speech processors. The induction coil is operational when the input selection switch is on the 'T' setting. The main purpose of the induction coil is the reception of magnetic fields from special induction loops. Such loop systems are common in churches and public buildings and in some telephones (Gilmore in Tyler and Schum, 1995).

Audio input

Most audio units (for example television, radio, and so forth) could be connected electrically via a cable connection or acoustically via a microphone directly to the loudspeaker. An acoustic or audio signal can then be picked up directly without distortion from the signal source. However, there will be some loss of the high frequency speech components and background noise will not be picked up as much.

Hand-held microphone

This is designed to allow the hearing-impaired listener to be closer to the speaker (providing a better signal-to-noise ratio). The hand-held microphone is connected via a cable to the audio input to enable better understanding under noisy conditions.

FM system

An FM system consists of a microphone, FM transmitter, and FM receiver. It is suitable for group amplification systems in schools as well as for personal use in meetings and conferences. The microphone picks up the speech directly from the speaker, and therefore the speaking distance is less than 20 cm (Lewis in Tyler and Schum, 1995).

Telephone assistive devices

A range of 'alerting devices' and amplification devices are available. These include replacement handsets, built-in amplifiers, in-line amplifiers, portable audio amplifiers and teletext and telecommunication devices (Slager in Tyler and Schum, 1995).

Wearing the device

Technology is improving and becoming more accessible, but this is worthless if the device is not actually worn. Huge numbers of devices end up in drawers, forgotten or broken and are never used. Adult hearing-aid candidates have reported anxieties about mechanical faults and their rejection of a device (Reiter in Sandlin, 1995). The following section will focus on children, however the information will also be useful for thinking about services for young people and adults too.

There are a number of reasons why people do not wear their device:

* painful or uncomfortable;
* not useful – for example, noisy, or does not help hearing;
* not working properly, ran out of batteries, leads, ear moulds, and so forth;
* embarrassment, body image, self-image difficulties;
* do not believe they need it, children not aware that hearing can be useful

The role of the clinical psychologist in the audiology team is important here for both individual work with a client (and/or their family) or as a consultant to the team when an individual does not wear a device. Consultation may include observing an audiology session to see how the client reacts to sound, alterations to their device, and concentration and understanding of what is happening to them. It may be possible to offer suggestions to the audiologist, which may help the individual in relation to this difficulty. With individual work with clients, an audiologist or teacher of the deaf would usually help a child to wear a device and an audiologist or hearing therapist would help an adult. Only if serious concerns arouse would they refer on to clinical psychology.

In the case of children, the child and family need to be assessed, by a team member and possibly the clinical psychologist, as prescriptive interventions will probably have been tried and failed at this point. Thus, interventions will have to be tailored to meet the individual needs of each child and family. From our clinical work, emotional reactions to deafness and parenting seem to be the two main reasons for difficulties in establishing the wearing of devices in nursery- and primary-school aged children. When children reach secondary level, factors often also include self-esteem, a feeling of difference, body image and peer pressure.

It is important that children and adults feel comfortable about wearing a device. If the devices are not worn, all technology is worthless. Establishing routines linked to a positive sense of self from childhood, will hopefully enable everyone who wants to wear a device for hearing to do so.

Establishing a routine for children wearing a device

For some children, it is difficult to establish a routine about wearing a device. Perseverance on the part of parents and professionals is important, and well-established techniques help in our work.

The following suggestions are aimed at motivating the younger child to use their device:

- *Routine.* Establish a routine around putting the device on and off. Let the children know what will happen during the day and what is expected of them in relation to wearing the device. Keep the device visible but in a safe place (e.g. help the children make a special box to keep the device in beside their bed). When the children are old enough, help them to take responsibility for putting it on and taking it off themselves. If a child is not wearing a device, keep the device visible to make sure that it remains a part of every day life, and not forgotten.
- *Communication.* If there is no formal language available to the child, use visual prompts to let them know what is expected of them (for instance, show them the device before putting it on, or show a battery before changing them). Always ask permission or tell the child what you are going to do to the device, or ear, before you do so. A device is seen as part of a child's body, and thus an integral part of the child, so permission from an adult to touch or change the device is paramount.

- *Emotion.* When establishing wearing, take emotion out of interactions related to the device. Act in a neutral way. This will help the child not to pick up on parental feelings, and associate any indirect negativity about the device.
- *Behaviour.* For those working with parents, it is worth considering how the children's behaviour is managed in other aspects of life. This will give an indication of how they are managing the device wearing, and will allow advice to be tailored appropriately. Consistency between parents and professionals is crucial. Parents and professionals should praise children for all behaviours that they would like to see more of, although it is best to praise an action (for example, wearing) rather than listening or hearing. If a child will wear a part of a device, or wear the device but turned off, keep this up so that the device remains a part of every day routines.

Integration of the device into everyday life

Children's integration of a device into their everyday lives does not seem to have been studied. A review of the literature on a child's acceptance of prosthetic devices is also remarkably small. From clinical practice, those children who integrate the device into their lives (hearing aid or cochlear implant) seem to take an increased personal benefit from the device.

Behaviourally, integrating a device into their lives might involve:

- taking responsibility for it;
- asking for it in the mornings;
- keeping it safe;
- changing batteries;
- noting faults;
- willingly wearing the device at home after school and weekends.

Helping children to take care of, and have pride in, their device is important by all those who support them. This will potentially benefit their esteem and self-image.

If possible, it is important for parents to set boundaries in terms of use of the device, for the child to get benefit from it initially. Giving choices often makes if easier for children to feel that they have some control over the situation. For example, asking them whether they would like to wear the device now or after breakfast gives them the choice of *when* to put on the device, not *whether* to put it on. Manufacturers of hearing aids, ear moulds and cochlear implant (speech processors) have developed colourful options and stickers to individualize the devices: sparkly ear moulds and moulds in the colours of favourite football teams can now be made.

Child-centred approach

A fundamental underpinning to successful interventions with children is to make a genuine and meaningful attempt to join them in their view of the world. This can be more challenging than it first appears, particularly when hearing adults attempt to understand deaf children. A useful starting point can be to step outside our own perspective and accept that reality for the child may be very different. For example, it is generally not the goal of a small child to want to hear (Lynch, Craddock and Crocker, 1999).

The aims between professionals, parents and children can all be very different, which will probably result in poor outcomes of any intervention. The following ideas may help in thinking about service delivery:

• Communication and cognitive style of the deaf child.

  – Do deaf children understand what is happening to them? If not, how can we augment the communication to help them with this (for instance, use of picture sequences, or sign language)?
  – Due to poor language skills with many young deaf children, the need for routine and predictability is crucial. This will enable them to know what is happening and therefore feel safe and give the children a sense of control (Dawaliby, Burke and McKee, 1983).

• Optimizing the approach and environment.

  – As in most situations, by using positive coping strategies (Peterson and Shigatomi, 1981), positive reinforcement and praise (Lansdown and Sokel, 1993), a child will more readily respond to audiological tasks and interventions.
  – For new experiences, modelling, play and rehearsal of events will prove invaluable in enabling a child to feel confident about procedures (Anderson and Masur, 1983).
  – Presenting the device to the child in a way that is non-threatening and gives the child time to explore it will help a child 'bond' to it more easily. For example, allowing children to take a new device out of a box in their own time, rather that putting it straight on them, and giving them time to explore the device without pressure, will save audiological time in the long run.
  – Direct communication with audiologists (being in the same room), and being able to see what they are doing will enable children to have an increased sense of what is happening to them, and be less frightening.
  – Wearing a device for a few days without it being switched on may help some children to get used to the physical sensations of the

device, and the routines around wearing it before having to also get used to listening, and taking meaning from sound.

- A child should always be warned before a device is switched on.
- Reducing any negative parental emotions so that they can pass on positive or neutral feelings to a child about wearing a device. For this to occur, the parents must be provided with enough information and time to ask questions (Jay et al., 1993).

• Monitoring psycho-social outcomes.

- Exploring a child's feelings about a device (through play, drawing and language).
- Monitoring a child's behaviour for distress, comfort or reaction to change.
- Monitoring a child's self esteem and body image if the child is old enough, to see their responses to having a hearing loss, and integration of a hearing device into their sense of self, for example by using 'My World' pictures (Hobday and Ollier, 2000).

Summary

This chapter has discussed the different hearing devices available for hearing-impaired people, with an emphasis on device fitting with children. The choice of device is usually made based on diagnostic or medical and audiological information. The fitting of a hearing instrument is merely the start of the road to (re)habilitation and does not 'normalize' hearing as spectacles can 'normalize' vision. There are many other factors such as the motivation of the client, mode and level of communication ability, age and support that are crucial in the successful outcome of the (re)habilitation process.

It is important to realise that a hearing impaired person with a hearing instrument is not a 'normally' hearing adult or child. This is due to the fact that almost any form of deafness, for which a hearing device is indicated, involves some less desirable effects, such as recruitment, amplification of background noise or loss of discrimination. In addition the hearing device itself still shows some imperfections, such as limited frequency range and small distortions of sound waves.

Ideas about fitting of the device with children, and making audiology services child centred, will hopefully go some way towards helping children integrate a device into their everyday lives. The role of the clinical psychologist is vital to assess the individual factors that might be present with the adult or child wearing a hearing device, and to tailor interventions accordingly. Services have an obligation to think about how their approach to adults or children aids their esteem and body image. Asking permission and informing a person before making any changes is imperative in this process.

References

Alpiner JG, McCarthy PA (1987) Rehabilitative Audiology: Children and Adults. Baltimore MD: Williams & Wilkins.

Anderson KO, Masu FT III (1983) Psychological preparation for invasive medical and dental procedures. Journal of Behavioural Medicine 6: 1–40.

Chute PM, Nevins ME (2002) The Parent's Guide to Cochlear Implants. Washington DC: Gallaudet University Press.

Crandell CC, Smalindo JJ (1995) The importance of room acoustics. In: Tyler RS, Schum DJ, Assistive Devices for Persons with Hearing Impairment. Boston MA: Allyn and Bacon.

Davis JM, Hardick EJ (1986) Rehabilitative Audiology for Children and Adults. London: Collier MacMillan.

Dawaliby FJ, Burke NE, McKee BG (1983) A comparison of hearing impaired and normally hearing students on locus of control, people orientation and study habits and attitudes. American Annals of the Deaf 128: 53–9.

Erber NP (1993) Communication and Adult Hearing Loss. Australia: Clavis Publishing.

Hobday A, Ollier K (2000) Activities with Children and Adolescents. BPS Books: The British Psychological Society.

Jay SM, Elliot CH, Ozolins M, Olson R (1993) Behavioural Management of Children's Distress during Painful Medical Procedures. Unpublished manuscript.

Katz J (1985) Handbook of Clinical Audiology. 3 edn. Baltimore MD: Williams & Wilkins.

Lansdown R, Sokel B (1993) Commissioned review: Approaches to pain management in children. ACPP Review and Newsletter 15(3): 105–11.

Ling D (1976) Speech and the Hearing Impaired Child: Theory and Practice. Washington DC: Alexander Graham Bell Association for the Deaf.

Lynch C, Craddock LC, Crocker SR (1999) Developing a child-centred approach for paediatric audiologists; a model in the context of cochlear implant programming. The Ear 1: 10–16.

Northern JL, Downs MP (2002) Hearing in Children. 5 edn. Baltimore MD: Williams & Wilkins.

Peterson L, Shigatomi C (1981) The use of coping techniques to minimise anxiety in hospitilised children. Behaviour Therapy 12: 1–14.

Pollack MC (1975) Amplification for the Hearing Impaired. New York: Grune & Stratton.

Sandlin RE (1995) Handbook of Hearing Aid Amplification. Clinical considerations and Fitting Practices. Volume 11. London: Singular.

Tietze L, Papsin B (2000). Utilization of bone-anchored hearing aids in children. International Journal of Pediatric Otorhinolaryngology 58: 75–80.

Tye-Murray N (1998) Foundations of Aural Rehabilitation. Children, Adults and their Family Members. London: Singular.

Tyler RS, Schum DJ (1995) Assistive Devices for Persons with Hearing Impairment. Boston MA: Allyn and Bacon.

Webster DB (1983) Identification of hearing loss in infancy and early childhood. In Alpines JG, McCarthy PA (1987) Rehabilitative Audiology: Children and Adults. Baltimore MD: Williams and Wilkins.

PART 2
PSYCHOLOGICAL MODELS
APPLIED TO DEAFNESS

CHAPTER 5

Psychodynamic considerations in working with people who are deaf

JANET FERNANDO

> I don't know who I am. I'm not allowed to be me. (A patient)

Introduction

Psychodynamic therapy is a psychological treatment that can help patients discover their true selves and is used to treat a wide range of mental health problems including depression. It stems from the work of Freud and psychoanalysis and has produced many offshoots as detailed by Brown and Peddar (1993).

In 1919 Freud wrote *Lines of Advance in Psychoanalytic Therapy*, in which he stated that in order to make treatment available to a wider range of people 'we shall be faced with the task of adapting our technique' and we are still doing this, the task of adapting it for deaf people being the focus of this chapter. Throughout, the author uses the term 'deaf' regardless of audiological or cultural status.

Psychodynamic theory

Psychodynamic refers to the psyche and implies a propensity for movement and change. Psychodynamic therapy explores a patient's anxieties through the patient's reactions to the therapist in the present. The overlap between many different models of psychodynamic theory and practice currently used means that there can be some confusion. For the author, who offers *psychoanalytic psychotherapy* once, twice and sometimes three times weekly over months and sometimes years, object relations theory, as developed in much of the work of Bion, Klein and Winnicott, provides a relevant conceptual framework. Central to this theory is the belief that human beings' prime motivation is to form relationships with other people rather than as Freud originally thought, the instinctual search for pleasure and the avoidance of pain. In object relations theory each person is seen to have an internal world containing a core self, versions of other people perceived by this core self (internal objects) and a network of relationships between these internal objects. The character of this matrix is determined by an infant's earliest experiences of communication and empathy with its mother, and significant others, including such experiences as feeding and holding. The experience of being deaf will inevitably influence this.

The psychodynamic relationship

A detailed and excellent account of the psychodynamic relationship and process is to be found in Chapter 8 of *Introduction to Psychoanalysis* by Bateman and Holmes (1995). The essence of what is written is encapsulated below and interspersed with the author's thoughts specific to working with people who are deaf.

The idea of a therapeutic relationship is present in a patient's mind before therapy begins. A potential patient knows something is wrong and wonders how it can be put right and begins to talk to professionals or friends. A potential patient begins to form a sense of the type of therapist he or she is seeking. This may be a therapist who is male or female, deaf or hearing, black or white, and so on.

The psychodynamic relationship starts when patient and therapist meet, form a contract and begin treatment. The therapist must explain what treatment involves, how long it is likely to last, the risks and possible benefits. Many deaf patients are particularly concerned about confidentiality, maybe more so than non-deaf patients, often because the deaf community is small and they feel there is not the same privacy that is guaranteed to hearing patients. It is often helpful to have a frank discussion about confidentiality rather than interpret their anxiety although this should not always be ruled out. Likewise, it is often important to prepare a deaf patient for the possibility of meeting his or her therapist in a social setting, especially if the therapist is deaf. Ideally it is better if the patient and therapist do not meet in social settings but clearly this is not always possible if both the therapist and the patient are members of the deaf community. What is important, however, is that both patient and therapist are clear about their objectives and expectations so the work can continue unhindered by external factors.

Bateman and Holmes (1995) remind us that it is the spirit of the therapeutic contract that is important. A patient who asks to change a session may be offered an alternative, if the therapist can accommodate the request and if the patient has an unavoidable commitment. Both patient and therapist must adhere to their arrangements as agreed when setting up the contract and only vary them through joint discussion. This places an obligation on both the patient and the therapist not to unilaterally alter the framework of the treatment.

The therapeutic setting

Bateman and Holmes (1995) describe the therapeutic setting as a set of counterpoised themes: attachment and separation; opening up and closure; holding/containment and frustration. Weekly and sometimes more frequent sessions encourage attachment and curiosity. An open-ended contract and adherence to the agreed arrangements, especially by the therapist, provides a holding function whereas protecting the therapeutic hour from interruption provides the necessary containment. The therapeutic setting is ordered so that it can become, or contain, a process and changes to the setting should be avoided if possible. Inevitable changes such as illness, meaning the patient or therapist is not able to attend, or lateness on either part may stimulate new material and the setting allows these events to be explored usefully. Their meaning is highlighted within the firm boundaries of the orderly contract.

The psychodynamic process

Once the boundaries of the therapeutic relationship have been set up treatment can begin. Initially patients feel anxious and often explain a great deal about themselves. Then, as they increase in confidence, they start to look to the therapist for clarification and help. Gradually doubt about the wisdom in embarking on therapy becomes evident. Patients begin to feel that therapists are not behaving in the expected or desired way and this increases their anxiety. The therapist's refusal to fulfil the increasing demands of the patient, for example to extend the finishing time of sessions, or the wish for physical contact, evokes disillusionment. The resulting frustration increases the probability of the patient reverting to earlier, more archaic patterns of relating and therapeutic regression begins to emerge. Wishes, phantasies, hopes, desires, disappointments, frustrations and longings of the patient's present and past become embodied in the therapeutic relationship and so provide an opportunity to study their origins, sometimes through dream work.

The secure setting and the attentiveness of the therapist provides an opportunity to develop trust and identify with a helpful, considerate object, which in turn enables a patient to be more thoughtful about him or herself and so listen to interpretations. The therapist's capacity to act as a container (Bion, 1959, 1962, 1963) facilitates this process. The therapist collects and integrates projected aspects of the patient's self. His or her capacity to understand, and to give meaning to the projected fragments, provides the containment that allows them to be transformed into a more tolerable form and reintrojected. The therapeutic encounter can become a 'holding environment' or transitional space in which the early experiences may be regressively reworked leading to greater creativity and increased awareness (Winnicott, 1971).

The re-experiencing of earlier difficulties is painful and many patients resist the regressive pull. They may use intellectualization and rationalization and other defensive styles in the hope of avoiding pain. Although a patient may long to change and be happier some of the thoughts, desires and needs he or she stumbles across lead to embarrassment and shame. The patient covers up and may even feel better with the symptoms than without them. The patient's anti-regressive function hardens and becomes a source of resistance (Sandler and Sandler, 1994).

Resistance, which is often a signpost of change, refers to the methods a patient uses to obstruct the process that is being relied on to bring about change. It takes on many forms, including the concealment of facts or unconsciously acting out, missing sessions or obsessively arriving on time, developing new symptoms or sometimes taking a flight into health. In all cases resistance should be the focus of interpretations.

The purpose of *interpretation* is to make something conscious that was previously unconscious. It will employ the use of *transference* and *counter-transference* experiences and enable patients to find meaning where there seemed to be none. *Transference* is a process that occurs during treatment when a patient unconsciously transfers onto the therapist feelings previously experienced in relation to significant others. *Counter-transference* applies to the thoughts and feelings that are experienced by the therapist and help to better understand a patient's inner world and so provide interpretations. Good interpretations restore balance, promote integration and lead to *insight* so that gradually the patient will feel ready to leave the therapist and begin to talk about ending treatment.

Endings of treatment take time and have been likened to mourning (Klein, 1950). They are difficult for both patient and therapist. The patient has to acknowledge the help that has been given as well as accept the loss of its on-going comfort, just as a baby gives up the breast when weaned. The patient also needs to accept the limitations of treatment and give up a desired but unattainable ideal. Throughout, therapists must follow the fluctuations between regression and integration and accept their own sadness about the ending of important relationships. They have to accept that they may never again hear about people with whom they have become so familiar, and reconcile themselves to areas of failure. Alongside their patients, they have to come to accept the therapy as 'good enough'.

Psychodynamics and deafness

As discussed in Chapter 1, definitions related to deafness shift constantly. Deaf people and their advocates have become more sensitive to negative terminology and insistent upon the use of language and descriptors they have chosen themselves (Meadow-Orlans and Erting, 2000). Those who identify exclusively with the Deaf culture have a sense of belonging, as do those who are deaf but see themselves as culturally hearing. There are some, however, who feel they do not fit into either hearing or deaf societies and their identities emerge as confused without clear notions of hearingness or deafness (Glickman, 1993). They may shift uncomfortably between hearing and deaf settings, unlike some who are bicultural and able to negotiate both settings and in doing so embrace Deaf culture and value hearing contacts.

Increasingly, people ask if there is a difference in working with people who are deaf compared to hearing people. Although not wishing to deny the different experiences of being deaf or hearing, it is the author's view that there is a tendency to overemphasize the differences and minimize the similarities. Why does this happen? Is it because there are more differences than similarities? Is it because over the years deaf people have been oppressed by hearing people who have denied the differences and in so doing forced deaf people to emphasize the differences themselves in order to establish an identity of their own? Whatever the reason, it is essential for deaf and non-deaf therapists to hold a transcultural model of practice in mind if therapy is to be effective. Therapists need to familiarize themselves with the growing literature of authors such as d'Ardenne and Mahtani (1989) who highlight the need for a good linguistic match between therapist and patient, as well as considering the cultural knowledge and experiences that both therapists and patients bring to the therapeutic setting. As well as acknowledging and valuing their patients' culture, however, it is also important to be aware of their own prejudices and those of their patients, and in so doing to provide an effective, sensitive and appropriate treatment.

The very nature of psychodynamic therapy – in that it is essentially based on the relationship between patient and therapist – lends itself to working in a transcultural way. It has, nevertheless, taken years to recognize that the reported and observed difficulties and failures in psychotherapy with deaf patients often reflected the therapists' skills and attitudes rather than the limitations of the deaf patient (Sussman and Brauer, 1999). The therapists themselves generally did not possess a working knowledge of deafness and were not able to communicate effectively with their patients. In recent years, a growing number of therapists, notably in the US and more recently in Britain, have applied psychodynamic therapy in the field of deafness. These therapists claim the nature of therapy with deaf patients is no different to psychotherapy with non-deaf patients. Nor is a new theoretical orientation needed despite earlier literature advocating this (Levine, 1960; Myklebust, 1960; Vernon and Andrews, 1990).

Culture

The implementation of effective psychotherapy clearly depends on the basic assumptions that both therapist and patient bring to the situation. This is particularly true if the patient and therapist are from different cultural backgrounds. It is important for therapists to be aware of and understand, and not pathologize, the differing factors that make up the disparity between themselves and their patients.

When there is a choice, deaf patients are more likely to select a deaf therapist. Deaf patients may consciously, or unconsciously, choose a deaf therapist whose cultural orientation reflects where the patient might eventually like to be (Harvey, 1989; Lytle and Lewis, 1996). Or it may be the bond of deafness and the perceived commonality of the deaf experience that prompts the choice. However, although the perceived commonality of deafness may facilitate the initial therapeutic alliance, difficulties may become apparent when one considers the various meanings and perceptions of deafness (Harvey, 1989) and caution should be exercised. The deaf therapist is not just deaf. He or she has his or her own defined perceptions of being deaf and these perceptions may or may not equate with the deaf patient's perceptions. Nonetheless, deaf culture identity parameters do affect therapist-patient attunement (Leigh and Lewis, 1999). Some, however, may consciously or unconsciously choose to work with a non-deaf therapist and hearing therapists will need to have explored their attitudes to deafness and motives for working with deaf people for treatment to be effective (Rebourg, 1992; Corker, 1994). Corker warns that hearing people may be afraid of deafness and deaf people. This would affect their behaviour towards deaf people, which in turn could be introjected by deaf patients, who would see the fear as part of themselves.

Language

The Babel of the Unconscious (Amati-Mehler, Argentieri, and Canestri, 1998) discusses the acquisition of language and differentiates polylinguism – the acquisition of various languages, often simultaneously, throughout childhood – from polyglotism. Polyglotism is the later learning of a new language based dominantly on translation and with far fewer emotional connotations than the early natural acquisition of several languages. Their work is based on the hearing population and focuses on mother tongue and foreign languages in the psychodynamic dimension. It does, however, raise interesting issues worthy of consideration, notably the advisability of undertaking therapy when the patient and therapist do not share the same mother tongue. They remind us:

> the unconscious has extraordinary ways of finding a new road to the 'other' when the usual roads are blocked; and linguistic limitations are important roadblocks. The analyst must signal to the patient his lack of understanding and explore the patient's ways of dealing with the experiences of not being understood. The unconscious usually finds its way; when it doesn't, corresponding defensive processes, invisible before, may become highlighted now, with the possibility of working through silent roadblocks previously ignored. (Kernberg, in the preface of Amati-Mehler, Argentieri and Canestri, 1998).

It is appropriate at this point to remind ourselves that not all people who are deaf learn, or choose, to sign. Those born to deaf parents more often than not become fluent in their 'mother language' – sign – and like those born to hearing parents may or may not become fluent in a second language, for example spoken English. But what about those who are born to non-deaf parents? Some as children are introduced to sign language – generally outside the family environment – and often report feeling better able to express themselves in sign and consider this to be their first language. For some, sign is the only communication mode that feels meaningful, whereas others comfortably switch from sign to speech, depending on the situation they find themselves in, as illustrated in the following.

Case study: The hearing child wants to be heard

A young woman came into treatment saying she was bilingual and preferred to work with a hearing therapist who could sign. She said she trusted deaf therapists but for her, working with a hearing person afforded greater privacy.

She was deafened at 4 years of age. Twelve months prior to this her mother was hospitalized for several weeks owing to a serious illness. She came into treatment saying she could not rely on others to be there for her and this made it difficult to maintain long-term relationships. Throughout her early sessions she signed in fluent British Sign Language.

Several weeks into treatment her session was cancelled at short notice and she arrived at the next session feeling tense and angry. She had had a difficult day at work and complained to her therapist about unreliable colleagues who were never around when needed. The therapist interpreted this as the patient feeling she was let down when the previous session had been cancelled. The young woman gave a relieved smile and went on to explain how much she had wanted to see the therapist the previous week and how upset she had felt when this had not been possible. Then after a silence she went on to talk about her mother being hospitalized when she was three years old. She was surprised to find herself thinking about this and became tearful and uttered verbally, 'Mummy, I want Mummy'. She was in touch with the painful memory of feeling abandoned by her mother. It was the hearing child in her that needed to be understood and she had unconsciously chosen a hearing therapist for this reason. It is the author's view, however, that a deaf psychotherapist could have helped her to get in touch with the 'hearing child' just as a hearing therapist can help deaf patients get in touch with the 'deaf child'. As long as there is a 'good enough' linguistic match, psychic growth can occur irrespective of whether a therapist is deaf or hearing as long as the hearingness or deafness of the therapist does not get in the way.

Deaf people in therapy

It is important to remember that there are more psychologically healthy deaf people than there are not and that these individuals live productive and satisfying lives (Lane, Hoffmeister and Bahan, 1996). Those who present for therapy are often successful in many aspects of their lives but are asking for help in resolving recurring anxieties that make them feel ill at ease. These anxieties may be rooted in early infantile experiences; for example, in the early mother/infant relationship during the first few weeks of life, or may belong to a later stage of psychic development. Like non-deaf individuals deaf people present for treatment for a variety of reasons: for example relationship problems with a partner, anxieties about becoming a parent, loss and bereavement, eating problems, difficulty in coping with a life change, general feelings of dissatisfaction or recurring bouts of depression. All these examples may or may not be directly associated to deafness although clearly the experience of being deaf must in some way play its part. The author has noted, however, that there are three clearly defined issues that arise more frequently in working with people who are deaf compared to hearing people. These three issues are anger, childhood sexual abuse and personal identity.

Anger

Anger is a human emotion experienced by everyone. However, 'Healthy Deaf Minds' (2002) indicated that deaf people might experience more anger than hearing people. ('Healthy Deaf Minds' is a series of talks, organized through the British Society for Mental Health and Deafness, about mental health with deaf people, their friends and families, and the professionals who work with them. They aim to inform deaf people about a broad range of mental health issues so as to empower deaf people to say what they want, based on their experiences and needs.) Possible reasons for this can be because of oppression, ignorance on the part of hearing people and because some deaf people do not know how to assert themselves in a way that will achieve a successful and appropriate outcome[1]. Many who come into treatment report feelings of overwhelming anger that they regard as unhealthy and want help understanding. Some, however, feel angry because they have never been able to express how they really feel and they experience hearing people as disabling.

Case study: fear of not being understood

A young man in his early twenties had an assessment interview with a hearing therapist. The assessor understood his sign language and recommended a treatment that was taken up with a successful outcome. It was clear, however, that the patient needed to monitor constantly that the assessor was following his sign. When this was raised he said he was not aware of any miscommunication but was enabled to express anxiety about working with a non-deaf therapist. He said he was fearful that if he became angry during the course of treatment a non-deaf person would not understand him and this would prevent him getting the help he really needed. It also emerged that he felt a non-deaf person would not understand his experience of being deaf, and it seemed clear that prior to the assessment interview he had made a conscious decision that he wanted a deaf therapist, and was disappointed and angry to discover the assessor was a hearing person. He had already received therapy from a non-deaf signing therapist in the past and terminated treatment as he experienced it as unhelpful. For him his fear of not being understood had been borne out and it was more likely than not that the hearingness of a hearing therapist would have got in the way of him being able to make use of a treatment, however proficient a hearing therapist may have been in sign. He was offered treatment with a deaf therapist.

Sexual abuse

It is well documented (and discussed in the final chapter of this book) that there is a higher incidence of childhood sexual abuse in the deaf community compared to the hearing community, so it is not surprising that issues associated with abuse present as often as they do. A range of complex emotions come about as a result of abuse but a recurring theme is the consequence of being understood.

Case study: fear of being understood

A young woman requested to see a non-deaf therapist for an assessment interview and it was evident from the outset a deaf therapist would provide a better communication match.

The young woman hoped therapy would help her understand herself better and take away the depression that often resulted in her taking time off work. When it was suggested she might prefer to work with a deaf therapist she insisted she felt more comfortable working with a hearing person as the deaf world is small and she did not want to run the risk of meeting her therapist in social situations.

During the early weeks of treatment she attempted to turn the therapist into a supervisor. She complained about her work situation saying people stopped her getting on with the work. When the therapist interpreted this as the young woman finding it difficult to allow the therapist to get on with her work and be a therapist, the young woman felt found out – her therapist had understood something more profound than her sign language – and she absented herself from her sessions.

There had been times when the therapist had not understood the patient's signed communications. When she returned to treatment it became important to explore what this meant to her and it quickly emerged that it made her feel safe. This was demonstrated powerfully in one particular session when there were constant shifts from one subject to another leaving the therapist feeling helpless and uncomfortable. Recognizing the discomfort as being something the patient was projecting into her – as opposed to the therapist's occasional discomfort about not actually understanding the signed communication – the therapist was able to reflect on the session and identify the point at which the shifting from one subject to another began. One example was when the patient had started to talk about an interaction at work. Someone had asked her how she felt about being deaf. She had not given the therapist her response and when the therapist drew her attention to this she blushed and looked away and for some time was unable to re-establish contact. When she eventually regained eye contact the therapist acknowledged the young woman's shame, which in turn evoked the response: 'I hate my deafness. I should feel proud but I don't. I feel ashamed, very, very ashamed. I could never admit this to a deaf person.'

She continued in once-weekly therapy for two years and as treatment progressed talked more and more about her mother. She explained that as a child she had wanted to talk to her mother about being deaf but sensed this caused upset and came to believe it was better to keep her thoughts to herself. There was, however, something else she had wanted to discuss with her mother – undisclosed sexual abuse

– and when she eventually attempted to do so a catastrophe occurred: her mother became seriously ill and she felt fully responsible for this. On coming into treatment it felt safer, albeit unconsciously so, to not be understood, hence her choice of a therapist. Over the weeks and months in treatment, however, she came to understand this and slowly internalized a therapist/ object who wanted to understand and could survive her unconscious aggressive impulses. She ended treatment feeling more comfortable with her deafness and relieved she had been able to disclose and talk about her feelings associated to the abuse.

Personal identity

Many people come into treatment saying they want to find themselves. They feel lost, they do not know who they are, or they feel they have been shaped into something they are not. This makes them feel angry – they do not know their true selves – and they go through life feeling confused and misunderstood and often experience feelings of shame.

Case study: I don't know who I am – I'm not allowed to be me

A woman in her thirties presented for treatment saying personal relationships were difficult. She felt consumed by overwhelming anger and experienced others – both deaf and hearing – as attempting to mould her into something she was not. Despite having a profound hearing loss she was educated in non-signing schools and bitterly remembers teachers 'showing her off' to visiting parents. Her speech was good and the school wanted to prove the merits of an oral education. She felt she was expected to behave as a hearing person, the only problem being she did not know what it was like to be hearing. She knew what it was like to be deaf but experienced other deaf people as denying her this experience: if she did not conform to their view of deafness then in their eyes she was not deaf. She felt as if there was a spring inside her. All the time it was becoming more and more tight. She wanted to feel calm and more in control of her own destiny. Throughout her treatment she spoke but asked the therapist to communicate using Sign Supported English.

During the early months of treatment she experienced her therapist as 'winding her up' and not doing her job properly and attacked the therapist in a relentless and self-righteous manner as if saying 'I have to be right and adequate and you have to be wrong and inadequate.' Then, one day she brought a dream.

She was on a bus. A passenger got on and started to argue in an unreasonable manner with the driver. The bus went nowhere. In an attempt to resolve the situation she tried to reason with the passenger and give a more constructive way of thinking. On waking she did not know what the dispute was about.

When asked for associations – thoughts linked to the dream – she said the unreasonable passenger made her think of herself but she was not sure why. In analysing the dream with her therapist, however, she came to realize that anger associated to the past often got in the way of her moving forward on her therapeutic journey. This insight caused great anxiety and she sat back in her chair and stared long and hard at the therapist. This had the affect of making the therapist feel hot and extremely uncomfortable. The patient demanded to know how her therapist was feeling but noticeably relaxed when the therapist said she thought she wanted her to understand how it felt to be her. She sensed the therapist had come to understand something that words could not explain. She was understanding her shame, a negative evaluative and emotional reaction to one's own being, which can develop during the early months of life through the 'unreflected' look in the eyes of an infant's mother (Ayers, 2003). The patient's difficulties in maintaining personal relationships were associated with her mother's depression and emotional unavailability during infancy and compounded by society's response to her deafness.

Additional difficulties

Psychodynamic therapy, as described by the author, requires psychological mindedness (Coltart, 1988) and is difficult for those with learning difficulties to access, although this is not to say that psychodynamic theory cannot be applied to work with people who have additional difficulties, as demonstrated in the work of Sinason (1992) and Hodges (2002). The author's view is that one of the arts therapies such as art therapy, dance and movement therapy, drama therapy and, in some cases, music therapy may be better suited to deaf individuals who have learning difficulties. It is important to note, however, that the arts therapies are not reserved for people with additional learning difficulties but rather the non-verbal nature of the arts therapies facilitates the expression and exploration of feelings that 'talk' therapies cannot always mobilise.

Summary

This chapter considered how psychodynamic theory can be applied to working with deaf people. It highlighted three recurring issues that are brought to treatment, anger, childhood sexual abuse and personal identity, and while acknowledging the importance of patients having access to deaf therapists, it demonstrated how valuable work can be undertaken when the patient/therapist dyad is deaf/non-deaf. Although the chapter focused mainly on patients who use sign language, it recognized the important fact that sign is not the preferred communication mode for all deaf people and that there are times when the 'hearing child' in deaf people needs to be heard.

Deafness *per se* does not mean that a person will experience conflict but rather that the experience of being deaf may impact on unresolved conflicts rooted in early infancy and childhood. These conflicts re-emerge in the therapeutic relationship and provide an opportunity for exploration and understanding, so that in time patients experience a greater sense of being their true selves.

Note

This was debated at 'Healthy Deaf Minds', a series of talks organized through the British Society for Mental Health and Deafness, about mental health with deaf people, their friends and families, and the professionals who work with them. Its aims are: to inform deaf people about a range of mental health issues, thereby empowering deaf people to say what they want, based on their experiences and needs.

References

Amati-Mehler J, Argentieri S, Canestri J (1998) The Babel of the Unconscious: Mother Tongues and Foreign Languages in the Psychoanalytic Dimension. New York: International Universities Press.

Ayers M (2003) Mother-Infant Attachment and Psychoanalysis: The Eyes of Shame. London: Routledge.

Bateman A, Holmes J (1995) Introduction to Psychoanalysis: Contemporary Theory and Practice. London: Routledge.

Bion WB (1959) Attacks on linking. In Bion WB, Second Thoughts. London: Heinemann, pp. 93–109.

Bion WB (1962) Learning from Experience. London: Heinemann.

Bion WB (1963) Elements of Psychoanalysis. London: Heinemann.

Brown D, Pedder J (1993) Introduction to Psychotherapy: An Outline of Psychodynamic Principles and Practice. 2 edn. London: Routledge.

Coltart N (1988) Diagnosis and assessment for suitability for psycho-analytic psychotherapy. British Journal of Psychotherapy 4: 127–34.

Corker M (1994) Counselling: The Deaf Challenge. London: Jessica Kingsley.

d'Ardenne P, Mahtani A (1989) Transcultural Counselling in Action. 2 edn. London: Sage.

Freud S (1919) Lines of Advance in Psychoanalytic Therapy. London: Hogarth.

Glickman N (1993) Measuring Deaf cultural identities: a preliminary investigation. Rehabilitation Psychology 38: 275–83.

Harvey MA (1989) Psychotherapy with Deaf and Hard of Hearing Persons: A Systemic Model. Hillsdale NJ: Lawrence Erlbaum.

Healthy Deaf Minds (2002) Why are deaf people so angry? British Society for Mental Health and Deafness. Unpublished proceedings reported by Roger Beeson.

Hodges S (2002) Working with People with Learning Difficulties and Psychoanalysis. London: Tavistock.

Klein M (1950) On the criteria of the termination of psychoanalysis. International Journal of Psychoanalysis 31: 78–80.

Lane H, Hoffmeister R,Bahan B (1996) A Journey into the Deaf-world. San Diego CA: Dawn Sign Press.

Leigh IW, Lewis JW (1999) Deaf therapists and the deaf community: how the twain meet. In Leigh IW (ed.) Psychotherapy with Deaf Clients from Diverse Groups. Washington DC: Gallaudet University Press, pp. 45–65.

Levine ES (1960) The Psychology of Deafness. New York: Columbia University Press.

Lytle L, Lewis J (1996) Deaf therapists, deaf clients and the therapeutic relationship. In Glickman NS, Harvey MA (eds) Culturally Affirmative Psychotherapy with Deaf Persons. Mahwah NJ: Lawrence Erlbaum, pp. 262–76.

Meadow-Orlans K, Erting C (2000) Deaf people in Society. In Hindley P, Kitson N (eds) Mental Health and Deafness. London: Whurr, pp. 3–24.

Myklebust H (1960) The Psychology of Deafness. New York: Grune & Stratton.

Rebourg F (1992) Which way are individual therapies with Deaf people original? Proceedings, Second International Congress, European Society of Mental Health and Deafness, Namur, Belgium.

Sandler J, Sandler AM (1994) Theoretical and technical comments on regression and anti-regression. International Journal of Psychoanalysis 75: 431–9.

Sinason V (1992) Mental handicap and the Human Condition: New Approaches from the Tavistock. London: Free Association Books.

Sussman A, Brauer B (1999) On being a psychotherapist with deaf clients in Leigh IW (ed.) Psychotherapy with Deaf Clients form Diverse Groups. Washington DC: Gallaudet University Press, pp. 3–22.

Vernon M, Andrew J (1990) Psychology of Deafness. New York: Longman.

Winnicott D (1971) Playing and Reality. London: Penguin.

CHAPTER 6

Working systemically with deaf people and their families

SUSAN CROCKER

Introduction

This chapter will look at the application of systemic therapy principles with families where there is an individual who is deaf. The term 'deaf' will be used for all people with a hearing loss, whatever the level, and all styles of communication and cultural principles. Systemic therapy looks at beliefs and meaning for the individual, therefore defining cultural difference is not necessary, as it should always be addressed in the therapy.

There will be a brief overview of the main schools of therapy and the basic principles that underpin the work. The case examples will be on children and young people, as this is the author's field of work. However, systemic research and literature will be explored for both children and adults, with clinical implications discussed.

Systemic theory: brief historical overview

An understanding of systemic principles would be useful for this chapter, however, a brief outline of the main schools of therapy will follow. Systemic therapy is the general term that many practitioners use to refer to three main schools of theory: structural, strategic and systemic. Along with the term 'systemic therapy', people often also refer to this field of practice as 'family therapy'. Family systems therapy developed out of earlier therapeutic thinking, for example, Freud and Bowlby, and an understanding of how systems worked in the natural world. In the 1950s Gregory Bateson and colleagues started to explore communication patterns in families with a member suffering from schizophrenia (Bateson, 1972). Subsequent studies looked at communication processes and the first family therapy centre was opened in the late 1950s. From here different forms of family therapy developed and continue to evolve.

Main systemic schools explained

There are three main schools of thought in family therapy that share similar foundations although they differ at the level of methodology, focus, and approach to therapy.

Structural

Minuchin (1974) developed the structural school of family therapy. This framework suggests that families form structures within which they relate (to carry out roles and functions). These structures are an invisible set of rules that organize people's behaviour. Minuchin highlights the fact that subsystems form within families where, for example, shared interests and cultures exist. Also, boundaries exist around these sub-systems, the family and outside world. This school of thought purports that a 'functional' family must have clear boundaries, appropriate hierarchies and alignments, be able to adjust to change and allow for individuation. All families undergo periods of transition in their life cycles requiring reorganization of roles, and inflexibility would not allow this to happen. The goal of therapy is to create greater flexibility of thinking by joining the family, and by accommodating the family's culture, language and so on. By 'joining', it means that the therapist must not assume to understand the meaning of word used by individuals or families. Therefore asking about meaning is paramount, and using the exact word that the person uses, enables joining with the family. By asking for the meaning of words used in therapy, flexibility of thinking can come about through questioning the beliefs behind the meaning.

Strategic

Within this model there are two broad schools: brief therapy (Haley, 1978) and a mixture of strategic and structural family therapy (Madanes, 1981). Strategic therapists believe that families organize themselves according to a particular sequence of repetitive interaction, and that they will respond to a disruption to family life according to this interaction pattern. Thus, vicious cycles may be played out in this situation. A family often presents with one member displaying the symptoms. Strategic therapists are interested in how the family is organized around these symptoms, rather than labelling one member with the problem. Strategic family therapists tend to be pragmatic and directive in their approach, and often use the technique of reframing (redefining a problem to give new meaning, thus challenging a family's perceptions). With brief therapy, the therapists do not look on families as pathological; rather they view them as having a limited range of solutions. Therefore the therapist looks for existing solutions to amplify unique outcomes (White and Epston, 1989). The idea is that families are sometimes using solutions effectively, and it is the therapist's role to help them identify when this happens and to bring this more into everyday life.

Systemic

Primarily, the systemic therapists have included the Milan Group (Palazzoli et al., 1980). Central to their work are the three concepts of circularity, hypothesizing and neutrality. The therapist is included as part of the system, and looks at the meaning a family gives to the symptom and relates this to all parts of the system. Difficulties in relationships are seen as triggered by difference in relationships (or the perception of difference), and located in the interaction, not the individual (Sanders, 1985). Difference comes about when one part of a system changes and the others in the system do not change. In a family this might be when a child is born with a hearing loss, meaning that there are many appointments to attend. The mother or father may have to significantly change their working practice and home life to accommodate this. If only one parent makes changes, then a difference will occur between the parents that may end up in arguments, feeling unsupported, believing that one parent does not care and so on. Thus, both the interaction and relationship will change.

Systemic therapy principles in brief

One significant premise of systemic therapy is neutrality. This is neutrality towards family members (fairness to all people, checking that the therapist is not taking sides with any one person) and beliefs (non-judgemental stance to all people). Also, neutrality towards the symptom (non-judgemental about the type of symptom that the therapist is presented with) and change (neutral towards the outcome of assessment and therapy) (Palazzoli et al., 1980).

It is important to note that, within systemic understanding, there is no absolute reality – reality is relative, and meaning is gained through relationships and context. In order to understand the meanings that individuals attribute to their relationships, a systemic therapist hypothesizes and, taking a stance of curiosity and not knowing, asks questions. Hypothesizing begins from the time when a referral is discussed or made. For example, asking 'how can my team or speciality be helpful?' 'Who should I/we invite to the consultation?' Hypothesizing happens at many levels – for example stage of lifecycle of the family members, or the protective function of the symptom in relation to the system, and asking 'why now?'. Hypothesizing will occur continually, and is circular in that it connects all parts of the system (Cecchin, 1987).

Cybernetic epistemology is discussed in the systemic literature. It means that the therapist examines meaning given to a symptom or problem and relates it to all parts of the system (of which the therapist is a part). Therefore, systemic thinking enables a move from the individual to the interpersonal, with systemic therapists locating difficulties in the pattern of interaction rather than in the individual. This is a very freeing experience for individuals and families and encourages exploration and reflexivity. Use of impersonal language allows this to happen (for example describing a problem as 'the problem' rather than 'your problem') and comes from the literature on externalizing (White, 1988). This enables the problem to be seen as located outside of the individual, and therefore more able to be changed by the individual. Any change by an individual requires change within the whole system or change will not be sustainable.

Reflecting teams can be inside the room or can look on the therapy session through a two-way screen. The purpose of these teams is to reflect to the interviewer via a conversation, on the family's conversations. These conversations are positively connotated, with tentative speculative comments about the verbal and non-verbal material. The ideas in the reflection should show curiosity and be new to the family but not unusual (Anderson, 1987).

Using questions in therapy

The use of questions is paramount in systemic therapy. They connect information not previously related (enabling links to be made between behaviour, meaning and beliefs held by individuals and systems). Initially, questions are often collaborative, mapping relationships within the system, for example, between professionals, friends and family. Within these questions, ideas about what has been helpful before are useful to set the scene. These questions can be posed to all parts of the system (Reder and Fredman, 1996). This leads into questions about 'what could we do differently?', opening up the forum for the individual and family to let us know what they hope to achieve from the session, or from therapy, thus making sure that expectations for work are discussed and that there is consent for therapy.

The next style of questions that will often be used in therapy are termed 'triadic' and refer to circular questions. These are used so that the family observes its own system, for example, 'What does your dad think about . . .?', 'Who would be most surprised to hear that you were able to tackle . . .?' Circular questions in themselves may bring about change as people reflect on the questions and therefore independently challenges their own belief (Tomm, 1988).

Contextual questions are also useful to think about beliefs relating to school, family, race, religion, culture, medicine, media and so on. Other styles of questions used are deconstruction questions (for example, 'What gets in the way of developing . . .?'), opening space questions (for example, 'Has there ever been a time when . . . could have taken control of your relationships but didn't?'), meaning questions (for example, 'What does it mean to you that your daughter would do this?') and preference questions (for example, 'Does this idea suit you? Why?'). When defining the problem, story development questions look at process, detail, time and so on (for example, 'Where did this happen? What was going on at the time?') (Fredman and Coombs, 1996). Questions enable unique outcomes to emerge from problem-saturated narratives (White, 1988).

As part of understanding individuals' or families' beliefs, understanding the meaning of the words used is paramount. Therefore, using the language of the client (joining the vocabulary) is necessary for shared meaning. With a client using a language that is different from that of the therapist this will require feedback from interpreters as to the translation of the discourse.

Systemic therapy with deaf people

The deaf systemic literature is sparse, although it spans almost 30 years. Much of the literature is dominated by the writings of one man, Professor Michael Harvey from Gallaudet and Boston Universities (see Harvey, 1989). Harvey explains that to provide effective treatment to a family with a deaf member, then the paradigms of both deafness and systemic therapy must be used to hold the communicative needs of the therapist and all family members (Harvey, 1985).

There are many ideas about when a systemic approach might be a helpful way of working, particularly with deaf people from hearing families, although a few papers also highlight its use with deaf parents (for example, Sloman and Springer, 1987). In the following sections, the ideas of a systemic application to grief and denial, implications of communication and language development, and use of interpreters in therapy, will be discussed. Transitions within the family are often times when family difficulties come to the attention of professionals, as highlighted in the case examples.

Use of interpreters

A central theme for systemic work, which has been acknowledged previously in this chapter, is the very specific use and wording of questions in therapy. There is always a difficulty, when working with interpreters of any language, that the specific style of the questions may change in translation. One also has to be careful to check that certain words can be directly translated from one language to another. Here, more than ever, the need to check the meaning of grammar is paramount.

When working with interpreters using a systemic framework for therapy, it is useful to meet with the interpreter before the session to discuss, in particular, the premise behind the use and style of questioning. Also, considerations for the use of a team, lighting and seating need to be thought about (Warner in Hindley and Kitson, 2000).

Interpreters in systemic sessions do not only 'interpret' for a family, but become a part of the system, and therefore influence the therapy in a number of ways (Harvey, 1984):

- Seeking permission from families about inviting an interpreter to be present for appointments immediately confronts the issue of communication. Depending on the family's response, this allows for a dialogue to take place about the deaf person's language abilities, communication within the family and family's communication skills and approach.
- Interpreters confront homeostasis: they highlight that an individual is deaf and requires support to enable communication.
- It may be that some hearing families are not used to including a deaf child or adult into all conversations, and this may highlight feelings of denial related to a deaf child's difference within a particular family.
- It may be the first time that a deaf child or adult will be party to *all* conversations with the family. This may be difficult for the family, which has become accustomed to talking in front of the deaf person about topics that they would not discuss if the person were hearing.
- Having an interpreter who is able to break down communication barriers may be challenging to a family. Thus, hierarchical power in a family can be confronted, as families have to listen to the interpreter voice the feelings and opinions of the deaf member.

In some cases, a hearing therapist will have sign language skills good enough not to require an interpreter. The therapist needs to consider whether to use these skills, rather than utilize an interpreter. This may affect relationships with particular family members (Harvey, 1986). If the therapist has signing skills and decides to use them, the therapist will have to remember to sign *all* conversations when seeing a deaf person with hearing family members. This is particularly challenging when talking at the same time, as the languages are not a literal translation of each other. This is particularly pertinent when working with children, as it can be easy to address the parents and not the child, particularly young children who may be playing. Even if a child is playing and his or her back is turned (not communicating as they cannot see) then it is still important that the therapist signs all communication so that a child has access to the communication. If the child were hearing then he or she would be able to 'overhear' even if playing. It also highlights to the family the need to include the child in all conversations and allows for the opening of discussions about communication.

Denial

Due to denial of deafness, some hearing parents do not learn to sign at all, or learn to sign only to a level that allows them to communicate in a rudimentary way. In an as yet unpublished study looking at hearing parents with a child who has received a cochlear implant for up to 4 years, denial (in relation to their child's deafness) was experienced most by fathers (Anagnostou, Crocker and Graham, in preparation). Sloman, Springer and Vachon (1993) state that unresolved grieving about having a deaf child gets in the way of parents accepting the deafness and leads to communication problems between the parents and child, mainly due to not facilitating a manual communication system between the child and family. Thus, denial often pushes children into certain educational and communication modalities, which affects all areas of development and options for adulthood.

Case study

A young deaf child with significant additional learning and medical difficulties had a cochlear implant. The cochlear implant was the best hearing aid available to the child and it was offered within the understanding that her other needs were equally important. Expectations for the use of the implant were fairly low due to the additional difficulties, and this was explained to the family. However, after implantation, both the family and the local education team pushed for the girl to be placed in a mainstream school, denying her other learning, social and language needs by believing that all were the result of her hearing difficulties, and would now be remedied by the implant.

Grief

Sloman, Springer and Vachon (1993) hypothesized that dysfunctional communication in deaf families is preserved by its circular relationship to unresolved grief. Grief is often a result of not accepting that a child is deaf, and looking for cures and possibilities to enable a child to lead a 'normal' life. Parents may therefore cling to hard-to-achieve goals and seek out 'therapies' and 'technologies', and in doing so mask their grief. Sign language heightens the visual awareness that a child is deaf, with some families feeling self-conscious about signing in public. This is likely to block helpful communication, and families can become accustomed to not communicating well with their deaf member, leading to particular difficulties at points of transition. In the same study of hearing parents with children with cochlear implants, Anagnostou, Crocker and Graham (in preparation) found that grief was the strongest emotional condition that parents continued to experience over the years.

Case study

I was asked to meet with a young lady due to concerns that she was not wearing her hearing device and thus not reaching her potential with her hearing and speech.

The young lady came from a hearing Muslim family and went to a school for the deaf where her first language was British Sign Language (BSL). At home the family spoke Arabic, with English spoken outside of the home. The young lady's mother had stage 1 BSL skills, but her father could not sign. She had one deaf and two hearing siblings. To begin hypothesizing, the question of 'why now?' in relation to accessing help was asked. Through discussions it emerged that the young lady's age meant that access to her family's faith and culture was now important. Her mother was unable to tell her daughter about their faith herself, as her signing skills were not adequate. In the sessions we were able to discuss all of the ideas through an interpreter, highlighting that it was possible to discuss cultural and religious beliefs in BSL. This opened up conversations about gender and culture, which were related to acceptance of deafness and a desire for oral skills in the young lady as a solution. In the family's culture, beliefs about God, disability and gender meant that the mother felt unable to sign in public, and the father did not want to learn to sign at all. By asking respectful questions about their god and cultural beliefs, dialogues were opened about this.

Communication and theory of mind

It is clear from the literature that linguistic difficulties are highlighted as the cause of many problems in families with a deaf member (for example, Sloman, Perry and Frankenberg, 1987). This may be for a number of reasons. However, it is only fairly recently that the implications of a delayed theory of mind has been linked to cognitive, emotional and linguistic development. Theory of mind (ToM) is the ability to put yourself in someone else's shoes. A network of mental states governs behaviour, thus the idea that people have different views from us is fundamental to developing abstract thought and creativity in our thinking. It is generally felt that these skills emerge in the pre-school years, predominantly through interaction where a child can learn about mental states and how these relate to behaviour (Peterson and Siegal, 1995).

It is understood from the literature that deaf children of hearing families are very late in developing these skills. In a study by Peterson (2002) only 14% of the deaf 4–12 year olds assessed passed a test to identify a ToM, compared to 85% of 3–5-year-old hearing children. There was still a high failure rate in the deaf 13–16 year group, with 40% not completing the task successfully. This is only applicable to deaf children of hearing families (not deaf children with deaf parents, who perform more like hearing children).

If a child or young person does not have a theory of mind, then thinking systemically will be compromised, as the premise of circular questioning is the ability to answer what you think another person thinks, for example, 'Would your dad think differently about that compared with . . .'? Thus, direct work with the child or adult with a poor theory of mind within family therapy is very difficult.

Case study

A young deaf person aged 14, and her hearing mother met with me to discuss the difficulties they were having in their relationship. The mother was shouting at her daughter and not wanting to spend time with her as she felt that she was rude and not listening to her. The girl's parents had divorced in the preceding year, and the young person had moved with her mother far away leaving behind her school with a hearing impaired unit and her friends. She had been at her new local mainstream school for two terms by the time she met with me. This young deaf person had been brought up orally, aided with a cochlear implant.

As part of my work with this family, I worked alongside a speech and language therapy colleague who, with the family's permission, was able to assess the young person's language skills. Through this assessment we were able to ascertain that she was managing orally at the level of a 6-year- old. This was reflected in the fact that she was unable to understand my circular questions, and covered up by continuing on the topic of conversation that was last discussed. This perseveration with the previous topic of conversation was found to be the cause of her mother's anger, as she felt that her daughter was not listening to her. In highlighting the struggles with language that her daughter was having, and allowing the young person to let us know that this was a difficulty, we were able to open up new conversations about her communication and educational needs. We were also able to think of how language and communication caused difficulties in their relationship.

Due to this young person's relatively low language abilities compared with her age, her skills in understanding that people can think and feel differently from herself are also very delayed and will affect the style of questions and therapy that can be used.

Children with additional difficulties

Approximately one third of deaf people have additional difficulties (see Flathouse, 1979). Others have language delay either in English, sign language or both (Marschark, 1993). Another concern is the deaf child or adult's emotional vocabulary. It is documented that many deaf people have a very limited emotional vocabulary due to linguistic restrictions (Rieffe and Terwogt, 2000). These all make the use of any therapy challenging as the child's understanding and ability to partake in therapy is limited. Thus, a systemic perspective enables reflections on a child's behaviour, interaction, play (for example, drawing) and so on to be included in therapeutic conversations. Behaviour is a form of communication, therefore an understanding of behaviours observed across situations can be explored alongside the family and wider system concerns.

Implications for working systemically with families with a deaf member

In hearing families with a deaf member, it is argued that two distinct cultures are represented (Harvey, 1984). However, in many families there are more than just the two cultures of hearing and deaf due to diversity in language, culture, religion (and so on). These need to be thought about, as in any therapeutic situation.

Working therapeutically across more than one culture (for example, working with deaf people from hearing families) raises many issues that this chapter does not have scope to address in full. However, as the premise of systemic therapy is that meaning is created within relationships, systemic thinking enables curiosity rather than blame in relation to differences, whether concerned with cultural, linguistic or other paradigms.

To be able to facilitate change in families with a deaf member, it is important that the systemic therapist has a good understanding of deafness from a cultural, linguistic and developmental perspective. An understanding of theory of mind in deaf children is crucial. Most systemic therapists will not be able to sign, so knowledge about the linguistic properties of sign language and the utilisation of interpreters in therapy is paramount. Understanding the limitations of certain questions will certainly be an area of consideration for the therapist.

There are currently very few specialist or generic services that are able to offer the combined knowledge of deafness and family therapy. With the onset of 'Sign of the Times' (Department of Health, 2002), a document highlighting the mental health service needs of deaf people in the UK, access to therapy will need further exploration in the months and years to come, as will the training needs of health professionals and interpreters.

Systemic therapy allows the therapist to join all parts of the system and to bring systemic principles within the therapist's team's thinking. As such, it is important that the therapist's team is able to acknowledge and be flexible to systemic thinking. In order for this to happen the therapist may need to work directly to educate the team as well as work clinically with the child and family.

Summary

This chapter has summarized the impact of working systemically with ideas around grief, denial, beliefs about deafness, communication, language and theory of mind, and additional difficulties. Similarly, the challenges in using systemic questions are discussed, along with considerations for the use of interpretation within therapy. Ultimately, systemic therapy enables all family members to feel heard within therapy, while accounting for differences in culture and beliefs between individual family members.

References

Anagnostou F, Crocker SR, Graham JM (in preparation) Parental emotions following cochlear implantation. Unpublished report. Paediatric Cochlear Implant Programme, Royal National Throat Nose and Ear Hospital, London.
Anderson T (1987) The reflecting team: dialogue and meta-dialogue in clinical work. Family Process 26: 415–28.
Bateson G (1972) Steps to an Ecology of Mind. New York: Ballantine Books.
Cecchin G (1987) Hypothesising, curiosity, and neutrality revisited: an invitation to curiosity. Family Process 28: 405-413.

Department of Health (2002) A Sign of the Times: Modernising Mental Health Services for People who are Deaf. London: Department of Health.

Flathouse VE (1979) Multihandicapped deaf children and public law 94-142. Exceptional Children 45: 560–5.

Fredman J, Coombs G (1996) Narrative Therapy. The Social Construction of Preferred Realities. New York: WW Norton.

Haley J (1978) Problem Solving Therapy. New York: Harper & Row.

Harvey M (1984) Family Therapy with deaf persons: the systemic utilization of an interpreter. Family Process 23: 205–13.

Harvey M (1985) Towards a dialogue between the paradigms of family therapy and deafness. American Annals of the Deaf 130: 305–14.

Harvey M (1986) The magnifying mirror: family therapy for deaf persons. Family Systems Medicine 4(4): 408–20.

Harvey M (1989) Psychotherapy with Deaf and Hard-of-Hearing Persons: A Systemic Model. Hillsdale NJ: Erlbaum.

Madanes C (1981) Strategic Family Therapy. San Francisco CA: Jossey Bass.

Marschark M (1993) Psychological Development of Deaf Children. New York: Oxford University Press.

Minuchin S (1974) Families and Family Therapy. London: Tavistock.

Palazzoli M, Boscolo L, Cecchin G, Prata G (1980) Hypothesising – circularity – neutrality: three guidelines for the conductor of the session. Family Process 19: 3–12.

Peterson CC, Siegal M (1995) Deafness and theory of mind. Journal of Child Psychology and Psychiatry 36(3): 458–74.

Peterson CC (2002) Drawing insight from pictures: the development of concepts of false belief in children with deafness, normal hearing, and autism. Child development, 73(5): 1442–59.

Reder P, Fredman G (1996) The relationship to help: interacting beliefs about the treatment process. Clinical Child Psychology and Psychiatry 1(3): 457–67.

Rieffe C, Terwogt MM (2000) Deaf children's understanding of emotions: desires take precedence. Journal of Child Psychology and Psychiatry and Allied Disciplines 41(5): 601–8.

Sanders C (1985) 'Now I see the difference' – the use of visual news of difference in clinical practice. Australian and New Zealand Journal of Family Therapy 6: 23–9.

Sloman L, Springer S (1987) Strategic family therapy interventions with deaf member families. Canadian Journal of Psychiatry 32: 558–62.

Sloman L, Perry A, Frankenburg F (1987) Family therapy with deaf member families. The American Journal of Family Therapy 15(3): 242–52.

Sloman L, Springer S, Vachon LS (1993) Disordered communication and grieving in deaf member families. Family Process 32: 171–81.

Tomm K (1988) Interventive Interviewing: Part III. Intending to ask lineal, circular, strategic, or reflexive questions? Family Process 27: 1–15.

Warner B (2000) Family therapy with families with deaf members. In Hindley P, Kitson N (eds) (2000) Mental Health and Deafness. London: Whurr, pp. 361–81.

White M (1988) The externalising of the problem and the re-authoring of lives and relationships. Dulwich Centre Newsletter 5–28.

White M, Epston D (1989) Literate means to therapeutic ends. Adelaide: Dulwich Centre.

CHAPTER 7

Cognitive behavioural models in deafness and audiology

SALLY AUSTEN

Introduction

Throughout the brief history of mental health and deafness, one question seems to come up time and again: 'Is there a psychology of deafness?' This chapter argues that the only way to answer this question in the affirmative is to reframe the question to: 'Is there a psychology of how the people perceive their deafness?'

Although a proportion of the d/Deaf community report being troubled by their deafness, others say they are not. Person 'A' may be extremely distressed by a mild hearing impairment whereas person 'B' finds little issue with profound loss. So who is right? Answer: both. The impact of deafness is dependent on self-cognition: how one *thinks* about one's deafness will determine how one *feels* about one's deafness. Furthermore, how one feels about one's *deafness* may differ from how one feels about an issue that is associated with the deafness.

This chapter attempts to elucidate the potential difficulties associated with deafness, and the variation in response to these, using the World Health Organization classifications of impairment, disability and handicap alongside the cognitive behavioural model. It will be argued that the 'psychology of deafness' is rooted, not in impairment or disability, but in handicap, largely the result of negative cognitions.

Potential difficulties associated with deafness

Each person's hearing loss will vary by degree and type. Each person will also have a unique cohort of physical, cognitive and emotional strengths and weaknesses. Thus, each person's difficulties and potential difficulties will be unique. Although there are some that report having nothing but positive experiences, difficulties reported by d/Deaf people collectively span a number of categories.

Practical difficulties

A huge variety of activities are rendered harder or impossible depending on degree and type of hearing loss: hearing oncoming traffic, listening to the radio, being aware of a fire alarm, playing the guitar, correcting your children's reading, hearing a coin drop, knowing from engine revs when it is time to change gear. Whereas technological or human assistance can help compensate for some such difficulties, the absence of normal hearing can have a real impact.

Painful and life-threatening conditions

Deafness can be caused by a number of factors (such as head injuries following road traffic accidents). They might be associated with other medical conditions (for example, acoustic neuroma), or the result of treatment for painful and life threatening conditions (certain drug treatments for HIV/AIDS). Some members of the Deaf community would consider their deafness a lifestyle choice, but deafness in the context of painful or life threatening conditions would not be considered in this way. Meningitis, which sometimes results in deafness, is still meningitis, a life threatening condition, with the potential to cause lasting physical, cognitive and sensory damage, which is terrifying for patients and their loved ones.

Communication and isolation

Reduced ability to hear or speak means that taking part in conversations presents difficulties, which can have detrimental effects on personal and professional lives. Communication on an individual level can often be difficult and at a group level can be impossible. Background noise, distracting visual environments and speakers who do not take their share of the responsibility for successful communication can make being deaf a frustrating and lonely experience. Isolation and reduced contact with people have practical and emotional repercussions.

Loss or restriction of role

We each have a number of broad roles: friend, parent, child, employee and other more subtle roles: the helper, the listener, the fixer, the joker, the organizer and so forth. Deafness can prevent people from either fulfilling their potential roles or can take away people's ability or confidence to do so. For example, many women regard their listening ability when friends have problems as fundamental to their identity and, as a result of an acquired hearing loss, feel less of a 'friend'. Likewise many men regard their ability to be the breadwinner as paramount: for them, hearing loss can mean feeling less of a 'man'.

Discrimination and inequity of opportunity

Like restriction of role, discrimination can occur on a broad or more subtle level. Broadly, research has shown that, as a group, d/Deaf people experience underemployment, financial inequality and restricted access to educational facilities (Harris, Anderson and Novak, 1995). Limitation of opportunity tends to have a cumulative effect. Lack of educational opportunity reduces job opportunities; lack of initial job opportunities lead to less experience and less impressive CVs, which reduce the opportunity for promotion and so on. Hogan (2001) reports that advancement in the workplace may also be blocked because of discriminatory attitudes.

On a day-to-day basis many d/Deaf people experience stigmatisation and ill treatment, as a result of their deafness (Higgins, 1980; RNID, 1998).

Associated disabilities

Discussed in more depth in other chapters in this book, deafness is often associated with other disabilities. Thus, the d/Deaf person will also have thoughts and feelings about any other difficulties they have, whether they are physical, neurological or associated with a specific or global learning disability. It may be that a d/Deaf person has no negative perception of their deafness but experiences distress in relation to another disability.

Associated audiological difficulties

For many people who are d/Deaf, other audiological difficulties trouble them. McKenna, Hallam and Hinchcliffe (1991) found that 42% of those attending an audiological rehabilitation centre needed psychological intervention. Tinnitus (the perception of sound in the absence of external auditory stimulation) and balance problems affect many of the d/Deaf population. Tinnitus troubles 50% of patients with a sudden sensorineural hearing loss, 70% of those with presbyacusis (deafness due to the ageing process) and 100% (by definition) of those with Menière's disease (Spoendlin, 1987). These and other audiological conditions such as recurrent ear infections, allergic or painful reactions to the ear moulds of hearing aids, hyperacusis (where noise is perceived as painfully loud) are commonly treated by psychologists in audiological services.

World Health Organization (WHO) definitions and deafness

Arnold (1998) reports that it is the differences in the subjective experience of deafness and its related difficulties that have lead to an interest in the categories of impairment, disability and handicap (WHO, 1980). Debate surrounds any classification system and as a result is seems sensible to assume there will be some blurring of the distinction between these categories.

The general WHO (1980) definitions describe the following:

* impairment – any loss or abnormality of physiological structure or function;
* disability – a consequence of the impairment, is a restriction or lack of ability to perform an activity in a way that is considered statistically normal for a human being;
* handicap – resulting from an impairment or a disability, refers to the disadvantages that limit or prevent the fulfilment of a role that is normal for that individual.

Impairment and audiology

According to the WHO system, 'disease or disorder' causes 'impairment'. In terms of audiology, Stephens and Hētu (1991, p. 187) say that impairment is defined as

> a defective function which may be measured using psychoacoustical or physiological techniques . . . which reflects the underlying dysfunction resulting from pathological changes in the auditory system. While there may be temporary impairment, it is essentially independent of psychosocial factors . . . It reflects the potentialities of the individual rather than his actual auditory behaviour in a real life environment.

Examples of audiological impairment could include damage or malformation of the outer, middle or inner ear.

Disability and audiology

Disability represents the patients' reports of auditory difficulties or consequences experienced as a result of the impairment of audiological structure or function. For example, an individual may experience tinnitus, or have difficulty hearing speech in a noisy place or maintaining balance in the dark. For the purposes of labelling, the WHO definitions compare the person's lack of ability to perform an activity with that which is statistically normal for a human being. Although a statistical norm exists for human beings in general, there are also statistical norms for sub-groups of humans. This may account for the displeasure that some people in the Deaf community (for whom being Deaf is the social norm) express when described as 'disabled'. For those Deaf people whose families have been predominantly Deaf for many generations, the statistical norm of their subgroup (their extended family) is deafness. Indeed, in such families the hearing members may be the ones who feel handicapped.

Handicap and audiology

Handicap, in this context, represents 'non-auditory problems' that result from hearing impairment and audiological disability (Stephens and Hētu, 1991). Thus, the disability in listening to speech negatively affects social integration so the individual may be handicapped, for example, by isolation, marital stress or reduced promotion prospects. While it is often argued that handicap is imposed upon people with disabilities by the unaccommodating society, the inconsistency of individual experience implies that some other variable must also be at work here. That is, there may be something about individuals that influences whether they experience their impairment or disability as handicapping or not.

McKenna (1993) reports a low correlation between degree of hearing loss and degree of disability; thus, people with similar impairments may have different degrees of disability. Likewise people with the same degrees of disability may have different degrees of handicap.

Treatment of audiological conditions

Treatment of audiological conditions may focus on the impairment, disability or handicap. An ear, nose and throat (ENT) surgeon might attempt to correct an impairment through surgery – for example, by removing an acoustic neuroma that is negatively affecting balance, hearing and life expectancy. An audiologist may attempt to reduce the disability of not being able to hear speech by fitting a hearing aid or a cochlear implant. Whereas impairment and disability are related by degree and can be treated directly, handicap is related to the other two by environment and attribution. Treatment may attempt to alter the environment directly – for example noise enrichment to distract from tinnitus – or it may attempt to influence others (sociopolitically) to affect the environment. For example, the introduction of the Disability Discrimination Act aims to improve access for people with audiological problems in the workplace or teaching hearing children to sign ensuring that the one Deaf child in a class is less linguistically isolated. The alternative is to affect the individual's attributions. For someone who is handicapped by social isolation associated with their hearing loss, treatment would attempt to facilitate a change in the individual's beliefs about their communication situation such that they feel less isolated.

Paradoxically, improvement in one of the three (impairment, disability or handicap) does not guarantee improvement in the others. For example, many people with mild to severe deafness prefer to struggle with reduced hearing rather than wearing a hearing aid with which they have negative associations. Although the hearing aid may reduce *disability* by helping the person hear more, if they have negative attributions about hearing aids and experience embarrassment or shame, the *handicap* may be increased. In such situations extremely negative beliefs can lead to depression or suicidal ideation. The benefits of hearing better would be outweighed by the increase in negative affect.

Arnold (1998, p265) reports that an increased understanding of the processes linking impairment, disability and handicap could 'help to reconcile more hearing-impaired adults to acquire and use hearing aids...to counsel them to come to realistic terms with their hearing loss and yet to reject any negative attitudes imposed by others.' This chapter proposes that it is the cognitive behavioural model that is crucial to understanding the link between impairment, disability and handicap and to being able to 'reject any negative attitudes'.

Cognitive behavioural model

Hollon and Beck (1986: 443) defined cognitive behavioural therapy (CBT) as 'those approaches that attempt to modify existing or anticipated disorders by virtue of altering cognitions or cognitive processes'. Cognitive theorists believe that people actively direct their behaviour through internal representations and personal interpretations of external reality, that humans have the capacity for self-control, and that cognitive processes are viewed as interacting causally with learning experiences to affect feeling and behaviours. Thus, according to cognitive behavioural theories it is not the situation but our thoughts *about* the situation that are paramount.

The cognitive behavioural model does not deny that some situations in life are more difficult than others – indeed, that some are horrific. However, Beck (1976) believed that negative thoughts and negatively biased perceptions could result in depressed or anxious affect and that these negative cognitions could be about oneself, the world or about the future. These negative thoughts may be linked to unfortunate past experiences but take on an automatic quality of repetition and intrusion in the present. They also have an indisputable quality, which implies that they are based on fact when they are often based instead on uncorroborated assumption. Cognitive behavioural therapy requires patients to examine their thought processes critically and to observe any connections between erroneous beliefs and inappropriate or unwanted emotional reactions. In brief, negative thinking can cause low mood, depression, anxiety and so on. Challenging and changing the thoughts can therefore change the mood and symptoms.

Beck (1976) outlined various types of distorted thought process that increase the likelihood of negative appraisal of events and thus negative affect. The next section gives examples of these and illustrates them with case vignettes.

Cognitive behavioural therapy and deafness

O'Rourke (in Hindley and Kitson, 2000) described CBT as a helpful model for using with Deaf people. She said that it allows the therapist to be creative, to use a variety of media (for example, drawing, writing, video) and to adapt their techniques according to the needs of the patient, giving it a particularly wide application to patients from other cultures or who had difficulty communicating.

It is likely that the Deaf patient's therapist will often be hearing and, given that many Deaf people will have experienced oppression from hearing people, the explicit agenda, rules and treatment goals of CBT are beneficial in that they establish equality between therapist and patient.

O'Rourke (in Hindley and Kitson, 2000) said that most patients referred to mental health services have low self esteem and that feelings of worthlessness often relate to difficulties in accepting their deafness or resolving issues of identity in relation to deafness. She added that some of the Deaf person's negative beliefs and assumptions might reflect the position of Deaf people in hearing society. When a thought or belief reflects actual fact it should not be challenged, as this would only serve to invalidate the patient's feelings or experience. However, thoughts that are only partially related to fact can be scrutinized for degree, universality or implication of the fact. For example, if a Deaf person thinks 'Hearing people ignore me and think I am stupid', CBT could usefully challenge whether *all* people ignore the patient *all* of the time and whether, if the patient was ignored, this definitely means that the hearing person thinks the Deaf person is stupid.

Negative thinking, audiology and handicap

Crucial to this section is the fact that not all people experience the 'handicap' associated with deafness in the same way. Stephens and Hētu (1991) explain that disability is not necessarily a bad thing and can be good. For example, it has advantages such as not being bothered by noise and a sense of camaraderie with other deaf people. Thus, positive or negative appraisal of the situation seems to determine whether the person is handicapped by their disability or not.

Jumping to conclusions

The individual interprets a situation negatively even though there is no evidence to support the conclusions. This comes in two forms: 'fortune telling' and 'mind reading'.

Fortune telling

Mr G was a 55-year-old man with Menière's disease and severe and unpredictable episodes of balance problems. His social life had become extremely limited and he had stopped going to the shops. He was depressed and hopeless. His negative thinking included fortune telling examples such as 'If I go out I will lose my balance, people will think I am drunk, they will hate me and I won't be able to cope.' Treatment involved challenging these thoughts on every level and seeking evidence to either prove the negative assumption (in which case harm minimization or problem solving techniques can be enlisted) or, more likely, disprove the negative assumptions in which case the feelings of low mood and hopelessness will also shift. Mr G was asked to find evidence to support or reject his belief that he would definitely lose his balance if he went out, that people would definitely interpret balance difficulties as him being drunk, that if they thought he was drunk that they would definitely hate him, or that if people hated him he would definitely not be able to cope with that. Because Mr G believed categorically that bad things would happen if he went out, then staying at home was a logical conclusion. However, once Mr G believed that none of these negative outcomes was definite he felt more able to go out and in doing so gathered more evidence that the bad things didn't always happen. And when, on the few occasions, bad things did happen, he gathered evidence that he could cope effectively with this.

Mind reading

Mrs J had a profound acquired hearing loss and felt extremely handicapped by her inability to join in conversations at dinner parties like she used to. She was particularly upset that one friend had stopped asking her to events. She described negative thoughts that included mind reading: 'My friend doesn't invite me any more because she is embarrassed by my deafness and finds organizing the seating around my hearing loss too much trouble.' Negative thoughts of the mind-reading type are one of the simplest to address as you can ask the person whose mind you are attempting to read whether your negative assumption is correct or not. If it is proven, then nothing is any worse than it was before you sought clarification. However, the likelihood is that the assumption will be disproved. Mrs J was encouraged to ask her friend if her assumption was correct and found that she couldn't be further from the truth. Her friend had some worries that her parties were not very entertaining and had not wanted to put pressure on Mrs J to attend if she did not enjoy them. The friend missed Mrs J's company but thought she was helping by not inviting her. As a result they discussed together how to maximize Mrs J's communication by planning the seating and lighting and by adjusting background music.

All-or-nothing thinking

This type of thinking discredits any good thoughts or experiences by categorizing everything as either black or white. When treating people with tinnitus one's aim is less to reduce its presence and more to reduce its negative impact. Mr B had had tinnitus and low-grade chronic depression for 18 years. He was socially isolated and spent many hours each day ruminating on how bad his tinnitus was and how handicapped he was by it. Treatment involved the use of antidepressant medication, sleep hygiene, and behavioural activity scheduling. As he slept better and went out more he reported increasing periods when he was not aware of the tinnitus or was aware of it but was not distressed by it. His low mood, however, was reinforced by the thought 'But I still have tinnitus'. Mr B's complete thought was along the lines of 'If I still have tinnitus it means I am not getting better, that it will get worse again, and that something is obviously wrong.' The challenge to this thought requires explanation of what is normal for this situation, which is usually defined by a shade of grey. With further discussion it became clear to Mr B that his expectation that tinnitus would go completely and forever was unrealistic and that his improvement was already impressive. As a result his thinking changed and his mood improved.

Overgeneralization

Ms A had a severe progressive hearing loss. In her late 20s, she was successful in career and social life. She asserted her communication needs to her friends and colleagues in such a way that she rarely felt handicapped by her hearing loss. However, she had become concerned that she was 'less of a woman' as a result of the effect her hearing loss had had on her sexual relationship with her partner. If she kept her hearing aids on during sex, they would whistle which they both found distracting; but without them she couldn't hear what he was saying. She used generalization (and some fortune telling) to fuel her negative thinking: 'Since I am less spontaneous and relaxed about talking during sex, I have lost my sensuality and am less of a woman. My boyfriend will go off me.' Cognitive behavioural therapy involves the therapist teaching the patients the theory and techniques of the model so that they become their own therapist. In this case the patient was able to spot and challenge her own generalizations and reframed her thinking to, 'We may not talk in bed like we used to, but there are lots of other ways of communicating. I am still very sexy and my partner is very satisfied.'

Personalization or blame

Mrs V was a profoundly prelingually Deaf, British Sign Language user. She had been seriously sexually abused throughout her childhood by a family friend and when her parents found out they blamed her and accused her of encouraging the man. Mrs V required long-term inpatient psychiatric care as a result of her experiences and was treated for post-traumatic stress disorder with concurrent psychotic symptoms and depression. There was a sense that Mrs V thought it was her fault that she was Deaf, that she believed being Deaf meant that she was stupid and worthless and that it was also her fault that she was sexually abused. Although the childhood abuse from the family friend had stopped, she continued to mentally abuse herself. This degree of personalization made progress difficult as she was in effect discrediting the very resource – herself – that she was going to need in her recovery. To challenge her belief that it was all her fault she was helped to tease out who was responsible for her deafness, her safety as a child, starting the abuse, stopping the abuse, and helping her recover from the abuse. As a result she was more able to harness the survival skills that had seen her through her childhood and apply them to her present psychiatric difficulties. Although still needing psychiatric support Mrs V has been able to return home and is clear she is not to blame for either her abuse or her deafness.

All my problems would be solved if . . .

One of the challenges for CBT is to help patients to identify their primary problem. Often people focus all of their energy or concern on one issue while being unaware, or deliberately avoiding, the real issue. For example, psychologists on cochlear implant teams are often asked to assess candidates' expectations of an implant. It is relatively common to come across people who perceive their deafness as being the root of all their difficulties – their marital difficulties, their teenagers' unruliness, their low mood – and who therefore see a cochlear implant as the solution to all of their difficulties. Often, however, these problems exist independent of the deafness and improved hearing would not bring the solutions that the candidate expects. The result is that the actual problems remain and the candidate is disappointed with the implant.

Cole (1989) found that Deaf teenagers tended to think that all of their problems were because they were Deaf. For example, they thought that their hearing peers did not have similar troubles with relationships or with school being boring.

In the following handout the author uses the analogies of 'smoke screens' and 'coat hooks' to help patients identify and prioritize their problems. For those people who have been troubled by tinnitus for a long time and for whom many treatments have proved ineffective, it may be that tinnitus is not the 'real' problem. The handout was used with great effect in a CBT-based group. In this case the coat hooks and smoke screens are connected with tinnitus, but they could just as easily be connected with deafness, balance problems, or any other supposedly obvious problems.

TINNITUS COAT HOOKS AND EMOTIONAL SMOKE SCREENS

What can coat hooks and smoke screens have to do with tinnitus treatments? Well, quite a lot sometimes.

Have you ever listened to someone whose marriage you knew was in trouble complain about their boss, or someone who you knew was grieving for a loved one convince you that their life would be perfect if only they moved house? Maybe what you are noticing is an emotional smokescreen. They have a priority problem (dealing with the troubled marriage or going through the grieving process) but they are avoiding it by focusing on the lesser priority problem.

Perhaps you know people who bring all of their problems back to one cause: 'I didn't get good school results because my parents divorced, I can't get a job because my parents divorced, I married a violent man because my parents got divorced, I drink because . . .' Whilst the divorce of parents can be emotionally traumatic they are using a 'divorce coat hook' to hang all their problems on.

The smoke screen helps us avoid admitting the problems; the coat hook helps us avoid taking responsibility for finding solutions to the problems.

I've overdone the example to make the point that sometimes the things we say we are upset about are not entirely the case. That is not to say that we lie or are trying to deceive people, on the contrary, what we are saying is the problem is very true. It is just that if we deal with our problems in order of greatest effect (or severity) we may make it easier to deal with subsequent problems and may take away the need to sort out the subsequent problems.

We all do this at some time and it is easy to see why. See if you can think of some reasons why people might avoid the really important issues for them (e.g. why they might use emotional smoke screens)...?

The 'real' issue might

- feel too painful e.g. loneliness or childlessness
- feel too embarrassing e.g. incontinence
- feel too confusing e.g. identity and sexuality issues
- feel too scary e.g. leaving a violent partner or just a partner of long standing
- make us feel guilty e.g. when we need to be assertive with a difficult relative
- be less available to us (to describe, to remember) e.g. depression or childhood traumas, where other things might be easier to conceptualise or to talk about.

Can you think of reasons why people might use 'Tinnitus Coat Hooks' . . .?

- Most likely is that it has just become a habit
- Other people have started to expect us to describe all problems in terms of the tinnitus
- The tinnitus might as well have some benefits
- It's less time consuming to blame tinnitus
- It can be less scary to think you have to find just one solution (to the tinnitus) than to find 7 solutions (to the dog fleas, the lazy teenagers, the noisy neighbours, the...and so on).

Taking some time to look at your own issues and motivations is crucial. If you have an underlying problem of loneliness then no end of tinnitus treatment will make you feel better. You may need to consider getting help to address the loneliness and to make some lifestyle changes. If you feel unappreciated, unfulfilled or you are being treated badly by someone then you may well have to tackle these problems before tackling the tinnitus.

This might not apply to you or you may disagree with the contents but give it some thought and keep this paper handy in case you have any thoughts related to it.

Conclusion

Deafness, difficulties associated with deafness and other audiological conditions may or may not be experienced as handicapping. Whereas what is happening biologically to us is important, the degree of impairment may bear little resemblance to our degree of handicap. Indeed, efforts to reduce impairment or disability may actually increase handicap.

Although handicap can result from a discrepancy between what the individual needs and what the environment can provide, it is also the case that the individual's attributions influence degree of handicap. In relation to handicap, the difficulty (whether it be audiological issues such as deafness and tinnitus or associated issues such as brain injury or unemployment) is less important than one's perceptions of the difficulty.

Cognitive behavioural therapy (CBT) is therefore a very effective way of reducing handicap by altering the negative perceptions of the individual to his or her situation. Some patients may find it difficult to identify the issues that are most important to them and may require help to do so before starting work to change thinking processes.

References

Arnold P (1998) Is there still a consensus on impairment, disability and handicap in audiology? British Journal of Audiology 32: 265–71.

Beck AT (1976) Cognitive Therapy and the Emotional Disorders. New York: International Universities Press.

Cole SH (1989) Cultural Identity and Coping in Deafness: A Study of Deaf Adolescents' Problems and Self-Perceptions. Unpublished thesis. University of Guildford, UK.

Harris JP, Anderson JP, Novak R (1995) An outcome study of cochlear implants in deaf patients. Archives of Otolaryngology, Head and Neck Surgery 121: 398–404.

Higgins PC (1980) Outsiders in a Hearing World – A Sociology of Deafness. Beverley Hills CA: Sage.

Hogan A (2001) Hearing Rehabilitation for Deafened Adults. A Psychosocial Approach. London: Whurr.

Hollon SD, Beck AT (1986) Cognitive and cognitive-behavioral therapies. In Garfield SL, Bergin AE (eds) Handbook of Psychotherapy and Behaviour Change. 3 edn. New York: Wiley, pp. 443–82.

McKenna L (1993) Some psychological aspects of deafness. In J Ballantyne, MC Martin, A Martin (eds) Deafness. 5 edn. London: Whurr, pp. 237–8.

McKenna L, Hallam RS, Hinchcliffe (1991) The prevalence of psychological disturbance in neuro-otology outpatients. Clinical Otolaryngology 16: 452–56.

O'Rourke S (2000) Behavioural and Cognitive Approaches. Hindley P, Kitson N (eds) Mental Health and Deafness. London: Whurr, pp. 383–99.

RNID (1998) Breaking the Sound Barrier. London: Royal National Institute for Deaf People.

Spoendlin H (1987) (ed.) Inner ear pathology and tinnitus. In Feldmann H (ed.) (1987) Proceedings of the Third International Tinnitus Seminar. Munster: Harsch Verlag Karlsrehe, pp. 42–52.

Stephens D, Hētu R (1991) Impairment, disability and handicap in audiology: towards a consensus. Audiology 30: 185–200.

World Health Organization (1980) World Health Organization: International Classification of Impairments, Disabilities and Handicaps. Geneva: World Heath Organization.

CHAPTER 8

Deaf wellness explored

MARY GRIGGS

Introduction

The field of psychology is slowly acknowledging the need to reflect cultural diversity within its client group. Traditionally mental health professionals have used normative criteria to define mental health and illness, and in doing so have seen normality and deviance through the cultural lens of the dominant group in society. Within the mental health field, an increasingly strong lobby is illuminating the ethnocentric and racist bias of Western psychiatry and psychology (see, for example, Fernando, 2002).

The notion of cultural deafness draws on the existence of collective beliefs and experiences within the deaf community. Deaf people's identity is rooted with those who have a similar life orientation and worldview and who share the same rich and meaningful cultural heritage (Chovaz, in Kazarian and Evans, 1998).

How then does this understanding apply to mental health? The limited data on epidemiology of mental disorder among deaf people presents a complex picture, often reflecting inappropriate assessment and diagnosis procedures. Higher rates of diagnosed illness have been recorded, particularly for affective disorder (see, for example, Hindley et al., 1994; Griggs, 1998). In seeking to make sense of these findings, it should be noted that, as with members of minority ethnic communities, the expression and understanding of (mental) illness among deaf people is thought to be unique, reflecting cultural and linguistic characteristics of the community. Within the mental health services, hearing professionals have demonstrated only limited appreciation of a deaf cultural experience of mental health.

Mental health services

As a starting point, deaf people are still seldom visible nationally in a professional capacity within the mental health services. Moreover as Klein and Kitson (in Hindley and Kitson, 2000) point out, deaf roles within the mental health field have traditionally been seen as a resource in the fields of entertainment or recreation, rather than any more qualified positions.

Within the specialist mental health services for deaf people, the need at least to balance the ratio of professionally qualified deaf to hearing staff is of particular concern. This desire is based upon an acknowledgement of the value of professional training and crucially, of a cultural insider understanding of deafness. Indeed Silo (1991) categorically states that hearing people, regardless of their level of training or experience cannot function well as mental health workers with deaf children and adults because of their preconceived ideas about what constitutes 'normal'. Concerns surrounding cultural misinterpretation have been reinforced by suggestions that deaf people mistrust hearing professionals who do not know sign language and do not understand the crosscultural implications inherent in deafness (Farrugia, 1988). Findings such as these add another dimension to existing data demonstrating low take up of mental health services within the deaf community (Checinski, 1991). Steinberg (1991) estimates that 90% of the deaf population's mental health needs remain unserved. Quite simply deaf people have rarely been involved in defining and delivering a service based upon their own cultural understanding of health and illness.

Returning to the notion of dominant Western models of mental health and illness, traditional focus has been on problems of a psychological nature (psychopathology); attempts to understand the processes by which they come about (pathogenesis); and seeking better ways to address them (for example, psychotherapy) (Cowen, 1994). This approach rests upon a universalist position that individuals share more similarities than differences. Underlying this philosophy is the tendency to focus on illness symptoms rather than physical or emotional wellbeing.

An opposing school of thought puts forward the belief that an understanding of mental health can only be reached from a cultural relativist or 'constructionist' position. Within this framework, experiences of health and illness are perceived as culturally mediated, leading to the existence of multiple constructions of reality. In order to explore this experience fully, we can turn to wellness theory. Rather than locating individual or community experience within a constructed 'pathology' framework, wellness theory instead explores what goes *right* in psychological development and adjustment, seeking to identify the factors that are perceived by the individual and by communities to create such an outcome.

Allowing for cultural diversity wellness is described as:

> a state of harmony, energy, positive productivity, and well-being in an individual's mind, body, emotions and spirit. The state of wellness also extends to the relationship between the individual and his or her family and other interpersonal connections as well as the relationships between the person and his or her physical environment, community, and larger society. Wellness does not preclude having a disability or experiencing positive stress. (Jones and Kilpatrick, 1996: 259)

As Cowen (1994) suggests, wellness is more than the simple absence of disease, rather it is defined by the presence of positive characteristics of adjustment. Drawn primarily from constructivist thinking, every person is viewed within a unique context of personhood, relationships with others, and relationship with the environment and attention is paid to the reciprocity and fluidity of these relationships and interactions (Jones and Kilpatrick, 1996).

Wellness theory, mental health and deafness

So why is wellness theory useful when thinking about mental health and deafness?

- Wellness theory focuses on positive indicators of adjustment and coping. Clearly many perspectives on deafness and mental health focus almost entirely on the existence and impact of pathology either within the individual or within the environment. Few approaches incorporate the expression and interpretation of signs of positive adjustment.
- Wellness theory is independent of traditional approaches (beliefs grounded in a medical model of deafness and mental health, or traditional notions of deafness and disability).
- Wellness theory can be explored at both an individual level and on a collective, community basis. Clearly while the effects of deafness are essentially individual, the experience of deafness for many is deep-rooted in a cultural deaf community.
- Wellness theory describes wellness as a process – that is, the nature and dynamic of the journey towards a state of wellbeing. Cowen (1994) identifies five main pathways to wellness, namely: a) forming wholesome early attachments b) acquiring age-appropriate competencies c) exposure to settings that favour wellness outcomes d) having the (empowering) sense of being in control of one's fate e) coping effectively with stress. This aspect of wellness suits certain features of cultural deafness, for example making a transition from the culture of hearing parents to cultural affiliation with deaf people.

A critical assumption is that a full understanding of deaf people's experience of mental health is obtained when researchers draw on the beliefs and understandings of deaf people themselves, rather than relying exclusively on dominant medical theories of deafness, health and illness.

Deafness and wellness theory

The following section details an exploration into how deafness relates to wellness theory. Essentially it is an attempt to demonstrate a construction of deaf wellness and in so doing to understand how the deaf community has come to establish a culturally negotiated understanding of what represents health and illness.

Several focus groups took place over a 2 month period. Participants were all members of the deaf community who identified themselves as being culturally deaf and were prepared to talk about it. This was the primary selection criterion. Respondents within each of the two main groups shared other socio-economic features, that is, they were of similar age and occupational status. A series of discussions explored a range of subjects including their experiences of family and community, as well as more direct observations of health and illness. Discussions in BSL were transcribed and cross-checked by a deaf BSL user.

As a cultural construction, an essential element within the model is its relationship to the dominant cultural construction of deafness and mental health. Thus Table 8.1 presents deaf wellness in relation to dominant traditional notions of mental health and deafness. Six key elements to the model emerged and each will be discussed in turn.

Deaf wellness is a process

Wellness is described both as a process and as possessing properties of an outcome measure. Crucially, as a process, deaf wellness incorporates the possibility of change and transition.

Psychological theories are extremely powerful. The prevailing medical perspective links deafness and pathology, fixing ideologically dominant beliefs about normal and abnormal. The 'different' is taken to be both pathological and deviant. Within this framework it is no surprise that deaf people are more likely to be mentally ill. In addition, the expectation of illness, sustained by proponents of the dominant ideology, is satisfied.

Traditional points of reference in considering deafness and mental health have constituted measures of illness. Deaf people are collectively assessed in comparison to hearing people, and are therefore thought to be worse off in terms of mental health. Whether this outcome results from

Table 8.1 Features of dominant theoretical framework of mental health and deafness against features of the model of deaf wellness

Dominant hearing ideology	Deaf wellness
1) Poor mental health is an inevitable outcome of deafness.	Wellness is a process as much as an outcome.
2) Deaf people experience a lower level of health than that which hearing people may expect.	Wellness occurs in a stable system. It does not require perfect health
3) Mental health symbolizes a permanent state of stress-free functioning.	Deaf wellness means coping.
4) Mental health in deaf people is predicted by their deviance from hearing norms of health.	Deaf wellness is identified against that which is perceived, in deaf people, to be unwell.
5) Deaf people have the best chance of health if they are looked after by knowledgeable professionals.	Wellness is an expression of reclaiming deafness.
6) The isolation of deafness necessitates that deaf people associate with one another.	Deaf wellness is a celebration of deafness

intrinsic pathology, or from experience, a ceiling is placed upon the degree of mental health a deaf person is expected to experience.

However, from this study it is clear that, for deaf people, the most meaningful points of reference for mental health were other deaf people, not hearing people. Furthermore, when respondents discussed aspects of their shared experience, they did not perceive their own mental health to be static, nor did they identify with the limitations placed upon their experience of mental health by hearing professionals.

The recognition of deaf wellness as a *process* is set against the tendency in dominant culture to equate good mental health with achieving a positive healthy outcome. While allowances are made for slips and periods of mental distress, the goal of mental health is clear, and the hope is that the 'goal state' is maintained. In contrast, deaf people described the shifts they make away from influences they perceived to be threatening. At times, these shifts were shorter term and reactive in nature, and at other times, shifts constituted longer-term responses, as in the emergence of coping strategies. By far the most profound and often dramatic shift was away from the family culture to cultural affiliation with other deaf people. This was specifically identified with a state of wellness.

Wellness necessitated engaging in such shifts, and awarding significance to the perception of wellness as a process as opposed to a 'well'
static endpoint.

Deaf wellness represents system stability

Deaf wellness is not a state of perfect mental health but a state of system
stability, or homeostasis.

A model of deaf wellness, first and foremost, does not deny the existence of mental distress, nor does it deny the fact that many more deaf
people suffer from mental distress than do hearing people. However,
while 'normal' distributions of health prevail, the deaf community is located at the lower end, peaking at a point below that for hearing people.
However, while beliefs and behaviour generally are awarded different
significance by deaf and hearing people, such baselines obscure a full
understanding of mental health and illness and what it means to those
who operate outside normal cultural constructions.

Certainly, a discrepancy emerges between quantitative data, collected
using procedures standardized on normal populations and the accounts
of deaf people themselves. Comparative data succeed in locating both
deaf and hearing people in relation to a gold standard of health, but deaf
people's *wellness* behaviour is seriously misrepresented. For example,
hearing standard measure assessments are sensitive to indicators of stress.
A deaf cultural 'baseline' would assume a certain degree of stress and
would rate the ability to cope or not with that stress as a positive indicator of adjustment. Furthermore, the recognition of a certain amount of
stress actually appears to free the individual to negotiate the process of
wellness. Those deaf people who attempted to 'pass' in hearing society
demonstrated behaviour that disguised stress to such an extent that pre-
carious coping mechanisms emerged.

Within this understanding, a state of perfect health, as anticipated by
hearing people is not the goal of deaf wellness behaviour, rather wellness
is expressed in the ability to negotiate and control a system which is constantly under assault.

Deaf wellness means coping

The concept of coping is critical to distinguish those who have achieved
deaf wellness from those who have not. If an individual can cope with
stress, then the deaf community recognises that he or she is well. Mental
illness is therefore described, first and foremost, as a state in which an
individual cannot cope.

For those outside the deaf community, the notion of coping appears
to have several interpretations. Coping may be associated with low

expectation, or of 'getting by' with something. As such, seeking merely 'to cope' may be thought to allude to the existence of internalized oppression among deaf people, a tradition of oppression having created low expectations among deaf people themselves with regards to mental health. Qualitative evidence suggests that this explanation may account for negative coping, however to deaf people a deeper significance is bestowed on the ability to cope.

Coping is also considered within a stress-coping framework, that is, as reactive behaviour that naturally seeks a dynamic equilibrium. While this may represent the status quo for hearing people, to many deaf people, a deeper and more positive significance is awarded to the expressed ability to cope. The knowledge of being able to cope constitutes a significant feature of the wellness identity.

Coping strategies may be positive or negative, active or inactive. Clearly negative coping, by its very nature, may sustain a system that does not benefit the individual in an adjustive sense, despite being long term. This situation begs the question as to whether individuals in the latter category who demonstrate coping strategies, albeit negative, can be thought to experience deaf wellness? In response, there is a strong sense in which deaf wellness has several components, including a degree of identification with other deaf people. For the most part, individuals who described particularly *inactive* styles of negative coping did not identify with their own deafness in any positive way, and, related to this, rarely desired contact with other deaf people. Positive coping, on the other hand, appears to have more adjustive qualities.

While coping skills may not always be thoroughly effective, there is a conscious awareness that they nonetheless form part of a process that constitutes adjustment. In the same manner, wellness theory does not necessarily equate to a state of perfect health but rather represents a collection of adjustive responses.

Deaf wellness versus deaf unwellness

Within a model of deaf wellness, respondents define wellness against characteristics deemed to represent an unwell state. An awareness of who is outside the central core of the deaf community confirms the placement of those inside membership boundaries. Likewise, recognition of those who are perceived not to cope certifies the coping skills of those who are well.

Medical perspectives on deafness and mental health essentially register deviation from a 'normal' state. Traditionally this has led to support for a 'deaf personality', characterized for example by increased impulsivity and aggression (Lane, 1992). Social perspectives, in contradiction, locate the causes of ill health predominantly within the social or developmental environment.

Cultural perspectives on mental health within the deaf community prescribe an approach that supposes, first and foremost, that the expression and interpretation of mental illness is exclusive to different cultural communities. Wellness behaviour is defined against 'ill' behaviour within the deaf community, rather than against any hearing standards. Consequently, wellness represents the opposite of that which is perceived to be unwell.

In the first instance, those who are well acknowledge this location against those who are unwell. The designation of 'outsider' groups however, holds a deeper symbolic value. There is a need to reinforce the position of wellness by creating a distance and positively rejecting those who are unwell.

At this point, it is pertinent to take a step back to consider the evolution of the cultural deaf community. The testimonies of deaf respondents suggest that a significant aspect of becoming a culturally independent community is the rejection of oppressive structures in which decisions are made by cultural outsiders as to who is well and who is ill. In this respect, consequences of moving from an oppressed state to an 'unoppressed' state are twofold, in that judgements are necessarily both strong and clear cut, and also represent a public statement of autonomy.

A consideration of the exclusion of certain deaf people from insider membership of the deaf community illustrates this process. While the process of exclusion serves to confirm insider status and reclaim wellness on deaf terms, it appears to be harshly exclusive at times. For example, deaf people with additional needs may be designated outsiders and incapable of independent coping. Clearly this has implications for their potential or actual achievement of wellness. From the data it is also apparent that exclusionary tactics often emerge at the interface between traditional nurturing professional practice and more recent initiatives among deaf people to promote cultural independence and change. A need to reclaim wellness necessitates the rejection of professional 'outsider' attempts to judge wellness or decide how to most appropriately restore wellness.

Wellness is an expression of reclaiming deafness

In recognition that judgements are often made by cultural outsiders concerning the beliefs and behaviour thought to represent mental health in deaf people, the need to 'claim back' cultural territory is identified. The process of reclaiming deaf wellness has necessitated identifying what deaf people themselves recognize to be well and unwell, placing certain groups firmly outside a constructed boundary of deaf wellness.

Medical perspectives on deafness constitute a common ideology within the medical and educational fields. The restitution narrative (Frank, 1995), underlying medical perspectives, supposes that in their best interests deaf people should be 'repatriated' to hearing society. It is clear that such a culture of paternalism runs through many of the institutions that directly impact on deaf people's lives. An effect of this cultural climate is to constrain the expression of difference and of cultural deafness.

Increasing dissatisfaction among deaf people both with decisions made on their behalf and with the ideological structures that command them, has instigated growing resistance. Combined with the knowledge that most decisions are made by people who at least are cultural outsiders, and at worst are ill-informed or under-informed as to the nature of deafness and the deaf community, this resistance is felt strongly. The knowledge that deaf people often fundamentally disagree with beliefs and decisions concerning them only corroborates this dissatisfaction.

Cultural perspectives on deafness rest on the belief that the deaf community is a minority community, and in accordance with this belief, features of deaf wellness depart significantly from dominant notions of mental health. Thus deaf people's resistance may be framed as a process of reclaiming deafness.

The significance to deaf wellness is clear. Recognition of wellness depends on rejecting the goals and practices of a dominant ideology of health and 'operationalizing' their own independent understanding of wellness.

Deaf wellness is a celebration of deafness

Within a model of deaf wellness, wellness is created through the recognition and celebration of deaf culture, for example, through the common use of sign language or mutual recognition of identity.

Aspects of the deaf wellness model serve to distinguish those goals, which others have set up on behalf of deaf people, from the goals with which deaf people themselves identify. A corresponding feature of deaf wellness is, therefore, to create new culturally independent definitions.

Features of a deaf wellness model draw very much upon aspects of deaf people's lives that have been oppressed. For example, the use of sign language in schools has traditionally been not only banned but heavily stigmatized. The use of sign language is now presented as a point of reference in the celebration of deafness, and a central component in the definition of wellness. Strength and wellness at the level of the deaf community are rooted in a recognition of the traits necessary for survival as an independent community, for example, the ability to cope and to recognise a resilient deaf identity in one another.

Ultimately, deaf wellness can be seen as the celebration of deafness and of those aspects of the experience of deafness that promote a sense of cultural identity and belonging.

Conclusions

To summarize, a central theoretical conclusion of this study is that membership of the cultural deaf community does not necessarily protect the individual from experiencing stress. However the ability to cope with stress and to develop strategies with which to respond to stress takes on enormous symbolic value, which contributes to deaf wellness behaviour.

This model of deaf wellness is drawn from the beliefs and experiences of members of the cultural deaf community. Just as experiences differ, for example, between different age groups and across different locations, so too it is anticipated that a model of deaf wellness would reflect the same diversity in expression.

Features of wellness are not clear cut, in that those who could be described as 'well' did not necessarily identify with each component of the model. For example, deaf people preferring to communicate with speech would not identify with the cultural deaf community, and yet may still demonstrate high levels of association with other deaf people and a significant degree of wellness. They do not consider deafness to be a barrier to achieving health, and yet similarly turn to other deaf people to support them. In this respect the model constitutes a theoretical construction rather than a blueprint for the interpretation of beliefs and behaviour. In addition, it is not expected that the average deaf person identifies with deaf wellness as a conceptual basis for daily life. On the contrary, this exercise demonstrates that respondents did not immediately associate with the conceptual notion of wellness, rather basing their testimonies on the everyday experiences that motivate beliefs and behaviour.

Implications of the model

This study offers a new framework within which to explore mental health within the deaf community. In essence, the framework has emerged in response to perceived gaps in a traditional understanding of health and illness for deaf people and as such, implications are far reaching. Traditional or dominant beliefs about deafness are woven into the fabric of many organizations established to provide services to deaf people. Deaf people themselves eagerly identify those areas of their life in which they have felt, at best, misunderstood and, at worst, oppressed. This clearly has implications for the status of a minority community, crucially affecting the power base with which deaf people access education, employment or the health services.

While it is essential to accept that cultural diversity exists and that deaf people do not necessarily share the same world view as hearing people, deaf wellness takes this understanding one step further. In seeking to create a new style of response to understanding and working with the deaf community, it is necessary to allow new interpretative frameworks to emerge and a model of deaf wellness demonstrates a theoretical step in promoting this approach.

Returning to the mental health field, applying such an understanding to the delivery of mental health services has tangible implications. Research has demonstrated that the use of health services is more closely linked to how people feel about health services than to their actual medical condition. Specifically, Mechanic (1962) states that people seek services most often when they perceive, within their own cultural frames of reference, or on the judgement of significant others, that something is 'amiss'. This study has demonstrated that deaf people confirm their perceptions of health with other members of the cultural deaf community. While the culture of service delivery remains inappropriate, deaf people are likely to be put off from seeking treatment for mental health problems. This issue may be seen in the context that deaf people are known to be under-represented as recipients of mental health services (Checinski, 1991). Suspicion as to the 'culture' of service delivery is potentially generated and affirmed at a community level leading to more widespread distrust of mental health services.

The issue of appropriate service delivery is increasingly being challenged. Mental health professionals have been typecast as 'guardians' of wellness – 'society's sanctioned repair agents for deficits in wellness' (Cowen, 1994: 150) – clearly reflecting the field's dominant 'fight pathology' orientation. Just as a need to reclaim deaf wellness is recognized, so mental health professionals have a distance to travel in developing a culture of collaboration in which the experience and expertise of the client is met with clinical skills flexible enough to negotiate supportive strategies and goals. In many spheres, notably the field of education, deaf people are slowly becoming service providers. Their value as language consultants and role models has been recognized and steps have been implemented to ensure that deaf professionals are the norm rather than the exception (Young, Griggs and Sutherland, 2000). However, particularly within the mental health field, a new framework of understanding necessitates that deaf professionals become more prominent. That is, that while they may yet not possess equal professional qualifications, their leadership in the construction of frameworks of understanding is prioritized.

References

Checinski K (1991) Conference Proceedings: Mental Health and Deafness, St George's Hospital School, Department of Mental Health Sciences Conference Unit. London: St George's Hospital Medical School.

Chovaz CJ (1998) Cultural Aspects of Deafness. In S Kazarian, D Evans (eds) Cultural Clinical Psychology: Theory, Research and Practice. Oxford: Oxford University Press.

Cowen EL (1994) The enhancement of psychological wellness: challenges and opportunities. American Journal of Community Psychology 22(2): 149–59.

Farrugia D (1988) Practical steps for access and delivery of mental health services to clients who are deaf. Journal of Applied Rehabilitation Counselling 20: 33–5.

Fernando S (2002) Mental Health, Race and Culture. New York: Palgrave.

Frank AW (1995) The Wounded Storyteller: Illness and Ethics. London: University of Chicago Press.

Griggs ML (1998) Deafness and Mental Health: Perceptions of Health within the Deaf Community. Doctoral dissertation, University of Bristol.

Hindley P, Hill P, McGuigan S, Kitson N (1994) Psychiatric disorder in deaf and hearing impaired children and young people: a prevalence study. Journal of Child Psychiatry 35: 917–34.

Hindley P, Kitson N (2000) Mental Health and Deafness. London: Whurr.

Jones GC, Kilpatrick AC (1996) Wellness theory: a discussion and application to clients with disabilities. Families in Society: Journal of Contemporary Human Services 77: 259–67.

Klein H, Kitson N (2000) Mental Health Workers: Deaf-Hearing Partnerships. In P Hindley, N Kitson (eds) Mental Health and Deafness. London: Whurr.

Lane H (1992) The Mask of Benevolence Disabling the Deaf Community. New York: Vintage Books.

Mechanic D (1962) The concept of illness behaviour. Journal of Chronic Disorders 17: 189–94.

Silo J (1991) Teachers and Parents as Mental Health Workers: Partners or Rivals? In Conference Proceedings, British Society for Mental Health and Deafness, London, 1991. London: British Society for Mental Health and Deafness.

Steinberg A (1991) Issues in providing mental health services to hearing-impaired persons. Hospital and Community Psychiatry 42(4): 380–9.

Young AM, Griggs M., Sutherland H (2000) Deaf Child and Family Intervention Services Using Deaf Adult Role Models: A National Survey of Development, Practice and Progress. London: RNID.

CHAPTER 9

Neuropsychological development of hearing-impaired children

LINDSEY EDWARDS

Introduction

Research regarding the neuropsychological development of hearing-impaired children spans a number of centuries, although it is only more recently that the term 'neuropsychology' has become widely used. It covers a wide range of cognitive functions, and presents philosophical and methodological challenges. The complexity of the issues makes reviewing and summarizing them a difficult task. However, this said, this chapter will consider the development of hearing-impaired children from a neuropsychological perspective. Research comparing the general intellectual and specific cognitive functioning of hearing and hearing-impaired children will be reviewed. This will be followed by consideration of the main neurodevelopmental disorders of childhood in terms of assessment and diagnosis in hearing-impaired children.

Hearing-impairment, intellectual ability and cognitive functioning

Historically, deaf children (and adults) have been considered less intellectually able than their hearing peers, and early research appeared to support this suggestion. However, significant flaws in the research design and methodology of these studies led to a shift in emphasis of research to greater consideration of the relationship between IQ and scholastic achievement, rather than a simplistic comparison of verbal or performance IQ between the groups.

As the field of neuropsychology has moved on, so too has investigation of cognitive processes in deaf children. More recently, research has focused on the cognitive abilities of deaf children as being different from their hearing peers, rather than deficient. The role of language in cognitive development (including so-called non-verbal tasks) is complex and remains relatively poorly understood despite considerable research interest.

When considering the validity and generalizability of the results of studies in this area a number of factors must be kept in mind. For example sample composition: issues such as age of participants, degree of hearing loss, hearing status of parents (and therefore access to sign language), etiology of deafness (genetic, syndromic, deafness due to meningitis and so forth), educational setting and approach (oral/aural, total communication or sign language) are all likely to influence performance on some cognitive tasks. The choice of test and administration style will also have an impact on deaf childrens' performance.

Intelligence tests

Braden (1991) conducted a meta-analytic review of IQ research with deaf people and concluded that on performance tests (requiring rapid manipulation of objects), deaf children/adults achieved IQs equivalent to the population average/standardized norms (M_M = 99.95). However, although he reports a significant difference between performance IQs, non-verbal IQs (non-verbal tasks with no manipulation), verbal IQs and other unclassified tests, he does not present the means for the non-verbal and verbal tests, making it difficult to interpret his findings.

Other studies have found the verbal IQ of deaf students to be significantly lower than their hearing peers (see, for example, Maller and Braden, 1993; Braden, 1994), but this is perhaps unsurprising given that the majority of deaf children have hearing parents, and therefore often do not have access to good language models until they enter formal education. Test bias is another possible explanation for these findings.

A number of studies have investigated the performance of hearing-impaired children on the Wechsler Intelligence Scale for Children, probably the most widely used test of intellectual ability (see, for example, Maller, 1996; Maller and Ferron, 1997). Differential item functioning was found between hearing and deaf students, indicating that deaf children simply do not perform at the level of younger hearing children. They conclude that verbal subtests cannot provide meaningful information regarding the comparative abilities of deaf and hearing children.

Given the inadequacies of tests of verbal intelligence for hearing-impaired children, most psychologists working with these children place greater emphasis on the results of non-verbal tests of ability, in terms of assessing general cognitive functioning. A number of such tests are available, and their validity and reliability (in hearing children) are reviewed by Athanasiou (2000) and for very young children, by Bradley-Johnson (2001). One of these, the Leiter International Performance Scale-Revised (LIPS-R), provides a comprehensive assessment of the visual perception, reasoning, memory and attention skills of children, including those with a hearing-impairment. Roid and Miller (1997) provide details of LIPS-R results for 69 severe to profoundly deaf children across the age range 2 years to 18 years. They report mean subtest scores of less than 10 (where 10 is average for all children) for all but one of the subtests (a mental rotation task), and mean composite and IQ scores of around one standard deviation below the norm (of 100) for the full standardization sample. However, it is not clear whether the sample was a 'pure' one – whether deafness was the only difficulty/disability experienced by these children. Indeed, results from Edwards (unpublished data), from a sample of 70 deaf children being assessed as part the decision regarding cochlear implantation, found the mean full non-verbal IQ to be 99.3.

Visual-spatial abilities

Anecdotally, deaf people have typically been attributed with enhanced visual and/or spatial skills, as a result of compensation of the visual system for the deficiencies in the auditory system, or as a result of the increased practice provided by a manual language. Research findings are more equivocal. The performance scale of the Wechsler Intelligence Scales includes a number of subtests that assess aspects of visuospatial ability: block design, object assembly and picture completion. Rush et al. (1991) reported mean standard scores for 72 deaf 16–18 year olds with no additional difficulties, for block design and object assembly of 12 and 11.77 respectively (where 10 is average, SD = 3). In contrast, Tomlinson-Keasey and Smith-Winberry (1990) found no significant difference between congenitally deaf students and their hearing peers on a block design task or a task involving mentally folding 2D diagrams to make 3D boxes. Conrad and Weiskrantz (1981) also failed to find any difference between deaf children of hearing parents and hearing children on the block design task. More recently, Parasnis et al. (1996) investigated whether deafness contributes to enhancement of visuospatial skills by looking at a group of deaf children aged 10–12 years who had never been exposed to sign language, and comparing them with hearing children. They found no differences between the groups on any of the visuospatial tests, but the deaf group did evidence shorter digit spans than the hearing group. They concluded that early exposure to sign language and consistent use of sign are critical for the differential development of visuospatial skills in deaf people.

Memory abilities

Memory function has been investigated extensively in deaf children and adults, probably because of the assumption that short-term memory

(STM) plays a crucial role in the development of aural-oral language. Despite many methodological problems a number of patterns are emerging. Deaf and hearing-impaired children are typically found to have poorer STM capacity/shorter memory spans for a variety of materials, but especially verbal material (see, for example, Waters and Doehring, 1990). Importantly, STM span, as measured by digit span, has been found to predict language and reading ability in deaf children, including those with cochlear implants (Pisoni and Geers, 2000).

Research into the memory functions of deaf children is far more complicated than a consideration of recall of verbal versus visual material. To focus on phonological or acoustic coding strategies for remembering material is to forget the role of visual codes in the encoding, storage and retrieval of information, particularly in those deaf individuals whose primary language is visual i.e. sign language. A number of studies have presented evidence that suggests that the 'signability' of a word influences how well it is learned and recalled by deaf signing adolescents but not hearing adolescents (for example, Bonvillian, 1983).

In terms of long-term memory (LTM) organization and strategies used for recall, the evidence base is complex and inconsistent. Some studies suggest that deaf children do not use the same strategies (for example, categorical organization) as hearing children to retrieve information from LTM, while others suggest that the same strategies are used, but less effectively, by the deaf children (Liben 1979; Bebko, 1984; Bebko and McKinnon, 1990). For a review of the literature in this area, see Marschark (1998).

Overall, it seems likely that there are differences between deaf and hearing children in terms of short-term and long-term memory functions, memory capacity, strategies and organization, relating to differences in verbal and non-verbal experiences, language medium and language fluency.

Attention abilities

Attention, in the sense of a cognitive function, is the ability to focus on one aspect of input or information (particularly but not exclusively, a visual or auditory stimulus), to the exclusion of other stimuli. Within this, 'attention' is also used to describe the process by which only one aspect of a specific input is focused on – for example, responding only to visual presentation of a circle in a stream of circles, squares, triangles, hexagons and rectangles. This is also known as selective attention. In the clinical sense, the term attention is used to describe the ability to remain 'on task' and not be distracted by extraneous stimuli, and will not be discussed further here, although clearly attentional abilities in the neurocognitive sense will translate into a behavioural picture in the individual child.

Attention skills, and in particular selective attention skills, develop over time as the child matures, from infancy through to adolescence. Clearly, there will be a significant difference in the ability to attend to auditory input between a child who can hear and a child who has no access to auditory information. However, Quittner et al. (1994) demonstrated that audition has an impact on the development of visual attention. Using a visual attention paradigm, requiring selective responses to specific stimuli, Quittner and her colleagues found that deaf children performed more poorly than hearing children. She also found that the rate of development of visual attention was faster for deaf children with a cochlear implant than those without. Following on from this study, Smith et al. (1998) found that visual attention abilities show a significant development between the ages of 7 years and 9 years, with only a slight delay in deaf children compared with their hearing peers. However, in contrast to these two studies, Tharpe, Ashmead and Rothpletz (2002) found no differences in visual attention between deaf and hearing children (or those with cochlear implants). They suggest that differences in non-verbal intelligence and age of the participants may be able to account for the discrepancies with the findings of previous studies.

Motor functions

Motor functions are included in this section on neuropsychological development because although nerves and muscles produce movements, ultimately it is the brain that instigates, organizes and coordinates those movements.

Several early studies have looked at gross motor development in hearing-impaired children. For example, Wiegersma and Van der Velde (1983) compared deaf children and hearing controls, and found that the former showed poorer general coordination and visual-motor coordination skills. In particular, they noted that deaf children execute movements more slowly than their hearing peers. Butterfield (1986) also investigated gross motor skills in deaf children and noted delays in acquisition of catching, kicking, jumping and hopping abilities. Motor skill performance was not related to the etiology of deafness. Savelsbergh, Netelenbos and Whiting (1991) also found that deaf children aged 10–13 years had difficulty catching a ball if it approached from outside their field of view compared with hearing children. However, a second experiment led them to conclude that this difference in performance was due to slower reaction times rather than slower movement times. Balance problems, and therefore delayed motor milestones and problems with gross motor coordination, are common in deaf children as a result of the link between the vestibular and auditory systems, particularly in the case of certain syndromes such as Usher syndrome.

Van Uden (1983) examined the link between a number of functions, including fine motor skill of the fingers and mouth, and the development of speech in deaf children. Van Uden described a constellation of abilities, comprising fine motor skills, memory for successively presented sequences and memory for rhythm, and labelled this the 'eupraxia/dyspraxia' factor, defined as the ability to quickly retrieve and automatize movements. Broesterhuizen (1997) extended the work of Van Uden to develop a diagnostic model to predict the development of speech reading skills and correct pronunciation of written words in young deaf children. However, Aplin (1987) was unable to replicate Van Uden's findings in a less homogeneous sample of hearing-impaired children, suggesting that a straightforward, reliable method for identifying children with dyspraxic-type difficulties has yet to be achieved.

Central auditory processing and phonological awareness

The study of what happens to auditory information once it has passed the peripheral auditory system (once it is travelling along the VIIIth nerve and reaches the auditory cortex and other 'higher' areas of the brain) is fraught with difficulties and some controversy. It is argued by some (for example, Cacace and McFarland, 1998) that the processes involved in accurately discriminating and understanding auditory input are crucial to the successful acquisition of language, and in particular reading skills. Unfortunately, central auditory processing (CAP) is a loosely defined concept with a number of subtly different ideas included within it – 'perception', 'discrimination', 'integration', 'selective listening', 'comprehension' and so on. However, perhaps the most functional definition of CAP is 'what is done with what is heard'. The situation becomes more complex when considering CAP in individuals who are hearing impaired. Clearly, a child who has a severe or profound hearing loss, even when appropriately amplified with conventional aids, may not have access to speech or other sounds, and therefore it does not make sense to talk about CAP in these individuals. However, there are a very large number of children who have a hearing loss of some degree, for whom processing of auditory information, and speech in particular, is of relevance. Children who have received a cochlear implant can be included in this group, as they typically achieve hearing levels in their implanted ear which give them access to the full range of speech sounds.

One approach to investigating CAP is the match-mismatch negativity (MMN) paradigm. Match-mismatch negativity is a brain response elicited by a discriminable change in any repetitive aspect of auditory stimulation in the absence of attention to the stimuli. In hearing children, abnormal MMN responses for speech stimuli but not tone stimuli have been found in children with specific language impairment or developmental dyslexia (Schulte-Korne et al., 1998; Uwer, Albrecht and Suchodoletz, 2002). This may lead to the problems in phonological processing experienced by children with specific reading disorders. Phonological or phonemic awareness has been argued to be important in the development of reading skills in both deaf and hearing children by Nielsen and Luetke-Stahlman (2002). However, Izzo (2002) reported that phonemic awareness, as measured by a word-to-word matching task, was not significantly correlated with reading ability, and did not contribute to the variance in reading ability in a group of 29 primary-school age deaf children.

Ponton et al. (2000) report that the MMN response is present in children who have been using a cochlear implant and have developed good spoken language. It seems likely that an abnormal MMN response in hearing-impaired children with mild-moderate losses, and those with cochlear implants, may indicate a neurodevelopmental disorder such as dyslexia. Unfortunately, the routine clinical use of MMN to help identify developmental dyslexia in hearing-impaired children is probably a long way off.

In an important development in this field, Samar, Parasnis and Berent (2002) used neuroimaging of the magnocellular visual system to detect deficits in functioning in adult deaf poor readers compared with deaf good readers. These deficits are the same as those reported in hearing dyslexics. The authors conclude that neural imaging may therefore eventually provide a useful tool in the differential diagnosis of developmental dyslexia in the deaf population.

Executive functions, higher order functions and reasoning

Executive functions can be conceptualized as having four components – goal formation, planning, carrying out the goal-directed plans and finally effective performance. Each of these components comprises many underlying functions, including processing of incoming sensory information, attention and impulse control, memory for past experiences/past learning, motor coordination and reasoning skills. Therefore it is difficult to differentiate those cognitive functions that are predominantly 'executive', from those that are more automatic or 'lower level' functions. However, in this section the focus will be on reasoning and planning skills, and how these relate to meta-cognitive abilities such as understanding the beliefs, intentions and desires of others, also known as 'theory of mind' abilities.

In the literature on hearing-impairment, executive function abilities have not generally been explored as a subject in their own right. Instead, they are subsumed within research on theory of mind (ToM) development. Jackson (2001) compared deaf children with signing parents, non-native signing children and children from a hearing-impaired unit on ToM tasks and four non-verbal executive function tasks. Jackson reported no difference between deaf and hearing children on the executive function tasks. Also, contrary to predictions they found that success on a series of false-belief ToM tasks did not increase with increased executive function performance. Woolfe, Want and Siegal (2002) also examined executive functions in relation to ToM in deaf children. They tested 39 deaf children (21 late signers and 18 native signers) using a version of the Wisconsin Card Sorting Test for young children, and found no difference between the two groups. In the combined sample, but not the two separate groups, executive function was significantly correlated with ToM. The authors therefore concluded that executive function ability could not account for the 'overwhelming advantage of native signers in ToM performance'.

Theory of mind research in deaf children is a highly complex area, with conflicting findings and various theoretical and methodological explanations proposed for these differences (Peterson and Siegal, 1998; Courtin, 2000; Rhys-Jones and Ellis, 2000; Marschark et al., 2000; Peterson, 2002).

A variety of neuropsychological tests are available to assess 'higher order' functions in adults. Relatively few have been specifically developed for children and an even smaller number have data available for hearing-impaired children. One example, the NEPSY, a developmental neuropsychological assessment battery, includes six subtests that assess executive functions. The NEPSY manual (Korkman, Kirk and Kemp, 1998) presents data from 32 hearing-impaired children on five of the six subtests. Differences between the hearing-impaired children and controls were found on only one subtest, named 'knock and tap'. Other traditional tests of executive function such as the Wisconsin Card Sorting Test and 'Tower of London' do not provide data on hearing-impaired children.

Disorders of neuropsychological development

Before considering each of the main neurodevelopmental disorders of childhood, and their assessment in deaf children, it is important to clarify a number of issues. Firstly, global intellectual difficulties/learning difficulties or global developmental delay will not be considered here. Although relatively common in the hearing-impaired group as a whole, due to the link with syndromal aetiologies of deafness, the focus of this chapter is on specific neurocognitive functions. Secondly, the distinction needs to be made between the specific neuropsychological/cognitive functions outlined above, and the clinical manifestations of these processes failing to work properly. Frequently the experimental paradigms used in exploring these processes, and the results they produce, appear to bear little relationship to the clinical problems as they present to professionals working with deaf children and adolescents. However, it is hoped that the reader will be able to identify the themes presented above as they appear in the following sections. Thirdly, the distinction also needs to be made between delay, and disorder or deficit in the context of neurocognitive processes. If the acquisition of a skill is delayed, it implies that the developmental trajectory for a particular individual is the same as for the general population but that development starts late and/or is slower than normal. If acquisition of the skill is disordered, or there is a deficit in that area, the pattern of development is substantially different for that individual compared with others of the same age. Finally, it is important to point out that although the assessment aspects of the following sections are written from the perspective of psychological practitioners, speech and language therapists and audiologists have crucial roles to play in the assessment of hearing-impaired children. Indeed, the most useful assessments derive from close collaboration between all professionals involved with a child, regardless of the nature of the presenting problem.

The diagnosis of a disorder of neuropsychological development in a deaf child is a particularly tricky challenge. Standard classification texts such as DSM IV and ICD 10 specifically state that most diagnoses should not be made where delays or distortion in function are a direct consequence of a hearing impairment. Therefore the diagnosis of a specific language or learning disorder can only be made where the hearing-impairment is not a sufficient explanation for the disorder – where there is disturbance in function over and above that expected as a result of the hearing impairment. Unfortunately, no specific guidelines are presented as to what constitutes a sufficiently large difference between what deaf children should be able to do and what they are doing in terms of a particular function. This is left entirely to the clinician's judgement! However, this is no reason to ignore the fact that some deaf children appear to have a greater struggle developing certain skills than other deaf children and, where appropriate, diagnosis of an additional disorder can open the door to the specific help needed to overcome their difficulties.

Specific disorders of speech and language

Several specific disorders are included in this section. Disorders of articulation, in the absence of any other difficulties, are evidenced by omissions of words in speech, distortions, substitutions and inconsistencies in pronunciation. Expressive language disorder is characterized by a restricted vocabulary, word substitutions, omissions of word endings and prefixes, syntactical errors and short sentences. Hearing children with a receptive language disorder will show lack of understanding of grammatical structure (for example negatives, questions and comparatives), difficulty following instructions, and also significant delay in expressive language. Non-verbal communication, including gesture, mime, demonstration and non-speech vocalisations are usually normal (WHO, 1992). However, therein lies the problem. The speech and verbal comprehension of hearing-impaired children is often characterized by errors of the kind described above, when there is no additional language disorder. The non-verbal communication of deaf children may not be completely typical of their hearing peers, but again this does not necessarily mean that they have a language, or any other, disorder. Also, language disorders are frequently associated with social, emotional and behavioural problems in hearing children, but there is a high rate of these difficulties in deaf children, even without language disorders. Thus distinguishing between the normal variations of the language (and behaviour) of hearing-impaired children, and the language (and behaviour) of a hearing-impaired child with a language disorder is very complex.

Assessment of language disorders in a hearing-impaired child is in many respects the same as in a hearing child, although the professionals involved should be experienced in communicating with and assessing hearing-impaired children. In accordance with diagnostic guidelines, language disorders must be assessed in the context of expectations appropriate for the child's 'mental age', or more specifically their non-verbal cognitive abilities. A detailed developmental history should always be taken, and videotaping the informal interactions and formal language assessment is helpful for subsequent detailed analysis of the child's language. In the absence of specific criteria, the clinician then has to decide, primarily on the basis of experience, whether the child's language is sufficiently more delayed or disordered than would be anticipated, given his or her degree of hearing loss and non-verbal cognitive abilities, to warrant a diagnosis of language disorder.

Obviously two major assumptions have been made throughout the preceding paragraph – that the children use oral language rather than sign language, and that they have sufficient language abilities to tackle formal assessments, even if they are not administered in the standardized fashion intended. This said, it must be theoretically possible for a child whose only language is manual to have a language disorder, but discussion of the issues that raises, although fascinating, is beyond the scope of this chapter.

Specific learning disorders, specific reading disorder, dyslexia

The terminology in this area is frequently confusing, because more than one label can be given to essentially the same disorder. 'Specific learning disorder' is often used to refer to specific disorders of reading and/or spelling, which are also known as 'dyslexia' or 'developmental dyslexia'. Children in this group have difficulty learning letter-sound correspondences and this is typically reflected in both their reading and spelling skills. They also usually show difficulties with speech sound discrimination, and may evidence auditory processing problems. Thus, diagnosis of dyslexia in hearing-impaired children is difficult, given that access to speech sounds is compromised to a greater or lesser extent, making it difficult to disentangle deafness-related difficulties from specific learning difficulties. However, as with specific language disorders, hearing-impaired children are not immune to additional difficulties and therefore some attempt at assessment and diagnosis is needed.

The first step, as always, is to establish the child's general cognitive abilities, particularly non-verbal abilities, to check whether there is a global delay or specific deficit. Following this, other tests are needed to build a picture of the child's difficulties. These include standardized tests of literacy, and qualitative observations of reading and spelling, tests of phoneme awareness (blending and deleting phonemes), verbal memory, naming speed, writing speed, and non-word reading. Children with dyslexia may also exhibit attention problems, and it can be useful to assess these. Finally, once again largely based on the clinician's experience in this area, a judgement must be made as to the degree of discrepancy between the child's actual reading and spelling attainments and those expected given their intellectual ability and level of hearing impairment, in the context of their language skills.

Central auditory processing disorder

Central auditory processing disorder (CAPD) is a deficit in 'what is done with what is heard'. Although it is most often diagnosed in children with normal intellectual abilities and normal hearing sensitivity, theoretically it can coexist with hearing loss or other cognitive or neurological impairments. It is characterized by a number of behavioural markers, for example poor concentration/attention span, difficulty following instructions, being easily distracted by auditory or visual stimuli, memory deficits, behaviour problems, frequent requests for repetitions of what is said, misunderstanding what is said, problems localizing sound, difficulty listening in background noise, language and learning deficits, and reliance on visual cues when communicating. Clearly, many of these difficulties are almost universal among hearing-impaired children, depending on the degree of hearing loss, once again making it difficult to be confident in diagnosing CAPD in hearing-impaired children. In children whose hearing loss is mild to moderate, it may be possible to undertake tests of speech in noise, auditory pattern perception, dichotic listening tasks (where different stimuli are presented simultaneously to each ear), auditory attention skills, auditory memory and language comprehension. Where available, MMN testing can be illuminating. However, regardless of degree of hearing loss, it is useful to observe the children's behaviour in clinic and classroom settings, to note their attention span, attention to structured and unstructured tasks, response to frustration, and the need for praise and encouragement to remain on task.

Specific developmental disorders of motor function/coordination

Dyspraxia refers to difficulty in planning and carrying out coordinated, voluntary movements. This can be movements of the large muscles of the body, the fine movements of the speech apparatus (lips, jaw, tongue, soft palate, larynx and muscles controlling breathing for speech), or both. Children with general motor dyspraxia are likely to have difficulty hopping, jumping, catching a ball, dressing, using buttons and zips, writing neatly and drawing. Verbal dyspraxia is characterized by difficulty in making speech sounds, sequencing them in words and sentences, difficulties controlling breathing when speaking, and problems in controlling pitch, intonation and rhythm in speech. Children with verbal dyspraxia also often have a history of feeding difficulties and great difficulty learning to blow their noses (WHO, 1992).

One of the most important steps in diagnosing dyspraxia in hearing-impaired children is to eliminate other possible causes of motor difficulties, for example, those related to specific aetiologies of deafness or medical and neurological disorders. Therefore a pediatrician's and/or neurologist's evaluation of the child is essential. Assessment by specialist speech and language therapists, occupational therapists and clinical or educational psychologists is also important to build up a comprehensive picture of the child's skills and difficulties. As usual, it is important to place any difficulties within the context of the child's developmental level and overall cognitive functioning, and be aware of the possibility that these difficulties may have had a negative impact on self-esteem and social relationships.

Autistic spectrum disorders

In order to consider assessment and diagnosis of autistic spectrum disorders (autism and Asperger syndrome) in hearing-impaired children it may be helpful first to consider the issues in hearing children. Autism is considered a 'pervasive developmental disorder' which is usually manifest by the age of three years, but certainly by 5 years of age. Evidence of a triad of areas of dysfunction needs to be observed for the diagnosis to be made:

abnormalities in social interactions, communication and restricted, stereotyped or repetitive behaviours (WHO, 1992). General cognitive delay is often, but not invariably, also present. The observed behaviours in autistic spectrum disorder include poor understanding of socio-emotional cues, poor use of social signs, lack of integration of social, emotional and communicative behaviours, impaired communication generally and impaired make-believe, social imitative and symbolic play.

The other primary area of behaviour disturbance in autism lies in restricted, repetitive and stereotyped patterns of behaviour, resulting in the child imposing rigidity and routine on a variety of play and other activities, any changes leading to anxiety and distress. Autistic children frequently have difficulties generalizing what they have learned from one situation to another, and they may also experience difficulties in integrating information gained from the different sense modalities. In addition to these specific areas of difficulty, autistic children also frequently show a range of other problems, such as sleeping and eating difficulties, fears or phobias, temper tantrums and aggressive behaviour (WHO, 1992).

Now the thorny issue of autistic spectrum disorder and deafness. The major problem facing the clinician working with hearing-impaired children is that many of the behaviours described above are apparent in hearing-impaired children to some degree, at some point during their early development. Clearly, children with a profound hearing loss, who do not have access to good language models from an early age, will evidence disordered patterns of communication. This can have a knock-on effect on all aspects of social-emotional communication, play skills and understanding of and response to others' verbal and non-verbal cues. In addition, deaf children may try to impose some kind of structure or order on their confusing world, resulting in restrictive behaviour patterns and the need for predictable routines. However, the fact that these behaviours are so common in hearing-impaired children generally, means that there is a real danger of over-diagnosing autism in this group. Conversely, as a result, caution over misdiagnosing autism in deaf children has led to children who do have genuine autistic-spectrum problems going unrecognized and therefore access to appropriate services is denied.

Perhaps the most useful indicators of significant autistic disorder in a deaf child are the absence of communicative intent and behavioural disturbance suggestive of disorder rather than simply delay. In other words, the child must show evidence of a lack of desire to communicate, rather than lack of understandable communication per se. Problems with the development of play skills, joint attention skills, understanding and response to others' emotions, and the need for routine and predictability, must be markedly different from those seen in the general population of hearing-impaired children, for a diagnosis of autistic spectrum disorder to be made. As with the diagnosis of any disorder of neuropsychological development, it is important to bear in mind any social and emotional factors that may be affecting the child's responses.

A number of assessment schedules and questionnaires are available, which can help guide diagnosis. Some are more useful than others in the hearing-impaired population. The Autism Diagnostic Observation Schedule-Generic (ADOS-G) (Lord et al., 2000) is a standardized, interactive schedule based on a series of structured and semi-structured situations in which the behavioural responses of the child are rated. The schedule is appropriate for children with no expressive language, through to verbally fluent, high-functioning adolescents and adults. However, even in the youngest children, some understanding of what the examiner is asking the child to do is required, and several of the items to be rated are directly dependent on the child's verbal communication skills.

The ADOS-G has been shown to have good validity, reliability and diagnostic utility, but as yet there are no studies specifically investigating its use in the hearing-impaired population.

A range of questionnaires is also available to aid in the assessment of autism. Unfortunately, the utility of these instruments in hearing-impaired children is questionable as they do not permit the differentiation of behaviours that could be attributable to either deafness or autism. In all cases, whenever assessment schedules or questionnaires are employed with hearing-impaired children, great care must be taken when interpreting the results, and a sound knowledge of the 'normal' communication and behaviour patterns of hearing-impaired children is essential.

Summary

The aim of this chapter has been to give an overview of the field of neuropsychological development as it relates to childhood deafness. A substantial literature has accumulated in many, but not all, of the areas of cognitive functioning which have been covered, and it has been possible only to give an indication of the complexity of the research findings. The assessment and diagnosis of neuropsychological disorders in hearing-impaired children is similarly complex, and this is an area where future research could usefully be focused. When working with hearing-impaired children it is important to remember that deafness has an impact on many aspects of functioning – a deaf child is not simply a hearing child without auditory input. In addition, hearing-impairment does not preclude the child from having a disorder of neuropsychological development, and great care must be taken not to assume that the child's deafness is a sufficient explanation for all manifest difficulties.

References

Aplin DY (1987) Classification of dyspraxia in hearing-impaired children using the Q-technique of factor analysis. Journal of Child Psychology and Psychiatry 28: 581–96.

Athanasiou MS (2000) Current nonverbal assessment instruments: a comparison of psychometric integrity and test fairness. Journal of Psychoeducational Assessment 18: 211–29.

Bebko JM (1984) Memory and rehearsal characteristics of profoundly deaf children. Journal of Experimental Child Psychology 38: 415–28.

Bebko JM, McKinnon EE (1990) The language experience of deaf children: its relationship to spontaneous rehearsal in a memory task. Child Development 61: 1744–52.

Bonvillian JD (1983) Effects of signability and imagery on word recall of deaf and hearing students. Perceptual and Motor Skills 56: 775–91.

Braden JP (1991) A meta-analytic review of IQ research with deaf persons. In Martin DS (ed) Advances in Cognition, Education and Deafness. Washington DC: Gallaudet University Press, pp. 56–61.

Braden JP (1994) Deafness, Deprivation and IQ. New York: Plenum Press.

Bradley-Johnson S (2001) Cognitive assessment for the youngest children: a critical review of tests. Journal of Psychoeducational Assessment 19: 19–44.

Broesterhuizen MLHM (1997) Psychological assessment of deaf children. Scandinavian Audiology 26, Suppl 46: 43–9.

Butterfield SA (1986) Gross motor profiles of deaf children. Perceptual and Motor Skills 62: 68–70.

Cacace AT, McFarland DJ (1998) Central auditory processing disorder in school-aged children: a critical review. Journal of Speech, Language and Hearing Research 41: 355–73.

Conrad R, Weiskrantz BC (1981) On the cognitive ability of deaf children with deaf parents. American Annals of the Deaf 126: 995–1003.

Courtin C (2000) The impact of sign language on cognitive development of deaf children: the case of theories of mind. Journal of Deaf Studies and Deaf Education 5: 266–76.

Izzo A (2002) Phonemic awareness and reading ability: an investigation with young readers who are deaf. American Annals of the Deaf 147: 18–28.

Jackson AL (2001) Language facility and theory of mind development in deaf children. Journal of Deaf Studies and Deaf Education 6: 161–76.

Korkman M, Kirk U, Kemp S (1998) NEPSY, A Developmental Neuropsychological Assessment Manual. New York: The Psychological Corporation.

Liben LS (1979) Free recall by deaf and hearing children: semantic clustering and recall in trained and untrained groups. Journal of Experimental Child Psychology 27: 105–19.

Lord C, Risi S, Lambrecht L, Cook EH Jr, Leventhal BL, DiLavore PC, Pickles A, Rutter M (2000) The autism diagnostic observation schedule-generic: a standard measure of social and communication deficits associated with the spectrum of autism. Journal of Autism and Developmental Disorders 30: 205–23.

Maller SJ (1996) WISC-III verbal item invariance across samples of deaf and hearing children of similar measured ability. Journal of Psychoeducational Assessment 14: 152–65.

Maller SJ, Braden JP (1993) The construct and criterion-related validity of the WISC-III with deaf adolescents. Journal of Psychoeducational Assessment, WISC-III Monograph: 105–13.

Maller SJ, Ferron J (1997) WISC III factor invariance across deaf and standardization samples. Educational and Psychological Measurement 57: 987–94.

Marschark M (1998) Memory for language in deaf adults and children. Scandinavian Audiology Suppl 49: 87–92.

Marschark M, Green V, Hindmarsh G, Walker S (2000) Understanding theory of mind in children who are deaf. Journal of Child Psychology and Psychiatry 41: 1067–73.

Nielsen DC, Luetke-Stahlman B (2002) Phonological awareness: one key to the reading proficiency of deaf children. American Annals of the Deaf 147: 11–19.

Parasnis I, Samar VJ, Bettger JG, Sathe K (1996) Does deafness lead to enhancement of visual spatial cognition in children? Negative evidence from deaf non-signers. Journal of Deaf Studies and Deaf Education 1: 145–52

Peterson CC (2002) Drawing insight from pictures: The development of concepts of false drawing and false belief in children with deafness, normal hearing, and autism. Child Development 73: 1442–59.

Peterson CC, Siegal M (1998) Changing focus on the representational mind: Deaf, autistic and normal children's concepts of false photos, false drawings and false beliefs. British Journal of Developmental Psychology 16: 301–20.

Pisoni DB, Geers AE (2000) Working memory in deaf children with cochlear implants: correlations between digit span and measures of spoken language processing. Annals of Otology, Rhinology and Laryngology Suppl 185: 92–3.

Ponton CW, Eggermont JJ, Don M, Waring MD, Kwong B, Cunningham J, Trautwein P (2000) Maturation of the mismatch negativity: effects of profound deafness and cochlear implant use. Audiology and Neuro-otology 5: 167–85.

Quittner AL, Smith LB, Osberger MJ, Mitchell TV, Katz DB (1994) The impact of audition on the development of visual attention. Psychological Science 5: 347–53.

Rhys-Jones SL, Ellis HD (2000) Theory of mind: deaf and hearing children's comprehension of picture stories and judgements of social situations. Journal of Deaf Studies and Deaf Education 5: 248–65.

Roid GH, Miller LJ (1997) Leiter International Performance Scale-Revised: Examiners Manual. Wood Dale IL: Stoelting.

Rush P, Blennerhassett L, Epstein K, Alexander D (1991) WAIS-R verbal and performance profiles of adolescents referred for atypical learning styles. In Martin DS (ed.) Advances in Cognition, Education and Deafness. Washington DC: Gallaudet University Press, pp. 82–8.

Samar VJ, Parasnis I, Berent GP (2002) Deaf poor readers' pattern reversal visual evoked potentials suggest magnocellular system deficits: Implications for diagnostic neuroimaging of dyslexia in deaf individuals. Brain and Language 80: 21–44.

Savelsbergh GJ, Netelenbos JB, Whiting HT (1991) Auditory perception and the control of spatially co-ordinated action of deaf and hearing children. Journal of Child Psychology and Psychiatry 32: 489–500.

Schulte-Korne G, Deimel W, Bartling J, Remschmidt H (1998) Auditory processing and dyslexia: evidence for a specific speech processing deficit. Neuroreport 9: 337–40.

Smith LB, Quittner AL, Osberger MJ, Miyamoto R (1998) Audition and visual attention: the developmental trajectory in deaf and hearing populations. Developmental Psychology 34: 840–50.

Tharpe AM, Ashmead DH, Rothpletz AM (2002) Visual attention in children with normal hearing, children with hearing aids and children with cochlear implants. Speech, Language and Hearing Research 45: 403–13.

Tomlinson-Keasey C, Smith-Winberry C (1990) Cognitive consequences of congenital deafness. The Journal of Genetic Psychology 151: 103–15.

Uwer R, Albrecht R, Von Suchodoletz W (2002) Automatic processing of tones and speech stimuli in children with specific language impairment. Developmental Medicine and Child Neurology 44: 527–32.

Van Uden AMJ (1983) Diagnostic testing of deaf children: the syndrome of dyspraxia. Lisse, Netherlands: Swets & Zeitlinger.

Waters GS, Doehring DG (1990) Reading acquisition in congenitally deaf children who communicate orally: insights from an analysis of component reading, language and memory skills. In Carr TH, Levy BA (eds) Reading and its Development. San Diego CA: Academic Press, pp. 323–73.

WHO (1992) The ICD-10 Classification of Mental and Behavioural Disorders: Clinical Descriptions and Diagnostic Guidelines. Geneva: World Health Organization.

Wiegersma PH, Van der Velde A (1983) Motor development of deaf children. Journal of Child Psychology and Psychiatry 24: 103–11.

Woolfe T, Want SC, Siegal M (2002) Signposts to development: theory of mind in deaf children. Child Development 73: 768–78.

PART 3
DEAFNESS AND
MENTAL HEALTH

CHAPTER **10**

Mental health services for Deaf people

NICK KITSON AND SALLY AUSTEN

Mental health services for Deaf people: past, present and future

This chapter considers the past, present and future of services whose prime function is to serve the mental health of their Deaf users. It will not discuss schools, theatres, jobs or Deaf clubs, or the services that family and friends provide, although these are also central to mental health and well being of Deaf people.

Data indicate that Deaf people have a greater overall prevalence of mental illness than the general population and that they stay in hospital for longer periods (Vernon and Daigle-King, 1999). It is acknowledged, however, that many Deaf patients in psychiatric hospitals have no psychiatric diagnosis, but have psychosocial or behaviour difficulties. However, there is a paucity of research in this area, and it is thought that misdiagnosis, particularly outside of specialist Deaf mental health services, is common.

The role of sign language in mental health and deafness has long been acknowledged. Lack of sign language in some schools has been associated with some of the non-psychiatric admissions (Denmark and Warren, 1972). Admission to hospitals where signing was not available is considered by Vernon and Daigle-King (1999) to represent 'antitherapeutic custodial isolation of the deaf patient'.

Past

As early as 1928 a Deaf Danish man Viggo C. Hansen, the then leader of the Danish Deaf Association, first recognized the plight of Deaf people in mental hospitals (Von der Leith, 2001). Although himself a painter, he was then leader of the Danish Deaf Association. However, specialist mental health services for Deaf people began in New York in 1955 under Dr Franz Kallmann (Rainer, Altshuler and Kallmann, 1963). Starting as an outpatient clinic, the University Mental Health Department of Genetics in the Columbia District of Manhattan Island, this service undertook an extensive survey of the Deaf community. Early services consisted of hearing psychiatrists and psychologists working alongside sign-language interpreters but gradually clinicians signed for themselves and Deaf clinicians were employed.

European services began with ward and community residential services in Denmark in 1967. From a general population of about 5 million, the service initially had enough patients to fill approximately 20 beds, which allowed a ward with signing staff, almost entirely dedicated to Deaf people. The Danish service, however, was a victim of its own success. As time went on the numbers of Deaf people requiring a mental hospital bed dwindled to an average of five beds and a full team of practitioners using sign language was no longer viable.

Services in the UK

Services started in a village near Preston in the northwest of England (Denmark and Warren, 1972). Dr John Denmark, a psychiatrist, happened to be the son of a headmaster of a school for Deaf children, and had learnt to sign. He was referred one Deaf psychiatric patient by a local GP and, realizing the need for psychiatrists who could sign, he created the first outpatient clinic, and by 1969 had the first inpatient facility in the UK.

As the result of a survey of Surrey Mental Hospitals by the Royal Association in Aid of the Deaf and Dumb (RADD), a day service was developed in Springfield Hospital, London in 1971. This grew to a centrally funded NHS inpatient service by 1978. Again, its establishment was by chance: the efforts of local charities combined with the presence of a psychiatric nurse whose parents were Deaf. The London service, described in detail by Kitson and Wilson (in Hindley and Kitson: 2000), with its base local population of about 10 million, was readily able to justify increasingly comprehensive services. The mid-1980s saw the establishment of community based services including a network of rehabilitation homes, day facilities for those needing ongoing support and a visiting service for patients able to maintain themselves in their own homes.

The third service in the United Kingdom, which opened in Birmingham in 1991, arose from another charity, the Birmingham Institute for the Deaf, and the chance presence of a deafened senior psychiatric trainee who had a strong interest in deafness.

It is interesting, and perhaps alarming, to note that none of these developments came from direct central planning by the NHS Executive or the Department of Health. Internationally, services developed in a similarly *ad hoc* fashion, with the exception of Dutch services, which developed from a central national plan in 1985 as the result of petitioning from a small group, led by a determined mother of a deaf child. It does seem, however, that national planning is beginning to take root: France now has an ambitious cradle-to-grave national plan and most recently the UK drafted its national plan in the form of a Department of Health consultation document entitled, *A Sign of the Times.*

In addition to the three United Kingdom NHS general mental health services for Deaf people and their associated community housing, there is also a specialist Deaf programme for the small number of Deaf people in Rampton High Security Hospital. For many years the policy of Deaf patients being nursed according to categories of mental disorder and degrees of disturbance meant that the approximately 10 patients were nursed on separate wards and met only in day facilities. However, as far as possible, the Deaf patients are now nursed on the same ward, resulting in improvements in the Deaf awareness and sign language use of their staff.

A further medium-secure forensic service for Deaf offenders with mental health problems opened in the north of England in 2001. Although privately run, it was developed through research performed in association with the Manchester Deaf mental health service (the upgraded version of the original Preston NHS service) and continues to have formal clinical staff input from there. A meeting of the British Society of Mental Health and Deafness in 2000, attended by service funders, concluded that figures probably justified two ten-bedded medium secure facilities, one in the north and one in the south.

There are also a number of stand-alone specialist mental health residential services as well as a few local counselling services for Deaf people.

Present

Good practice

The United Kingdom's three centres for Mental Health and Deafness have been the envy of European health providers. They are based in the largest most densely populated areas and provide a model for services in large cities with general populations in the millions. Nationally, they provide approximately 60 hospital inpatient beds and provide community based services for adults with acute mental illness, challenging behaviour and rehabilitation. They tend to provide a combination of medical, nursing and psychological therapies.

In 1995, the London service moved from outdated premises and in doing so demonstrated what could be achieved by multi-agency working. The new service was provided jointly by the National Health Service, the local government, the charity Sign Campaign (supporting Deaf people with mental health problems), Harding Housing Association and the local branch of the charity MIND (representing people with severe mental health problems). Moving out of the hospital campus to a four-storey suburban street site the service was able to provide a complex of 20 active treatment 'hospital' beds, six intensive long-term care beds, nominally 18 day places as well as office and clinic space. This became the hub of a network providing an additional 40 supported residential places in a variety of styles in the locality and a 20-place day centre. Patients who had moved on to ordinary housing and/or employment in the area local to the service continued to be supported. This service has become a model for good practice internationally.

Integrated versus specialist services

In the UK there is a clear practice of providing segregated non-mainstream specialist mental health services for Deaf people. Although some authors disagree with segregated care (Glow, 1989), Whitehouse, Sherman and Kozlowski (1991) claim that mainstream services are ineffective and costly, finding that the 'complexity of the disability and the isolation from the general population, which Deaf people uniquely experience, justify specialised services.'

Although, of course, good work can be achieved by hearing professionals using sign language interpreters, there are limitations. There is a great shortage of sign language interpreters in the UK and there is often debate about their funding. As a result, in a treatment setting, it would be likely that one-to-one sessions with particular professionals would be interpreted but peer group interaction and other vital, but less structured, interactions may not (Boros, 1981). The presence of an interpreter also affects, sometimes negatively, the therapeutic relationship. There will also be situations where, in the authors' opinion, only the professional signing for themselves could accurately assess the Deaf patient: for example, where the patient is displaying disordered language or thought disorder as a result of schizophrenia.

Whitehouse et al. (1991) recommend that services should have staff well trained in sign language and Deaf culture and affirmative action to employ deaf staff. A therapeutic environment is not just about translation between two languages: it is also about the meeting of two cultures. With this is mind, the three Deaf services in the UK, supported by the European Society for Mental Health and Deafness, follow an affirmative action policy to employ Deaf staff (Kitson and Monteiro, 1991).

Deaf patients in the UK tend to live and in some cases work in a Deaf signing environment, and segregated services better reflect Deaf people's choices. Ninety per cent of Deaf people, although born to hearing parents, marry Deaf partners (Rainer, Altshuler and Kallman, 1963) and seek each other's company in Deaf clubs (Phoenix, 1988). In a predominantly hearing world, provision of good communication in the patients' first/native/preferred language, and a culturally appropriate environment, is vital for maximizing emotional wellbeing and for respecting human rights. The London service describes its attempt to provide services 'for Deaf people, by Deaf people' (Kitson and Klein in Mayer, 1997).

Deaf staff's skill

Accused, at times, of creating Deaf ghettos, the congregation of sign language users with mental health problems has been a deliberate one. All the UK mental health services use sign language and up to 30% of their staff are Deaf sign-language users. In the associated community supported housing up to 60% of staff are Deaf sign language users and the clinical management in both levels of service is essentially Deaf centred.

Communication with patients is fundamental to mental health practice. Deaf people and hearing people brought up in Deaf families have a natural advantage with sign language as a first language and a deeper understanding of the cultural experience of Deaf people. Additionally, Deaf staff with good language skills tend to be able to use visual and tactile communication flexibly to communicate with Deaf people with different dialects or communication difficulties and to work with hearing people who have varying abilities in manual communication. In technical interpreting terminology, they have the ability to 'code switch' (Hoffmeister and Moores, 1987).

Staff members who have personal experience of deafness tend to have a greater credibility with Deaf clients. This can be used in specific therapy aimed at increasing cultural awareness and enhancing self-esteem and identity as a Deaf person (Sims, 1989). The 'Deaf way' or Deaf-centred approaches cannot be fully achieved without Deaf people as the cultural norm. Deaf staff provide appropriate role models and motivation to patients through both their professional behaviour and social lives. They demonstrate that Deaf people can achieve, can have families and can experience the usual variety of interests and lifestyles. They are best placed to encourage and support activities within local Deaf communities and this modelling also provides training for hearing staff. The example of Deaf staff to the local Deaf community in their normal daily life should also demystify mental health issues and reduce the stigma of mental health institutions (Rebourg, 1991).

In the authors' experience the Deaf person's natural visual skills can be particularly useful in psychiatric nursing observation, particularly when the patient is difficult to diagnose by simple psychiatric interview. In situations where either the diagnostician or the patient may have difficulty with sign language the psychiatric interview is likely to be impaired, so observation is all the more important.

The Deaf/hearing staff mix

Initially modest aims involved only the training of hearing mental health staff in deafness and communication skills (Denmark and Warren, 1972), however Kitson and Klein (in Mayer, 1997) report crucial gains from the systematic employment of Deaf mental health workers.

They recall a number of concerns when Deaf staff were first actively recruited. For example, there was some concern from hearing staff that, during incidents of challenging behaviour, that Deaf staff would not hear shouts for help. In fact the anecdotal evidence was that over the period when Deaf staff were employed, the number of serious incidents fell. The 'explosive rage' said to be characteristic of some Deaf patients proved to be much less common in an environment staffed by Deaf people. Additionally emergency warning system technology and Deaf staff's visual and vibration sensitivity enabled an appropriate response.

There was also anxiety amongst both service users and Deaf professionals about confidentiality issues. Deaf professionals and patients are more likely to meet or to have met each other socially. The experience of employing and training significant numbers of Deaf mental health workers in health and residential services showed that, when Deaf people learn professional codes of behaviour, they gain the respect of their clients and can model appropriate boundary setting.

Deaf people may be motivated to help other Deaf people as a result of their own life experiences but, just as in other specialities of mental health, overidentification with the patient can result in impaired clinical accuracy and poor boundary setting (Rebourg, 1991). Similarly Deaf staff may inflict their negative emotional baggage from their past experience on hearing staff, expecting discrimination in a prejudicial fashion and maybe causing it by defensive behaviours. However, hearing staff may also exhibit prejudice or ignorance of Deaf Culture, a fear of the unknown or negative assumptions about disability.

Mutual hostility and paranoia between Deaf and hearing staff can develop, as can splits between any two groups. Greater fluency of communication between the Deaf staff and Deaf patients can lead to exclusivity in relationships that can damage the team approach (Rebourg, 1991). Where Deaf and hearing staff work together hearing staff may feel linguistically deskilled. Their communication handicap, in a profession largely reliant on communication, is highlighted by the Deaf staff members' fluency. Consequently, in order to maintain 'superiority', the hearing staff may avoid sharing mental health skills or deny their communication handicap. However, Deaf/hearing status may in fact be an easy scapegoat onto which other splitting issues are projected. Emotional support and good teamwork are important to redress these issues.

Training Deaf professionals

Deaf people, despite ability and aptitude, continue to be at a disadvantage in education, and face significant obstacles in gaining recognized mental health qualifications, most of which at present require good oral and written English skills. Despite the authors' positive experiences of working with Deaf staff, attempts to encourage them into qualifying training have not been so positive.

In 1989, a respected counselling training organization in the UK agreed to provide a 2 year course conducted in sign language. Deaf graduates of the courses subsequently joined the teaching staff. Unfortunately, after a few years, funding failed and the courses ceased. However, similar courses followed in other British cities and several Deaf counsellors are now qualified to the level required for independent practice.

Until there are large groups of professionally qualified Deaf mental health workers, there is a danger of unqualified Deaf mental health workers being undervalued (lack of qualification can lead to assumed lack of ability) or overvalued (Deaf experience and fluent communication can lead to assumed ability).

Deaf sign language users who have achieved formal mental health qualifications remain rare throughout Europe, whereas in America equality of access to training is far more common. Considering that most of the mental healthcare professions espouse equality and promote models of rehabilitation, it is alarming how few exhibit this in their own professional training provision.

From the 1980s, a number of Deaf people in the UK completed social work training; a few have qualified as occupational therapists and the first two Deaf postgraduate clinical psychology trainees in the UK are presently being trained. Progress in training Deaf nurses has been slow. Salford University, with the support of the Manchester Deaf mental health service, has provided a registered mental health nurse training course for Deaf students since September 2000 (Sharples, 2001). Attempts at establishing National Vocational Qualifications (NVQ) for Deaf mental health workers initially floundered though there has been some success with training residential care workers (Vaughan, 1994). National Vocational Qualifications are largely practical and work based, and so should be ideal for those Deaf people who have difficulties with written language or have had poor educational opportunities.

Future provision of services

The authors' opinion on the best provision of services is encompassed in the policy statement of the London National Deaf Services: 'Deaf people have the same right to services and opportunities as hearing people . . . When Deaf people are disadvantaged by deafness or society's attitude to it, they have the right to additional services to overcome that disadvantage.' The goal of treatment is simply the best mental health possible for any individual. It is to be hoped that, where this is not currently happening, future services will develop to address this.

Geographical challenges

One of greatest challenges for future Deaf mental health service is addressing the geographical inequalities of service provision. At present the range of services one receives is dependent on proximity to Manchester, Birmingham or London. Satellite clinics and associated home visits to distant sites do operate but these are infrequent and do not provide the range of skills of a full mental health team. They are often only served by psychiatrists and community psychiatric nurses.

A locally based example of a mental health service for Deaf adults in Nottingham (general population 600,000) has been described (Chan, 2001). The Health Authority and local NHS Trust jointly established this pioneering service in February 1999. A community psychiatric nurse (CPN) was employed to work exclusively with Deaf people in the locality. The remit was to improve access to mainstream as well as specialist Deaf mental health services, to facilitate the local services in working with Deaf people, and to promote the general mental health of the Deaf community. Over 50% of the caseload did not have a formal mental illness diagnoses yet they were equally disabled by common mental health problems. Clients demonstrated significant social functioning deficits and levels of impairment comparable to hearing clients suffering from formal mental illness, therefore justifying the need for local mental health services for Deaf people. The Nottingham experience may provide a model for future services in smaller urban populations where reasonable access to one of the three specialist hospitals is impossible.

Service commissioning

Commissioning, planning and funding of Deaf mental health services in the UK have been a frustrating business, associated with a number of time-wasting changes, false starts and dashed hopes.

The NHS Health Advisory Service (HAS, 1998) report was commissioned following the campaign by the three services and the British Deaf Association to maintain central government funding. It proposed a tiered model incorporating graduated care from the general practitioner, the local psychiatrist, satellite services of the three services and from the three specialist hospitals themselves. It failed to recognize that the so-called 'specialist' mental health services for Deaf people were not specialist; rather they provide a wide ranging general mental health service, for a special population. Despite some flaws in the model, it did recognize Deaf people's needs and attempt to describe a systematic nationwide solution, yet there was no attempt by any national or regional authority to implement it.

As is so often the case, a disaster is required before notice is taken. A gory homicide by a Deaf mentally ill patient in 1998 looks set to fundamentally improve the political will. The homicide inquiry report (known informally as 'the DJ inquiry') was severely critical of the lack of a National Strategy on mental health services for Deaf people. It appears to have galvanized the Department of Health into action in the form of a national strategic framework for mental health and deafness for adults of working age. A government consultation document, *A Sign of the Times,* although expected by April 2000 was finally published in draft form in 2002 (Department of Health, 2002). The government's stated intent is to provide both a strategy and funding. The central theme of the consultation is how to balance local services, which may be inexpert and largely interpreter based, with the specialist services whose distance renders them less accessible.

Assertive outreach and other community based initiatives

Crisis resolution, home treatment and assertive outreach teams provide intensive community support. Their aim is to avoid admission to, or allow early discharge from, hospital. The key finding of the 'DJ inquiry' was the paradox that those with the skills to help a Deaf patient – the staff of specialist Deaf mental health services – are the least available when the Deaf patient is in crisis or requires assistance out of office hours.

Within months of the incident the number of consultant psychiatrists serving Deaf adults from London was doubled. Within days of the report the London service was advised to prepare to be given funding for an assertive community treatment team to cover those with severe mental illness, at home, over the whole of the London region. This was funded and set up from 2001 and can, if necessary, provide daily visits, for example to ensure medication compliance. This model is staff intensive and focused on the most needy, particularly those who are most difficult to engage with services. Similar developments are probably possible for all large dense conurbations with a population over 2 million.

Emergency beds

The three UK services function as tertiary services, which means that the local (mainstream) mental health teams have responsibility for Deaf patients in emergencies. Geographical distance, funding anomalies and long waiting lists for admission to Deaf mental health service prevent the use of tertiary beds for emergencies. At times of crisis, expert skills are required, particularly when assessments under the Mental Health Act are required, which may result in a patient being detained compulsorily.

The problem of how to spread expertise so wide as to enable expert emergency assessments remains. More local expert services are not yet available and probably will never be adequately viable. Telemedicine and interpreters may solve local communication problems but neither are ideal in emergencies when patients are most disturbed and the right interventions are most crucial.

Psychiatric specialties

Access to general Deaf mental health services can be problematic, but a further challenge is access to the range of psychiatric specialties in the UK. For example, despite evidence that Deaf people suffer to the same degree as hearing people, there is virtually no progress in providing addictions services to Deaf people (Austen and Checinski, in Hindley and Kitson, 2000). Services for the elderly are similarly neglected, unlike in the Netherlands, where the elderly receive high quality physical and mental health care services. In the UK, the three centres do some work in all these specialities, on a case-by-case basis, and receive some support from specialists serving the non-Deaf, specialist populations. From time to time there have been mental health professionals working in deafness who also have an interest in a particularly specialty or are dual qualified, but their presence is somewhat random.

Physical health and 'One-Stop Shops'

There has been a change of emphasis in the European Society for Mental

Health and Deafness from 'mental health and deafness' to general 'health and deafness'. This is only slowly gaining momentum.

Schatzimayr (2001) found significant numbers of previously undiagnosed or untreated high blood pressure, hypertension, dermatological diseases, neurological disorders, thyroid diseases, upper gastrointestinal tract disease and ophthalmologic diseases in a Deaf population. Fellinger and Holzinger (1999) noted that the Deaf population had an increased risk of metabolic disorders. Deaf people in mental health services may be especially prone to such diseases due to associations between the mental and physical symptoms of some causes of deafness, such as rubella, and the associations of some physical and behavioural disorders or impulsivity, like meningitis.

The Deaf Mental Health Services in Linz, Austria, have functioned within such a 'One-Stop Shop' in all but name since 1993. Bilingual practitioners mostly provide family medicine and mental health services whereas hospital specialities are provided via sign language interpreters, Schatzimayr (2001). Primary and secondary preventive medical checkups are routine for all Deaf people in the area and risk factors (work, general living situation, alcohol and nicotine) are routinely explored. The clinic is integrated into a modern general hospital such that patients can be admitted to the varied speciality wards with sign language users on the staff guaranteeing sufficient communication and accompanying the patients.

There had been a consortium bid in 2000 for a Deaf Healthy Living Centre for London, although it was rejected. One solution to services for small and sparsely spread populations would be to provide a very wide range of services via multi-skilled staff to enable viable numbers of users to be served. The feasibility of Healthy Living Centres and One-Stop Shops will probably be revisited as part of the Department of Health strategy. From such bases, distant expert services could be made more available locally, through telemedicine.

Telemedicine

Afrin and Critchfield (1999) pioneered the use of 'video-telepsychiatry' or 'telemedicine' with Deaf people in South Carolina from 1995. They provided both assessment and treatment in a way that could overcome both the dearth of sign-fluent mental health professionals and the logistics of having to serve such large geographical areas due to the dispersed nature of the Deaf population. Videophones were installed in three centres across the state. They reported that telepsychiatry by videophone could be used effectively stating that informal data indicated that it had been well received by staff and patients. Start-up costs were reported to have been recouped in 2 years by the saving of travel expenses alone. Despite the obvious advantages, it has not been widely adopted.

Some mental health professionals for Deaf people have expressed concern about the accuracy of telemedicine in that subtle innuendo or non-verbal behaviour, which is so much part of clinical risk assessment, may be missed. The lack of availability for physical examination is also a concern. The immediate impact of any mental health contact is unpredictable, especially in initial assessments, and the concern is that patients might be left distressed or suicidal. Practice protocols can, with the co-operation of local services, overcome most of these cautions. For example, a sign-language user with appropriate competence to de-escalate or ensure contact with local mental health practitioners could accompany the patient to the telemedicine consultation. Further research into the efficacy and safety of telepsychiatry is needed.

Conclusion

Services for Deaf people with mental health problems in the UK are well developed and the envy of many of our European peers. However, these services often emerge as a result, not of national strategy planning, but from the enthusiasm of a few key individuals. This has implications for recruitment and retention of staff and succession planning.

Present UK services aim to segregate Deaf people with mental health problems such that their language and culture is promoted. The value of training and employing Deaf professionals is noted.

The greatest challenge to providers of Deaf mental health services is a geographic one. A small number of patients are spread across vast areas. A recent homicide inquiry has resulted in the start of a national strategy and has highlighted a crucial paradox: those with the skills to help a Deaf patient, the staff of centralized Deaf mental health services, are the least available when the Deaf patient needs them most. We must expand services to include intensive community care, crisis care and out of office hours services in the patient's own locality if we are to provide Deaf people with equity of mental health services.

References

Afrin J, Critchfield B (1999) Telepsychiatry for the deaf in South Carolina: maximizing limited resources. In Brauer B, Marcus A, Morton D (eds) Proceedings of the First World Conference on Mental Health and Deafness. Vienna VA: Potiron Press, p. 27.

Austen S, Checkinski K (2000) Addictive behaviour and deafness. In Hindley P, Kitson N (eds) Mental Health and Deafness. London: Whurr, pp. 232–52.

Boros, A (1981) Alcoholism Intervention for the Deaf. Alcohol Health and Research World. The Multidisabled (special issue) 5(2): 26–30.

Chan E (2001) An innovation in the provision of a locally based mental health service for deaf adults – Nottingham model. In Hjortso T, Von der Lieth L, Carlsen C (eds) Proceedings of the Fifth European and Second World Conference on Mental Health and Deafness, pp. 235–39.

Denmark J, Warren F (1972) A psychiatric unit for the deaf. British Journal of Psychiatry 120: 423–8.

Department of Health (2002) A Sign of the Times: Modernising Mental Health Services for People who are Deaf. London: Department of Health.

Fellinger J, Holzinger D (1999) Deaf patients: a challenge in health care. In Brauer B, Marcus A, Morton D (eds) Proceedings of the First World Conference on Mental Health and Deafness. Vienna VA: Potiron Press, p. 29.

Glow BA (1989) Alcoholism, drugs and the disabled. In Lawson G, Lawson AW (1989) (eds) Alcoholism and Substance Abuse in Special Populations. Rockville: Aspen Publishers.

Health Advisory Service (1998) Forging New Channels: Commissioning and Delivering Mental Health Services for People who are Deaf. British Society for Mental Health and Deafness.

Hoffmeister R, Moores DF (1987) Code switching in deaf adults. American Annals of the Deaf 132 (1): 31-34.

Kitson N, Klein H (1997) Services for Deaf people, by Deaf people? In Leopold Mayer C, La Librairie (eds) Proceedings of the Third European Conference on Mental Health and Deafness Conference, pp. 145–8.

Kitson N, Monteiro B (1991) Policy on Deaf Mental Health Professionals. European Society for Mental Health and Deafness.

Kitson N, Wilson S (2000) Rehabilitation. In Hindley P, Kitson N (eds) Mental Health and Deafness. London: Whurr, pp. 414–34.

Phoenix S (1988) An Interim Report on a Pilot Survey of Deaf Adults in Northern Ireland. Northern Ireland Workshop with the Deaf.

Rainer JD, Altshuler KZ, Kallmann FJ (1963) Family and Mental Health Problems in a Deaf Population. New York: Columbia University.

Rebourg F (1991) Minutes of the meeting on the training of deaf professionals in mental health work in ESMHD. Proceedings of the Second European Conference on Mental Health and Deafness, pp. 423–33.

Schatzimayr W (2001) A special preventive medical provision for deaf people – an absolute necessity. In Hjortso T, Von der Lieth L, Carlsen C (eds) Proceedings of the Fifth European and Second World Conference on Mental Health and Deafness, pp. 247–53.

Sharples N (2001) Diversity in nurse education from rhetoric to action. In Hjortso T, Von der Lieth L, Carlsen C (eds) Proceedings of the Fifth European and Second World Conference on Mental Health and Deafness, pp. 396–402.

Sims J (1989) Breaking the silence. Nursing Times 84(24): 116–17.

Vaughan J (1994) Sign training initiatives. Annual Report to Sign Campaign, UK.

Vernon M, Daigle-King B (1999) Historical overview of inpatient care of mental patients who are deaf. American Annals of the Deaf 144(1): 51–61.

Von der Lieth LA (2001) European concept of mental health and deafness: a brief historical remark. In Hjortso T, Von der Lieth L, Carlsen C (eds) Proceedings of the Fifth European and Second World Conference on Mental Health and Deafness, pp. 31– 42.

Whitehouse A, Sherman RE, Kozlowski K (1991) The needs of deaf substance abusers in Illinois. American Journal of Drug and Alcohol Abuse 17(1): 103–13.

CHAPTER 11

The dynamic roles of interpreters and therapists

JEMINA NAPIER AND ANDY CORNES

Introduction

Therapy sessions provide challenges for all participants involved, regardless of audiological status. Counsellors perceive themselves as having a particular role, as do the recipients of therapy. Perceptions of role and therefore choice of role adopted intrinsically determine the dynamics of therapy, as in any form of human interaction. The quality of the relationship, individual fears, phantasies and drives are also paramount in any communication within therapy. Imagine, however, entering a therapeutic process, and accessing that 'rapport' via a third person – an interpreter. For deaf people – and in this chapter we use the term 'Deaf' when the Deaf community and its culture is the crucial issue, and the term 'deaf' to refer to deaf people who choose to use sign language as their preferred language of communication – access to therapy rarely takes place without the assistance of a sign language interpreter. Aside from the few exceptions where hearing therapists are fluent signers, or qualified therapists are deaf sign-language users themselves, deaf people are virtually guaranteed to have an additional person present at their therapy sessions.

Cross-cultural counselling encompasses any counselling situation that involves two or more participants being culturally different. Variables may include language, values, beliefs, customs, ethnicity, gender, sexuality, religion, disability and socio-economic status (SES). In most cases, the counsellor will belong to the majority group and the client will be a minority group member. In recent years, there has been a growing recognition of deaf individuals as constituting a linguistic minority with different cultural values and beliefs (see Woodward, 1972; Padden, 1980; Brennan, 1992; Power, 1996). This paradigm shift has informed clinicians how psychotherapy is framed with deaf clients (Harvey, 1985; Harvey, 1986; Sloman and Springer, 1987; Harvey 1989, Glickman, 1993; Corker,

1994; Glickman, 1996, Leigh, 1999) and has resulted in the emergence of a new discipline of specialization (Leigh et al., 1996; Pollard, 1996).

As a sign language interpreter experienced in working in therapeutic contexts and a therapist who regularly works with deaf people and sign language interpreters, our aim in writing this chapter is to discuss how the presence of an interpreter can impact on the therapeutic process for these people. Although the impact of sign language interpreters in clinical practice has been explored (Stansfield, 1981; Harvey, 1982; Harvey, 1985; DeMatteo, Vietri and Lee, 1986; Harvey, 1989; Frishberg, 1990), the nature of the relationship between interpreters and therapists remains uncertain. We aim to expand on some of the key issues raised by these authors based on our own clinical experience and provide recommendations for interpreters and therapists to work symbiotically. In Australia, where the authors work, 'there is a shortage of sign language interpreters in general, and few are familiar with psychiatric terminology and phenomenology' (Cornes and Wiltshire, 1999: 317).

By considering literature in the areas of interpreting, counselling, and mental health and deafness, and by drawing on our own experiences, we will provide recommendations as to how interpreters and therapists can consider the cultural dynamics of a deaf/hearing therapeutic milieu and the respective roles of the interpreter and therapist in this context, and how they can develop strategies to work together to provide optimal treatment and outcomes for deaf clients. For the purpose of this chapter, examples of therapy will come from a psychodynamic model, but the examples should be relevant and applicable to all styles of therapy.

Learning from spoken language interpreting

Issues in relation to linguistic and ethical challenges relating to signed language interpreting are also experienced by spoken language interpreters, hence references to spoken language interpreting literature will be found in this chapter. The notion of 'community interpreting', where interpreters are working with clients in community settings such as the legal, medical and employment fields (rather than conferences), has long been well-established in the sign language field, but has only been professionalized and discussed more recently in the spoken language field (Mikkelson, 1999). Therefore, although we can assume that interpreters are working in therapeutic settings with clients in languages other than spoken English, there is a dearth of research in this area. One of few references available is the discussion of the role of the interpreter working with people with aphasia in speech pathology sessions (Whitworth and Sjardin, 1993), with another paper discussing the need for qualified interpreters to work in therapeutic situations in hospital settings (Pochhacker and Kadric, 1999). By discussing various models of interpreting and the code of ethics adhered to by interpreters, it is possible to identify some of the potential challenges for interpreters working in therapy, with regards to their role and where issues may arise.

In the current climate, where more deaf people are training as therapists, the issues discussed in this chapter may also be applicable to situations where a deaf therapist is working with a hearing client and an interpreter. To date, there has been no research in this area, therefore any application can only be surmised.

Models of interpreting

When discussing the nature of the sign language interpreter's role in a therapeutic setting with a deaf person and a hearing therapist, it is necessary first of all to establish the interpreting role advocated within the sign language interpreting profession as a general guideline for any context.

The three most commonly referenced 'models' of interpreting are the helper model, the conduit model and the bilingual-bicultural model. The Deaf community has witnessed a pendulum swing from the helper model to the conduit model. Current consensus indicates that the bilingual-bicultural model is a balance between the two and is more appropriate to interpreting practice.

Helper model

The helper model was common in the earlier years of the interpreting profession, before interpreting was really recognized as a career. Traditionally, interpreting was usually carried out by missionaries or welfare workers for the deaf, who were heavily involved in all aspects of deaf people's lives. The model was embedded within a philosophy of vulnerability – the 'let me do it for you' approach (McIntire and Sanderson, 1993: 100) – and the welfare workers/interpreters would interact with hearing people on behalf of the deaf people, explain things and provide them with answers. People who functioned in this role were typically hearing people who had deaf family members, some of them working para-professionally as welfare workers. This model reflected the *zeitgeist* at that time, in the assumption that people with disabilities could not look after themselves, and had to be assisted and treated as 'special'. Welfare workers were eventually replaced by social workers with deaf people who soon discovered a significant proportion of their casework involved 'supportive counselling' for a range of problems they were not skilled to deal with. This initially led to referral to generic (hearing) therapists with interpreter support. As specialist mental health services were established, referral to therapists equipped with the requisite knowledge to work effectively with deaf clients was finally possible.

Acting in the role of 'helper' may, however, blur boundaries that are central to effective therapy, as stated by Hoyt, Siegelman and Schlesinger (1981: 810): 'Deaf patients may exercise a passivity or coercive dependency that results in therapists becoming excessively helpful out of a sense of guilt; rescue fantasies among therapists are common and usually counterproductive.' Consider the following case vignette.

Case study

BH was a 10-year-old profoundly deaf boy in ongoing individual and family therapy in the context of escalating violent behaviour at school. No problems were reported at home. He lived with his mother, a single parent, who was able to sign well. Family life was chaotic with inconsistent limit setting and harsh discipline, including verbal and physical abuse. Interpreters were present for family sessions. In one of the sessions, unexpectedly, BH's mother began to verbally abuse him. When the therapist checked to see if the interpreter was managing the situation, he was surprised to find her engaged in a pleasant conversation about what types of jams and preserves the boy liked to eat for breakfast. The dialogue had become too emotionally challenging for the interpreter and she had 'rescued' BH (and perhaps herself) from further psychological trauma. Post-session, the interpreter explained that BH had initiated the conversation, and stated that she had little recollection of what BH's mother was saying. She appeared to have little insight into what had transpired.

Conduit model

In line with the 'integration–segregation debate' within the disability movement, the 1980s saw the pendulum swing to the other extreme as deaf people began to demand access to information, rather than help. It was at this time that the role of the interpreter became separated from that of the welfare or social worker, with deaf people asserting that they could make decisions for themselves, as long as they had the correct information. The theory behind this model describes interpreters as conduits or machines, where they are completely impartial and have no impact on the communication of information whatsoever – 'I'll give you everything that's said so that you can do it' (McIntire and Sanderson, 1993: 100). The role of interpreters, when adhering to this model, is to ensure that they do not influence the communication process in any way. The premise is that interpreters should see themselves as some kind of vessel for the relaying of information. One analogy given is that interpreters could be considered as telephone links (Neumann Solow, 1981), that is, a channel for communication.

Frishberg (1990) quite rightly states that the model of interpreter as channel for communication is flawed. She asserts that the various metaphors that have been used, such as 'interpreter-as-window' and 'interpreter-as-bridge', have emphasized the role of the interpreter as a means to 'transport' information between languages, without acknowledging that the interpreter is a human being. According to this model, interpreters should behave as if they are 'invisible', and should be treated as such. Humphrey and Alcorn (1996: 167) have described interpreters adhering to this model as being 'rigid and inflexible', and 'insensitive to the human dynamics within the interpreting setting'. Although the authors recognize the limitations of this interpreting model, particularly in therapeutic settings, we acknowledge that this model may be best suited to psychiatric assessments where a Mental State Examination is needed, particularly if there are concerns that the client is presenting with a thought disorder or psychotic illness (see Roberts and Hindley, 1999).

Bilingual-bicultural model

This model emphasizes the attitudes and subsequent behaviour of interpreters while incorporating many elements from the preceding two models. The bilingual-bicultural approach (often shortened to *bi-bi,* or referred to as the 'ally' model) has developed as a consequence of greater understanding of the interpreting process, the interpreter's role, and the nature of the consumer/client relationship. Humphrey and Alcorn (1996: 70) summarize the concept of the bi-bi model in the following way:

> The interpreter continues to be sensitive to physical communication dynamics, indicating who is speaking, placing him/herself appropriately, etc. S/he is also keenly aware of the inherent differences in the languages, cultures, norms for social interaction and schema of the parties using interpreting services. Thus, interpretation is defined more broadly to include cultural and linguistic mediation while accomplishing speaker goals and maintaining dynamic equivalence.

Hence, rather than seeing the interpreter as being an entity who does not effect interaction, the interpreter is recognized as a human being who can influence, and is influenced by, the participants, languages, cultures and social norms of any interaction. Baker-Shenk (1986) and Metzger (1999) have stated that it is impossible for sign language interpreters to be completely neutral, either because they are members of the hearing majority, and therefore members of the society that has historically oppressed deaf people; or because they are present within the interaction, and therefore will obviously have an impact on it. The interpreter is regarded as an 'ally' of the Deaf community, who will take on the role of linguistic and cultural mediator to empower deaf people to gain equal access to information (McIntire and Sanderson, 1993; Page, 1993). Wadensjö (1998), in writing about spoken language interpreters, has also acknowledged that interpreters are present within any interaction, and will therefore influence the nature of the interaction.

To be able to mediate successfully between two cultures, one would have to possess a thorough knowledge of the interplay between them. For most individuals, therapy remains elusive, misunderstood and characterized by the image of Freud perched behind the couch taking notes. When one considers the range of psychotherapies available, each with its own language, rules and traditions, the task faced by interpreters to mediate between two cultures is considerable.

Interactive model

In considering the linguistic, socio-cultural, psychological, physiological and environmental factors within any therapeutic context, as well as the needs of the deaf person and therapist within that context, sign language interpreters may adopt a much more 'interactive' approach to interpreting (Stewart, Schein and Cartwright, 1998); that is, they function in whatever model is appropriate within the interactive-therapeutic setting in order to account for influencing factors, as shown in Figure 11.1.

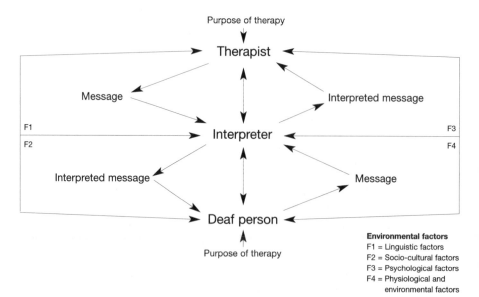

Figure 11.1 An interactive-therapeutic model of interpreting. Figure adapted from Stewart, Schein and Cartwright (1998) 'interactive model of interpreting'.

Heaton and Fowler (1997) suggest that interpreters should adopt a different model of interpreting, depending on the context of the interpreting assignment. An interactive-therapeutic approach allows for interpreters working with therapists to adopt whatever approach is deemed necessary at the time, in order to ensure successful communication. In other contexts, for example, an interpreter may become more of a 'helper' when interpreting for an elderly person at the doctor, a 'conduit' when interpreting for a bilingual university student in a lecture, and a bilingual-bicultural ally during a job interview.

This perception could be dangerous if the interpreter does not have a clear understanding of the therapeutic goal and the objectives of the therapist. Although as a bilingual-bicultural facilitator of communication, the interpreter is likely to be the only person in the room who could identify points of breakdown in communication, the interpreter should discuss carefully with the therapist what information they need to receive, and how it will assist the therapeutic process.

Another reason for the confusion around this dynamic is the existence of the interpreters' code of ethics, and the contradictory nature of the code when applied in a therapeutic setting.

Code of ethics

Once sign language interpreters become accredited/qualified, they are expected to abide by a Code of Ethics – usually endorsed by the sign language interpreters' association or governing body of the country (for example ASLIA – the Australian Sign Language Interpreters' Association, CACDP – the Council for the Advancement of Communication with Deaf People (UK) or RID – the Registry of Interpreters for the Deaf (USA)). Four key tenets of any interpreters' code are as follows:

* remain impartial;
* interpret faithfully and accurately;
* accept work within your own limitations;
* keep confidentiality.

Codes of ethics were developed around the time that the conduit model was popular, and few codes have been updated since that time. Turner (2001) discusses how interpreters who stick to a more conduit approach look to the code of ethics for 'instructions' on what their role allows them to do. Pollitt (1997: 24) states that interpreters often assume that they 'are individual failures because [they] may have cause to transgress the Code' – especially in situations such as therapeutic settings, where interpreters have to make decisions about how to interpret something, or how to interact with deaf clients, which is technically 'breaking' the code of ethics, and therefore stepping outside of their role.

These 'transgressions' do not only happen in therapeutic settings, but in many situations depending on the sensitivity of the context. Tate and Turner (1997) conducted a survey of British Sign Language (BSL) interpreters by presenting them with four scenarios and asking how they would deal with it, and what ethical decisions they would make. The majority of interpreters who responded to their survey indicated that most of the time they would make decisions based on morality and 'common sense alternatives' rather than the code alone.

In relation to working within a therapeutic situation, 'common sense alternatives' used by interpreters may include: commenting on a deaf client's linguistic ability to understand a therapist's questions; developing a relationship with a deaf client in order to engender trust within the therapy sessions; or explaining to a therapist about the concept of Deaf culture. As developing good relationships is central to effective counselling, as mentioned earlier, consultation between the interpreter and therapist is vital to ensure that setting parameters for working roles are set.

Establishing a therapeutic alliance

Whereas the interpreter translates the person through observable material, the therapist translates the person through observable and hidden material. In order to make these translations and formulate ideas about the client's world, the therapist has to possess a good knowledge of the client's culture, that is, his or her ways of 'being'.

In treating the deaf client, the role of the therapist can easily be confused. Common misunderstandings can centre on maintaining good eye contact (the deaf client will be looking mostly at the interpreter). Of course, the most useful tool a hearing therapist has is audition – listening skills. The process of joining the client in therapy is thought to be the single most important predictor of the success or failure of therapy, independent of the type of therapy offered and has been investigated extensively (Luborsky, McLellan, and Woody, 1985; Horvath and Symonds, 1991; Lambert, 1992; Horvath, 2000). Large-scale clinical trials have found that a positive alliance is a significant predictor of a successful outcome (Krupnick et al., 1996; Connors et al., 1997). This centralizes the role of the therapeutic relationship or as it is known in clinical practice, the 'therapeutic alliance' (the working relationship between the therapist and client). The therapeutic alliance can be conceptualized as bonding and agreement on tasks or goals (Bordin, 1994) or the client regarding the therapist as helpful and feeling that therapy is a collaborative process (Luborsky, 1994). Basic issues relating to establishing a therapeutic relationship with a deaf client has been explored previously (Lytle and Lewis, 1996).

Impartiality

There are various styles of therapy, however. In the tradition of psycho-analytical theory, therapists function as mirrors or blank screens on which clients project their emotional world. With the presence of an interpreter in therapy, who exactly is acting as the screen, the therapist or the inter-preter? In all interpreted interactions, the interpreter is the 'competitor' of the participants in a communicative event (Dimitrova, 1995), whereby his or her presence can influence the dynamics of interaction. Although the interpreter is technically not participating, just facilitating communi-cation, he or she needs allocated time with 'the talking stick' in order to convey the message of certain participants, and he or she is another phys-ical 'body' in the room competing (unintentionally) for space and attention. This phenomenon has a particularly direct impact on the dynamics of therapy.

Freud postulated that there are a number of ego defence mechanisms that protect the conscious mind from those aspects of reality it may find difficult to accept, including transference (a person transferring his or her feelings/behaviour onto another person and accusing him or her of feel-ing/ behaving that way) and counter-transference. A simplistic explanation of counter-transference is the therapist's emotional reactions to the client's material. As illustrated previously, the same is true for inter-preters, yet the emotional loading may be greater if they are part of the Deaf community. For example, many interpreters who are CODAs (chil-dren of deaf adults) and may over-identify and react more strongly to issues raised in therapy sessions related to the inequalities that deaf peo-ple experience as 'Codas, for example, have spent much of their childhood bearing witness to such oppression' (Hoffmeister and Harvey, 1996: 82). Therefore, how easy is it for interpreters to remain impartial?

Unconscious effects in therapy

A recent study found that sign language interpreters' moods were direct-ly influencing the moods of the deaf client in therapy via non-verbal behaviours (Brunson and Lawrence, 2002). The study also highlights inadequacies with the theories that underpin the conduit model of inter-preting. Our clinical experience leads us to hypothesize that deaf clients tend to forge stronger alliances with the interpreter, not the therapist. As the mediator of the alliance, the interpreter can unknowingly influence the content and manner of questioning, the framing of the question and the emotional context in which the messages are delivered. This dynamic is also true of spoken language interpreters, who have been found to influence courtroom interactions through the decisions made, and the consequent impressions created (Kadric, 2000). It is therefore essential that the deaf client does not overly identify with the interpreter as this will disrupt the process of establishing rapport with the therapist and shift alliances in therapy – as demonstrated in case vignette 1.

All interpreters have their own cultural, political, personal and pathological 'baggage' (Wiegand, 2000), regardless of what languages they use. Thus the potential transfer of feelings from interpreter to client has clear implications for training and raises questions about whom exactly the deaf client is joining in therapy. One could extrapolate that the interpreters' personal experiences will directly influence their reception and production.

Working in unison

Interpreters interacting with participants could be perceived as in direct contravention of the first interpreter ethic of 'impartiality', which presents the greatest challenge for interpreters working in therapeutic settings. For example, in studies of interpreted medical consultations, Metzger (1999) found that interpreters interact with participants in a way that could be regarded as not totally impartial.

Sign language researchers, such as Metzger (1999) and Roy (2000), and spoken language researchers, such as Wadensjö (1998) and Rosenberg (2001), assert that interpreter interventions (for example, responding to direct questions) are needed in order to accommodate cultural differences and individual needs. Within a therapeutic environment, the need for interpreters and therapists to recognize and incorporate these cultural considerations into their work together is paramount for the success of the therapeutic alliance. If a hearing therapist with little knowledge of deaf issues is hoping to develop a sense of the client's world, this process of 'filling in the gaps' is essential.

Faithful and accurate interpreting

Moving onto the second ethical tenet for interpreters – that of interpreting 'faithfully and accurately'. Typically, the notion of interpreting accurately requires interpreters to determine meaning of a concept in one language/culture, and identify the equivalent meaning in the other language/culture (Baker, 1992). Therefore, to interpret faithfully means not providing word-for-sign (or vice versa) interpretations, but a holistic interpretation of the message (free interpretation). Interpreters therefore will endeavour to make sense of an utterance. This ethical tenet can provide interpreters with a particular conflict in therapeutic situations if a therapist needs to hear the 'stream of consciousness' of a client, whereby the utterances will not necessarily make sense. However, as with other approaches, traditional psychoanalysis using free association, a process whereby clients say (or sign) the first thing that comes into their head without censorship, has not been widely used or evaluated with deaf clients. In this scenario, if the interpreter tries to make sense of what is being signed by a deaf client, the therapist may not be able to make an accurate diagnosis of the client's psychological status. Therefore what may be needed is a more literal, rather than free, interpretation. There may be points during the therapy session where the interpreter will need to use a more literal approach, and others when a freer approach is needed, depending on the goal of the interaction; as in other contexts, such as educational settings (Pollitt, 2000; Napier, 2001).

Alternatively, switching between free and literal methods may be required within an interpretation, especially when dealing with terminology. Napier (2001) identified that interpreters can effectively switch between free and literal interpretation methods as a linguistic strategy to cope with the interactive environment. In this instance, it is imperative for the interpreter and therapist to agree on what is needed from the interpretation, and whether the goal is to ascertain meaning in language, to establish psychological status or assess for psychiatric disorder.

Working within limitations

Being intellectually out of one's depth

In terms of the ethic of 'accepting work within own limitations', this typically refers to the fact that interpreters should consider whether their skills and experience are suitable for an interpreting assignment. Several writers have referred to the fact that the more familiar interpreters are with the content being discussed/delivered in any particular context, the better able they are to effectively interpret the message (Stewart, Schein and Cartwright, 1998; Neumann Solow, 2000; Napier, 2002).

Being emotionally out of one's depth

Another interpretation of this tenet, is that interpreters should only accept work that will not have a personal impact on them, for example, in situations that may result in them reacting emotionally. For example, spoken language interpreters in South Africa were found to become 'physically sick from trying to cope with the heavy load of other people's personal problems and their own fears' when interpreting in sensitive situations (Wiegand, 2000: 213).

This can be a problem, however, as interpreters are not always provided with the information necessary to make this kind of decision. When booked to interpret for a therapy session, interpreters may have no idea what the focus of the therapy will be, and whether the content of the session will be something confronting to them, and that they have difficulty interpreting. Harvey (1985: 307) explains that 'interpreters, as human beings, would be expected to perceive inaccurately and therefore interpret inaccurately content that is highly emotionally loaded for them'. Similarly, interpreters may be aware of the topic/focus of a therapy session, but may underestimate the impact the session will have on them. Harvey (2001) has highlighted the fact that sign language interpreters may experience vicarious emotional trauma working in clinical settings.

It is clear that human communication is distorted in direct relation to our emotions. The nature of therapy is layered with emotionally charged material. How then do interpreters avoid misinterpretations based on their own natural reactions to the psychic arena? This also relates back to the tenet of impartiality, and the recognition that interpreters will be affected by interpreting for emotionally challenging sessions, thus potentially compromising their position of neutrality. Consider the next case study.

Case study

An interpreter was working regularly with the same deaf girl (aged 16) and her parents in a family therapy session. The girl was diagnosed as anorexic and the therapy team is working with her and her family to improve communication strategies, and improve her self-esteem. The girl and the interpreter (who is a young woman in her early twenties) formed a bond, which led to the girl opening up and communicating well during the therapy sessions. As the weeks went by, the girl became thinner and thinner, until finally after one session the interpreter broke down crying – dismayed at how gaunt the girl had become, and how helpless she felt about the situation. The interpreter wanted to reassure the girl that she had so much to offer and it didn't matter that she was deaf, but feeling bound by her ethics, she felt a conflict in that she would be perceived as acting outside of her role, and breaching the code of ethics.

This scenario highlights the importance of interpreters and therapists working together for the best interests of all parties concerned. This would involve: identification of roles and responsibilities, discussion of content, process and goals of therapy sessions, establishment of appropriate interpreting approaches to be used, and arranging the opportunity for interpreters to debrief so that they can discuss emotional/adverse reactions to the content of sessions.

Confidentiality

The next ethical tenet of 'confidentiality' can be one of the more contro-versial issues in interpreting, especially in mental health settings (McCay and Miller, 2001). Interpreters may be presented with a dilemma if they have information about a deaf client that may impact upon the therapist's diagnosis or approach to treatment. Due to the fact that interpreters are often the only people in the room that fully understand both languages and cultures, they are therefore the only people who may identify when a situation may be skewed due to lack of understanding or disclosure of information. It is within these instances that cultural misunderstandings often arise, and as stated by Mindess (1999), interpreters are at the hub of intercultural, as well interlingual, communication, and should account for this within interpretations. This could mean, for example, providing the therapist with background information on a deaf client that could be vital to understanding particular behavioural manifestations. This is an extremely delicate issue, which both interpreters and therapists must treat with sensitivity. This is, therefore, another scenario that requires interpreters and therapists to work closely together to establish roles and responsibilities.

Recommendations

A review of the literature indicates there is little practical advice available on how interpreters and therapists may work collaboratively to achieve positive psychological change for their deaf clients. In addition to dis-cussing the roles of interpreters and therapists in working with deaf people, and considering some cultural dynamics at play, we make the fol-lowing recommendations drawn from our own clinical experience.

Prepare and debrief

Interpreters and therapists should take the time to prepare for sessions, and also take the opportunity to debrief after each session, to ensure that:

- therapeutic goals are clear,
- linguistic and cultural issues can be discussed, and
- emotional and psychological reactions can be revealed and discussed.

Use of second interpreter

The 'reflecting team model' (Andersen, 1987) in which family members observe therapists reflecting through a one-way mirror could be used by interpreters to comment on a fellow interpreter's performance. This may offer less threatening alternatives to 'shadowing' practices of re-interpretation, in that the co-interpreter does not actively take part in the actual interpreting and is hidden 'out of sight'.

Peer support and specialist code of ethics

In addition, the importance of peer support should not be underestimated. Therapists are often able to access a formal supervision system, where it is acceptable and expected for them to debrief with a peer or mentor. This kind of system, however, is not yet in place for interpreters. Anecdotal evidence suggests that generally interpreters are more comfortable discussing issues with other interpreters. As mentioned earlier, however, many interpreters may feel constrained by their code of ethics, and feel that they are breaking the code by discussing details with another interpreter.

Within the context of professional solidarity and support, it is suggested by the authors that allowances are made for interpreters to 'offload' to peers. Thus it may be necessary to develop a code of ethics specifically for interpreting in mental health settings, in the same vein of codes for interpreting in educational settings, as endorsed by the Registry of Interpreters for the Deaf (USA) and the Association of Sign Language Interpreters (UK).

Specialist training/education

Training of therapists and interpreters

Specialist training for therapists should include knowledge about the cognitive, social, emotional and psychological development of deaf people. Glickman's (1996) conceptual framework highlighting four key stages in the development of deaf identities – culturally hearing, culturally marginal, immersion in the deaf world and bicultural – would be an excellent tool for professional development.

Specialist training for interpreters would include counselling theories and practices, with opportunities to practise interpreting in therapeutic contexts. For example, under the auspices of the Deaf Education Network, a pilot course for Auslan interpreters was delivered in Sydney, Australia (Napier, 1999), which focused on interpreting in counselling situations. The key modules included:

- counselling issues
- socio-cultural contexts of interpreting;
- the interpreting process;
- coping strategies of interpreters; and
- a practicum.

Alongside the interpreter training, a course was also provided for coun-sellors (Cornes and Napier, 1999), with key modules on:

* the Australian Deaf community and its culture
* cross-cultural therapy – linguistic, cultural and behavioural differences;
* treating the deaf client in context;
* working effectively with interpreters;
* joining the deaf client in therapy

and also featured a practicum.

During the practicum, the interpreters and counsellors worked with deaf actors (who had been briefed) in role-plays of scenarios of deaf peo-ple presenting different problems in alternative therapeutic contexts. This *in vivo* experience enabled both the interpreters and counsellors to expe-rience working in a lifelike therapeutic environment, within a safe environment. The course facilitators (two interpreters and a therapist) discussed the role plays with the participants, eliciting how each of them felt with regards to the communication and interaction, and gave feed-back to the participants on language use, interaction and issues of transference/countertransference and projection (counsellors) and inter-pretation choices and communication control choices (interpreters). Evaluations received from the course participants were extremely posi-tive, stating that they felt more confident about working with deaf clients in therapy, as they had been given the opportunity to understand the the-ory, and apply it in practice. Elements from the course were used to develop further specialist training workshops for Auslan interpreters interested in mental health (Cornes, 2001a, 2001b).

Educating the Deaf community

Another recommendation is that in collaboration with Deaf community organizations, experienced therapists and interpreters could work to pro-vide information/psycho-education workshops to members of the Deaf community, to inform them of the role of the therapist; the purpose of, and techniques used in, therapy; and the role of interpreters and families in the therapeutic process.

Summary

We have highlighted key issues that demand investigation if interpreters and therapists are to assist deaf clients to access mental health services and to obtain optimal care. It is essential for the interpreter and the ther-apist to comment on the process, not simply the content, of the therapy.

Discussions around the process could include what is happening in the professionals' internal worlds and how this affects a therapy session. Dialogue about the content could include interpretations and therapeutic interventions, and could consider how language is framed and its effects. This dialogue would occur post-session, yet there may be scope to actively include interpreters in therapy by discussing them with the deaf client. This may draw out fantasies, wishes and fears that can be used as currency for psychological change.

Our experience in clinical settings strongly indicates that therapy can only be greatly enhanced by interpreters and therapists adopting flexible roles, working symbiotically and adopting clinical practices that reflect and respond to clients' individual needs. Central to this tenet is an ongoing commitment to specialized training, ideally with consumer and Deaf community involvement. As previously stated, such training has been piloted successfully in Australia and could be contextually adapted to 'fit' other geographical regions. Culturally appropriate therapeutic interventions are necessary to address existing difficulties to ensure they do not become enduring barriers to the attainment of social and emotional well-being.

References

Andersen T (1987) The reflecting team: dialogue and metadialogue in clinical work. Family Process 6: 5–20.

Baker-Shenk C (1986) Characteristics of oppressed and oppressor peoples: their effect on the interpreting context. In McIntire M (ed.) Interpreting: The Art of Cross-cultural Mediation. Silver Spring MD: RID Publications, pp. 43–53.

Baker M (1992) In Other Words: A Coursebook on Translation. London: Routledge.

Bordin ES (1994) Theory and research on the therapeutic working alliance: new directions. In Horvath AO, Greenberg L (eds) The Working Alliance: Theory, Research, and Practice. New York: John Wiley & Sons.

Brennan M (1992) The visual world of BSL: an introduction. In Brien D (ed) Dictionary of British Sign Language/English. London: Faber & Faber, pp.1–133.

Brunson JG, Lawrence PS (2002) Impact of sign language interpreter and therapist moods on deaf recipient mood. Professional Psychology – Research and Practice 33(6): 576–80.

Connors GJ, Carroll KM, DiClemente CC, Longabaugh R, Donovan DM (1997) The therapeutic alliance and its relationship to alcoholism treatment participation and outcome. J Consult Clin Psychol 65: 588–98.

Corker M (1994) Counselling – The Deaf Challenge. London: Jessica Kingsley.

Cornes AJ (2001a) Mental Health Interpreting – How the Hell Did I End Up in Therapy? Workshop presented at the Australian Sign Language Interpreters Association (ASLIA) Summer School, Canberra, 7–8 July 2001.

Cornes AJ (2001b) Mental Health Assessment of Deaf Children: Interpreting Issues. Workshop presented at the Tasmanian Sign Language Interpreters Association (TASLIA), Hobart, 1 December.

Cornes AJ, Napier J (1999) Working with Deaf Clients in Counselling Situations. Sydney: Deaf Education Network (curriculum).

Cornes AJ, Wiltshire CJ (1999) Still waiting to be heard: deaf children in Australia. Australasian Psychiatry 7(6): 313–18.

DeMatteo A, Vietri D, Lee, S (1986) The role of sign language interpreting in psychotherapy. In McIntire M (ed.) Interpreting: the Art of Cross-cultural Mediation. Silver Spring MD: RID, pp.183–206.

Dimitrova BE (1995) Degree of interpreter responsibility in the interaction process in community interpreting. In Carr SE, Roberts R, Dufour A, Steyn D (eds) The Critical Link: Interpreters in the Community. Amsterdam: John Benjamins, pp. 147–64.

Frishberg N (1990) Interpreting: An Introduction. 2 edn. Silver Spring MD: RID.

Glickman N (1993) A cross-cultural view of counseling with deaf clients. Journal of Rehabilitation of the Deaf 16(3): 4–14.

Glickman N (1996) The development of culturally deaf identities. In Glickman NS, Harvey MA (eds) Culturally Affirmative Psychotherapy with Deaf Persons. Hillsdale NJ: Lawrence Erlbaum Associates, pp. 115–53.

Harvey MA (1982) The influence and utilization of an interpreter for deaf persons in family therapy. American Annals of the Deaf 127: 821–7.

Harvey MA (1985) Toward a dialogue between the paradigms of family therapy and deafness. American Annals of the Deaf 130(4): 305–14.

Harvey MA (1986) The magnifying mirror: family therapy for deaf persons. Family Systems Medicine 4(4): 408–20.

Harvey MA (1989) Psychotherapy with Deaf and Hard of Hearing Persons: A Systemic Model. Hillsdale NJ: Lawrence Erlbaum.

Harvey MA (2001) Vicarious emotional trauma of interpreters: a clinical psychologist's perspective. Journal of Interpretation: 85–98.

Heaton M, Fowler D (1997) Aches, aspirins and aspirations: a Deaf perspective on interpreting service delivery. Deaf Worlds 13(3): 3–8.

Hoffmeister R, Harvey MA (1996) Is there a psychology of the hearing? In Glickman NS, Harvey MA (eds) Culturally affirmative psychotherapy with deaf persons. Hillsdale NJ: Lawrence Erlbaum Associates, pp. 73–97.

Horvath AO (2000) The therapeutic relationship: from transference to alliance. J Clin Psychol 56(2): 163–73.

Horvath AO, Symonds BD (1991) Relation between working alliance and outcome in psychotherapy: a meta-analysis. J Couns Psychol 38: 139–49.

Hoyt MF, Siegelman EY, Schlesinger MD (1981) Special issues regarding psychotherapy with the deaf. American Journal of Psychiatry 138(6): 807–11.

Humphrey J, Alcorn B (1996) So you want to be an interpreter? An introduction to sign language interpreting. Amarillo TX: H & H.

Kadric M (2000) Interpreting in the Austrian courtroom. In Roberts RP, Carr SE, Abraham D, Dufour A (eds) The Critical Link 2: Interpreters in the Community. Amsterdam: John Benjamins, pp. 153–65.

Krupnick JL, Sotsky SM, Simmens S, Moyer J, Elkin I, Watkins J, Pilkonis PA (1996) The role of the therapeutic alliance in psychotherapy and pharmacotherapy outcome: findings in the National Institute of Mental Health Treatment of Depression Collaborative Research Program. J Consult Clin Psychol 64: 532–9.

Lambert MJ (1992) Psychotherapy outcome research. In Norcross JC, Goldfried MR (eds) Handbook of Psychotherapy Integration. New York: Basic Books, pp. 94–129.

Leigh IW, Corbett CA, Gutman V, Morere DA (1996) Providing psychological services to Deaf individuals; a response to new perceptions of diversity. Professional Psychology: Research and Practice 27: 364–71.

Leigh IW (ed.)(1999) Psychotherapy with Deaf Clients from Diverse Groups. Washington DC: Gallaudet University Press.

Luborsky L, McLellan AT, Woody GE (1985) Therapist success and its determinants. Archives of General Psychiatry 42: 602–11.

Luborsky L (1994) Therapeutic alliances as predictors of psychotherapy outcomes: factors explaining the predictive success. In Horvath AO, Greenberg L (eds) The Working Alliance: Theory, Research, and Practice. New York: John Wiley & Sons.

Lytle LR, Lewis JW (1996) Deaf therapists, deaf clients, and the therapeutic relationship. In Glickman NS, Harvey MA (eds) Culturally Affirmative Psychotherapy with Deaf Persons. Hillsdale NJ: Lawrence Erlbaum Associates, pp. 261–76.

McCay V, Miller K (2001) Interpreting in mental health settings: issues and concerns. American Annals of the Deaf 146(5): 429–34.

McIntire M, Sanderson G (1993) Bye-Bye! Bi-Bi! Questions of empowerment and role in a confluence of diverse relationships in Proceedings of the Thirteenth National Convention of the Registry of Interpreters for the Deaf. Silver Spring MD: RID, pp. 94–118.

Metzger M (1999) Sign language interpreting: deconstructing the myth of neutrality. Washington DC: Gallaudet University Press.

Mikkelson H (1999) The professionalisation of community interpreting. Journal of Interpretation 119–133.

Mindess A (1999) Reading between the signs: intercultural communication for sign language interpreters. Yarmouth ME: Intercultural Press.

Napier J. (1999) Preparatory Auslan Interpreter Course in Liaison Interpreting (Counselling). Sydney: Deaf Education Network (curriculum).

Napier J (2001) Linguistic coping strategies of sign language interpreters. Unpublished doctoral dissertation, Macquarie University.

Napier J (2002) University interpreting: linguistic issues for consideration. Journal of Deaf Studies and Deaf Education 7(4): 281–301.

Neumann Solow S (1981) Sign Language Interpreting: A Basic Resource Book. Silver Spring, MD: National Association of the Deaf.

Neumann Solow S (2000) Sign Language Interpreting: A Basic Resource Book Revised edition. Burtonsville MD: Linstok Press.

Padden C (1980) The Deaf community and the culture of Deaf people. In Gregory S, Hartley G (eds) Constructing Deafness. Milton Keynes: Open University Press, pp.40–5.

Page J (1993) In the sandwich or on the side? Cultural variability and the interpreter's role. Journal of Interpretation 6: 107–26.

Pochhacker F, Kadric M (1999). The hospital cleaner as healthcare interpreter: a case study. The Translator 5(2): 161–78.

Pollard RQ (1996) Professional psychology and Deaf people: the emergence of a discipline. American Psychologist 51(4): 389–96.

Pollitt K (1997) The state we're in: some thoughts on professionalisation, professionalism and practice among the UK's sign language interpreters. Deaf Worlds 13(3): 21–6.

Pollitt K (2000) On babies, bathwater and approaches to interpreting. Deaf Worlds 16(2): 60–4.

Power D (1996) Language, Culture and Community: Deaf People and Sign Language in Australia. Occasional paper no. 4. Brisbane: Centre for Deafness Studies and Research, Griffith University.

Roberts C, Hindley P (1999) The assessment and treatment of deaf children with psychiatric disorders. Journal of Child Psychology and Psychiatry and Allied Disciplines 40(2): 151–67.

Rosenberg BA (2001) Describing the nature of interpreter-mediated doctor-patient communication: a quantitative discourse analysis of community interpreting. Unpublished doctoral dissertation, University of Texas, Austin.

Roy C (2000) Interpreting as a Discourse Process. Oxford: Oxford University Press.

Sloman L, Springer S (1987) Strategic family therapy interventions with Deaf family members. Canadian Journal of Psychiatry 32(7): 558–62.

Stansfield M (1981) Psychological issues in mental health counseling. Journal of Interpretation 1(1): 18–31.

Stewart D, Schein J, Cartwright B (1998) Sign Language Interpreting: Exploring its Art and Science. Boston MA: Allyn & Bacon.

Tate G, Turner G (1997) The code and the culture: Sign language interpreting - in search of the new breed's ethics. Deaf Worlds 13(3): 27–34.

Turner G (2001) Regulation and responsibility: the relationship between interpreters and Deaf people. In Harrington F, Turner G (eds) Interpreting Interpreting: Studies and Reflections on Sign Language Interpreting. Gloucestershire: Douglas McLean, pp. 34–42.

Wadensjö C (1998) Interpreting as Interaction. London: Longman.

Wiegand C (2000) Role of the interpreter in the healing of a nation: an emotional view. In Roberts RP, Carr SE, Abraham D, Dufour A (eds) The Critical Link 2: Interpreters in the Community. Amsterdam: John Benjamins, pp. 207–18.

Whitworth A, Sjardin H (1993) The bilingual person with aphasia: the Australian context. In Lafond D, Joanette Y, Ponzio J, Devigiovani R, Taylor SM (eds) Living with Aphasia: Psychosocial Issues. San Diego: Singular, pp. 130–49.

Woodward J (1972) Implications for sociolinguistics research among the Deaf. Sign Language Studies 1: 1–7.

CHAPTER 12

Substance use disorders and developing substance use services for Deaf people

BRUCE DAVIDSON, HELEN MILLER AND SYLVIA KENNETH

Introduction

The focus of this chapter is on substance use in the Deaf population. We examine the type and severity of problems that Deaf people can develop, how frequently they occur, and prevention and treatment issues. Access to services is discussed, as is 'comorbidity' (when substance use disorders occur simultaneously with other psychiatric disorders).

Here, we are really focusing on the Deaf community and Deaf people, where being (D)eaf: 'refers more to membership of a particular linguistic and cultural grouping than it does to the physical condition of deafness' (Brennan, in O'Brien, 1992). Currently the Deaf population is estimated as between 50,000 and 75,000 people across the UK (Department of Health, 2002b).

Defining substance use disorders

Substance use disorders (SUDs) can be defined as: 'mental and behavioural disorders resulting from psychoactive substance use' (WHO, 2001).

A psychoactive substance is any substance that has an effect on the mind (or psyche). It can be anything from very mild stimulants such as tea and coffee to street drugs such as heroin. In this chapter 'substance' refers to legal drugs like alcohol and tobacco, illegal drugs such as cocaine and heroin, and prescription drugs such as Valium.

Substance use disorders (SUDs) are subdivided into four categories according to severity of the disorder and its relationship to increased mortality and morbidity in substance users (WHO, 2001):

- 'Substance related problems'. Substance use that has resulted in domestic, legal or occupational problems; injuries resulting from substance use, or concerns expressed by others but does not meet the criteria for 'hazardous' use or formal diagnosis.

- 'Hazardous use'. An established pattern of use placing the user at greater risk of future damage to physical and mental health, but which has not yet resulted in significant medical or psychiatric consequences.
- 'Harmful use'. A pattern of substance use that has already caused damage to health, either physical or mental, but does not meet the criteria for a diagnosis of dependence.
- 'Dependent use'. A diagnosis of dependence is made if at least three of the following criteria relating to use have been met over the previous 12-month period:

  - strong desire or sense of compulsion to take the substance;
  - impaired capacity to control substance taking behaviour;
  - evidence of tolerance to effects of substances;
  - other interests being given up or reduced because of substance use;
  - evidence of tolerance to substance effects;
  - persistent use despite harmful consequences.

'Dependent use' is a term synonymous with 'addiction'.

The cultural context of Deaf peoples' substance use

Cochrane (in Brugrab and Cochrane, 2001) writes that culture 'refers to a concept which lies at the heart of how people think behave and define themselves, and how they perceive and react to other people'. Cultural factors influence the presentation and prevalence of mental health problems as well as access to services and to treatment approaches.

In recent years there has been increasing research activity into the substance use and misuse patterns of different ethnic and cultural minorities (Westermeyer, 1995). Emphasis has been placed upon the importance of socio-cultural factors impacting upon prevalence, incidence, pattern and course of SUDs:

> Cultures and ethnic groups within cultures prescribe, proscribe or tolerate the use of various psycho-active substances for social or personal purposes. These ethnic strictures vary widely. Ethnic enculturation into particular psychoactive substances can either decrease the risk of substance abuse or greatly increase this risk. (Westermeyer, 1995)

It is clear from research into non-Deaf cultural and ethnic groups that many complex biological, psychological and socioenvironmental factors influence the relative risk of individuals developing problems with substance use, and the course and severity of disorders. Very little of this research has involved Deaf people, but it appears probable that cultural factors can impact on Deaf peoples' patterns of substance use and misuse. Deaf people, for example, share a history of discrimination against, and proscription of, their alcohol consumption in public bars and clubs ('blanket bans' on members of a particular group) with other minorities such as Gypsies (Morris, 2001) and the gay community (John and Patrick, 1999).

Biological, psychological and social risk factors for development of SUDs in Deaf people.

There is a host of factors that, although not directly causative, have been suggested as influencing the level of risk of individuals developing SUDs. There is an extensive range of socioenvironmental, biological and psychological influences thought to be of importance in the genesis of SUDs (Bonner and Waterhouse, 1996). Here, however, we are focusing only on some of the factors that have been proposed as significant influences on Deaf people. It should be cautioned that these risk factors only have the status of 'educated' inferences, as there is little evidence to confirm or refute that they have a mediating role in the development of SUDs in Deaf people.

Isolation and discrimination

Particular stressors and difficulties associated with Deaf people's life experience may increase the relative likelihood of them misusing alcohol and drugs. Possible factors include isolation caused by the communication barriers that Deaf people face, feelings of loneliness, and continually dealing with prejudice (Kearns, 1989; Rendon, 1992). A survey of 1,507 Deaf and hard-of-hearing people found that 86% had suffered 'prejudice and ill-treatment from people they had just met' (RNID, 1998). Negative stereotypes of deafness continue to be common in society (Munoz-Baell and Ruiz, 2000). Cambra (1996) analysed 222 university students' attribution of personality characteristics to different groups and found Deaf people were viewed most negatively. These attitudes could have a pernicious effect on Deaf people's sense of self-worth and esteem, factors thought to increase susceptibility to SUDs (Shope et al., 1993).

Poverty

Poverty and social exclusion have been linked to increased risk of SUDs in the general population (Home Office, 1998). 'Sensory disabilities' including deafness are linked to poverty (Meadow-Orlans and Ehrting, in Hindley and Kitson, 2000). Deaf people are more likely to be in lower socio-economic groups and to be unemployed than the general population.

Negative childhood experiences

Traumatic experiences in childhood are associated with development of SUDs later in life. Sexual abuse is associated with greater risk of drug and alcohol disorders, starting at an earlier age and with more severity in the course of the disorders (Montcreiff et al., 1996, Montcreiff and Farmer, 1998). Childhood physical abuse has been similarly linked (Westermeyer, Wahmanholm and Thuras, 2001). Studies in the Deaf population have found higher rates of sexual abuse, physical abuse and neglect than occur in the general population (Sullivan, Brookhouser and Scanlan, in Hindley and Kitson, 2000).

Additional disability

Deafness can be viewed as a cultural phenomenon rather than a disability but there is a higher prevalence of additional disabilities in the Deaf population compared with the general population. This is partly because some conditions, which cause deafness, also cause other disabilities: visual problems, metabolic disorders, cardiovascular disorders and, of particular importance here, neurological disorders. Attention deficit disorders are one of the consequences of neurological damage and diagnoses of conduct disorder and attention deficit hyperkinetic disorder (ADHD) in childhood are associated with increased risk of developing SUDs in adulthood (Shubiner et al., 2000). A number of conditions, which are common causes of early onset deafness, are also causally related to ADHD, for example, rubella and meningitis.

Research issues

Researching substance misuse in the general population is a difficult undertaking. Baker (1999) comments: 'Assessing the prevalence of drug misuse in Britain is more like piecing together a jigsaw . . . with most of the pieces missing and the rest fitting poorly if not at all . . . than an exercise in statistics.' Therefore, the true prevalence of SUDs in the UK population is unknown.

It is perhaps not surprising that researchers have found researching SUDs in the Deaf community particularly challenging. Lack of information on the demographics of the Deaf population means that there is no convenient frame from which to draw representative samples for research (Austen and Checinski, in Hindley and Kitson, 2000).

Deaf people may not trust hearing researchers, especially if they lack knowledge and awareness of Deaf culture (Schroedel, 1984). Deaf people may collectively share a higher index of suspicion of researchers' intentions and have concerns over stigmatization if problems in the Deaf community, such as drug and alcohol use, are given greater weight and publicity (Lipton and Goldstein, 1997).

Difficulties researching SUDs in the Deaf population may be compounded by other significant problems known to occur in researching SUDs in the general population. For example, the illicit nature of many of the behaviours connected with substance use and the stigma associated with addictions can affect drug and alcohol users' willingness to participate in research. This in turn adds to the problems in achieving a representative sample of users.

Evidence of Deaf people's substance use and misuse

There is, for the reasons outlined above, a dearth of evidence on Deaf people's substance use. Some of the main findings are summarized here.

Two studies found no differences in rates of SUDs between Deaf and hearing people. Isaacs, Buckley and Martin (1979) compared alcohol use in 39 white Deaf men with data from two comparable non-Deaf samples, and found no significant differences between the deaf and non-Deaf samples in patterns of alcohol consumption. Similarly, a survey of drug and alcohol use amongst New York City's Deaf population suggested Deaf people experienced similar drinking and drug use patterns to the general population (Lipton and Goldstein, 1997).

In the UK, Dye and Kyle (2001) interviewed 236 Deaf adults about a range of health related issues including alcohol and tobacco use. They found 22% of Deaf men and 24% of Deaf women to be consuming alcohol at higher amounts than recommended safe limits. Forty-three per cent of women on higher incomes were drinking above the recommended limits. Deaf men aged 18 to 24 drank the most with the average weekly intake being over 30 units. These results can be compared to the findings of a recent survey of the general population (N = 8,000) where 38% of men and 15% of women were drinking at above recommended limits (Singleton, 2001).

Dye found that Deaf people over 25 years old were more likely to report never having smoked than hearing people of the same age. Barnett and Franks (1999) analysed American national survey data to examine tobacco use amongst deaf people. They found smoking prevalence among 'postlingually'deafened adults was not significantly different from that among hearing adults. 'Prelingually deafened' adults, however, were found to be less likely to smoke than hearing adults, even though they had less education and lower income: factors associated with higher smoking in other populations. Barnett and Franks hypothesized that the lower prevalence of smoking in the prelingually deaf group might be due to cultural differences or limited access to English advertising.

Comorbidity of SUDs and psychiatric disorders

After reviewing evidence in the general population, Rachbeisel, Scott and Dixon (1999) concluded: 'Although estimates of the prevalence of SUDs vary by population, a higher prevalence among persons with severe mental illness has been confirmed.'

The simultaneous presence of two or more disorders in an individual is termed 'comorbidity' or 'dual diagnosis' (Weaver et al., 1999). Comorbidity has been found to significantly worsen the course, severity and prognosis of both SUDs and psychiatric disorders. Increased suicidal and violent behaviour is associated with comorbidity (Department of Health, 2002a).

The interaction between SUDs and psychiatric illness is complicated and not currently well understood (Weaver et al., 1999). In the general population, people with a psychiatric illness are more likely to have a SUD than people with no psychiatric disorder. Similarly people with a SUD are more likely to have a psychiatric illness than people without a SUD (Department of Health, 2002a). The Epidemiological Catchment Area Study (USA) and British studies have identified alcohol and cannabis to be the substances most frequently used by individuals with mental health problems (Regier et al., 1990; Department of Health, 2002a). Alcohol misuse is the most common form of substance misuse, probably because alcohol is readily available and, where drug misuse occurs, it often coexists with alcohol misuse (Department of Health, 2002a).

Comorbidity in Deaf people

One recent study used an alcohol screening instrument – the Alcohol Use Disorders Identification Test (AUDIT) (Babor et al., 1992) – to investigate the alcohol use of Deaf psychiatric inpatients and outpatients (N = 69) in the south of England. It found 24% of all subjects had alcohol use disorders (Davidson, 2002). In mainstream community mental health teams the average prevalence of SUDs is between 8% and 15% (Department of Health, 2002a), with prevalence being higher in inpatient samples and in urban areas. A recent study of admissions to a south London hospital found a prevalence of 50% for alcohol use disorders (McCloud et al., 2003).

Davidson (2002) found Deaf male psychiatric patients were more likely than their female peers to have an alcohol use disorder and more likely to be drinking at higher levels with more adverse social, psychological and physical consequences. This finding mirrors those in the general population and in mainstream psychiatric populations (Singleton, 2001; Department of Health, 2002a).

In Davidson's (2002) study each of the subjects interviewed was offered an information sheet providing advice on sensible limits for alcohol consumption, and an opportunity to discuss this with their interviewer in his or her preferred language. The umbrella term for this type of treatment approach is 'brief interventions': a range of information giving and counselling techniques designed to be used in conjunction with screening instruments, usually in primary care environments, with a minimum of time and resource implications. Evidence of their effectiveness in reducing substance-related harm is very good (Babor and Grant, 1992). Subjects were followed up in routine outpatient appointments. Of 18 subjects who had tested positive for alcohol use disorders, four had significantly curtailed their alcohol consumption at followup (three had reduced their weekly intake to within recommended limits, and one had become abstinent). This is a noteworthy finding for two principal reasons:

- It suggests that an effective evidence-based treatment approach may be adaptable for use with Deaf people.
- All of the subjects had comorbidity with psychiatric disorders, which typically means that interventions to reduce substance-related harms are less likely to be effective (Department of Health, 2002a). This suggests that using brief interventions with Deaf people who do not have psychiatric disorders may be useful in a higher proportion of cases.

Treatment of SUDs in Deaf people

Substance use disorders occur in both Deaf people without mental illness and Deaf people who are mentally ill, so there is a need for treatment. The current system is outlined below.

Deaf people may receive treatment from their local community alcohol and drugs team or be admitted to their local alcohol and drugs treatment unit. If they have a psychiatric disorder as well, they may be treated in their local alcohol and drugs service and then transferred to their local community mental health team. This type of care involves sequential referrals to different services and puts patients at risk of receiving a fragmented service or of falling between services. Comorbid patients may receive parallel care, with both the SUD service and the mental health service engaging the patient at the same time. Finally, they may receive an integrated treatment that is delivered by one team, usually the local community mental health team, either as inpatients or outpatients. In integrated care, the community mental health team receives training and support from SUD services. Integrated care ensures continuity of care and appears to deliver better outcomes than serial or parallel care. There are also some specialist teams for people with comorbidity (Department of Health, 2002a).

All of the above options require the Deaf person to fit into mainstream services and this can be problematic for the Deaf person.

There are three specialist Deaf mental health services in the UK. These are based in London, Birmingham and Manchester. All provide inpatient and outpatient services. None of them have specialist SUD services and Deaf people who do not live near them have to travel if they wish to access the specialist Deaf service. There are no specific programmes aimed at improving Deaf people's access to mainstream alcohol services or specialist units for Deaf people with SUDs in the UK – and no immediate prospect of resource allocation to develop this. The British Deaf Association, a voluntary agency, does provide some counselling for Deaf people about alcohol and drug use, but resources are very limited.

Difficulties in accessing treatment

The difficulties Deaf people experience gaining access to generic medical and psychiatric services are well known, longstanding and ubiquitous in the UK health system and elsewhere (Steinberg, Sullivan and Loew, 1998; Reeves et al., 2002). Reeves et al. (2002) comment that Deaf people have 'substantially poorer access to primary care and Accident and Emergency services and experience difficulties at all stages of the health care process.'

Drug and Alcohol services are no exception in this respect and access problems are discussed extensively in the literature – see, for example, Austen and Checinski (2000). Some of the factors leading to poorer access include:

* Lack of resources and strategic planning for a geographically disparate minority population.
* Lack of provision of human and technological aids to communication.
* Lack of Deaf awareness and failure to adapt existing practices and materials to accommodate Deaf peoples' linguistic and cultural needs.

Problems specific to substance misuse services

Existing treatment facilities and treatment approaches were designed for the general population (or in some cases other non-Deaf minority groups) and interventions have not been modified, or resources provided, to take account of Deaf peoples' requirements. Although Deaf people can occasionally access detoxification and crisis intervention services, a broad range of longer term intensive group-based and individual treatment approaches and facilities are almost entirely inaccessible.

In the US, a number of specialist substance misuse facilities exist that cater for Deaf people and, more often, others that serve the general population have adapted to accommodate Deaf people in their treatment programmes (Guthmann and Blozis, 2001). Although there may be a temptation to look to the US practises that could be applied to a UK context for Deaf people, there are several arguments against this including:

- Financial and resource management structures are very different in the insurance-based US health care system and the UK's centrally funded and managed NHS. The mechanisms for initiating and maintaining services are not replicable.
- Programmes in the US frequently prioritize complete abstinence from substances as the overriding aim of treatment. Treatment for Deaf people in the US is dominated by the 12-step Minnesota Model, most commonly represented by Alcoholics Anonymous and its sister organisation Narcotics Anonymous. Whereas this may be entirely appropriate for many individuals who exhibit severe addictive behaviour, they represent a small proportion of the entire 'substance-using' population. Many other treatment approaches exist that have proven efficacy and that may incorporate a range of treatment goals, ranging from minimization of harm through to abstinence. It is of note that no treatment approach has yet been fully crossculturally validated for use with Deaf people.

A primary care model for delivery of substance use interventions to Deaf people

Rather than dwelling on what is lacking in terms of resources in the UK context, it may be more useful to consider possible directions for development of accessible SUD services for Deaf people.

In recent years recognition that substance misuse is a key component in many of the pressures facing health services at local level has led to the development of strategies to introduce effective evidence-based disease prevention and health promotion services into primary care. Since 1990, general practitioners or family doctors have a statutory responsibility (and receive financial incentives) to provide advice about the health significance of diet, exercise, smoking, alcohol consumption and use of drugs (Anderson, 1996).

It is now also policy for strategic health authorities and primary care trusts to address inequities in access to health care for minority groups.

In the case of the Deaf minority, this approach is underpinned by the Disability Discrimination Act 1995 (Part III) and is a major focus of the recent Deaf mental health consultation document, *Sign of the Times* (Department of Health, 2002b).

Sign of the Times outlines a number of proposals for the development of primary care services for Deaf people and improving access throughout the health care system – for example, introducing individuals, or teams specializing in Deaf mental health, into primary care at regional level. A key principle underpinning proposals is the coalescing of scarce expertise in deafness between agencies, to serve the geographically disparate Deaf minority more effectively. This is of particular relevance when focusing on very low incidence groups such as Deaf people with SUDs. The extremely low incidence of such people means that there is little likelihood that locally based SUD services will devote resources to their treatment, or identify a need to modify treatment to accommodate Deaf people's requirements.

Regional teams could become direct providers or enablers of substance use screening, prevention and treatment interventions for Deaf people. In reality, given the pervasiveness of the harmful social and health consequences of SUDs, Deaf primary care teams and mainstream providers would have to address SUDs in order to offer a more holistic, equitable and effective service.

Regional Deaf primary care teams could be in a superior position to develop links with specialist statutory and voluntary drug and alcohol services, making referrals, monitoring care pathways and assisting them in meeting their obligations to provide treatment access. Data collection and analysis by teams would provide more accurate information about the prevalence, incidence, course and severity of SUDs in Deaf people across regions and nationally. Over time this could create positive feedback into the process of establishing what forms of service provision and interventions are most effective for Deaf people with SUDs.

Conclusion

It is an unfortunate fact in the twenty-first century that a paucity of evidence means that discussion of Deaf people's substance use largely remains an exercise in supposition, inference and 'guesstimation'. This should not obscure the increasing concern that many Deaf people have about substance use in the Deaf community (Dodds, 1999). We would contend that it is possible to make some positive statements about the potential for change. In our opinion, delivery of treatment interventions and preventative strategies for the Deaf community through primary care is achievable and likely to be effective – particularly for individuals who have disorders of low to moderate severity. Severe and complex SUDs present challenges of a more serious magnitude and may need to be dealt with on a regional basis. Effective treatment requires skilled personnel, resources, activity and the highest order of cooperation, between disciplines and across agencies. The emphasis in recent proposals to enhance Deaf mental health services on primary care provision, multi-agency collaboration and cooperation, and providing for low-incidence conditions is entirely in keeping with this approach and appears to offer a viable framework for SUD interventions. Improving access to interventions will require the full attention of all stakeholders and most importantly the community of Deaf people themselves.

References

Anderson P (1996) Intervention in Alcohol and Primary Health Care. Geneva: World Health Organization.

Austen S, Checinski K (2000) Addictive behaviour and deafness. In Hindley P, Kitson N (eds) Mental Health and Deafness. London: Whurr, pp 232–52.

Babor T, Grant M (1992) Project on Identification and Management of Alcohol Related Problems. Report on Phase II: A Randomized Clinical Trial of Brief Interventions in Primary Health Care. Geneva: WHO.

Babor TF, De la Fuente JR, Saunders J, Grant M (1992) AUDIT: Alcohol Use Disorders Identification Test, Guidelines of Use in Primary Health Care. Geneva: World Health Organization. http://www.who.int/substance_abuse/docs/audit2.pdf.

Baker S (1999) Dual Diagnosis: A Report on Eight Mapping Projects. London: Alcohol Concern.

Barnett S, Franks P (1999) Smoking and deaf adults: association with age of onset of deafness. American Annals of the Deaf 144(1): 44–50.

Bonner A, Waterhouse J (1996) Addictive Behaviour. London: Macmillan.

Brennan M (1992) The Deaf community and its language. In Brien D (1992) Dictionary of British Sign Language. London: Faber & Faber, p. 10.

Cambra C (1996) A comparative study of personality descriptors attributed to the deaf, the blind, and individuals with no sensory disability. American Annals of the Deaf 141(1): 24–8.

Cochrane R (2001) Race, prejudice and ethnic identity. In Brugrab N, Cochrane R (eds) Psychiatry in Multicultural Britain. London: Gastell.

Davidson B (2002) Prevalence of Alcohol Use Disorders Among Deaf Psychiatric Patients. Unpublished MSc Dissertation, University of London, England.

Department of Health (2002a) Mental Health Policy Implementation Guide – Dual Diagnosis Good Practice Guide. London: HMSO.

Department of Health (2002b) A Sign of the Times – Modernising Mental Health Services for People who are Deaf. http://www.doh.gov.uk/mentalhealth/signofthetimes.

Disability Discrimination Act (1995) http://www.disability.gov.uk/dda

Dodds JK (1999) Drugs in the deaf community – an issue ignored. British Deaf News (February), p. 4.

Dye M, Kyle J (2001) Deaf people in the community: health and disability. Bristol: Deaf Studies Trust.

Guthmann B, Blozis SA (2001) Unique issues facing deaf individuals entering substance abuse treatment and following discharge. American Annals of the Deaf 146(3): 294–304.

Home Office (1998) Tackling Drugs to Build a Better Britain. UK Anti-Drugs Co-ordinating Unit, Cabinet Office. London: HMSO.

Isaacs M, Buckley G, Martin D (1979) Patterns of drinking among the deaf. American Journal of Alcohol Abuse 6(4): 463–9.

John S, Patrick A (1999) Poverty and Social Exclusion of Lesbians and Gay Men in Glasgow. http://www.lapa.org.uk.

Kearns GA (1989) Hearing impaired alcoholics – an underserved community. Alcohol Health and Research World 13(2): 103–10.

Lipton DS, Goldstein MF (1997) Measuring substance abuse among the deaf. Journal of Drug Issues 27(4): 733–54.

McCloud A, Barnaby B, Omu N, Drummond C, Aboud A (2003) The relationship between alcohol misuse and suicidality in a psychiatric population: findings from an inpatient prevalence study. Unpublished report of the Bipps Project, Springfield Hospital Academic Programme, February.

Meadow-Orlands K, Erting C (2000) Deaf people in society. In Hindley P, Kitson N (eds) Mental Health and Deafness. London: Whurr, pp. 3–24.

Montcreiff J, Drummond CD, Candy B, Checinski K, Farmer R (1996) Sexual abuse in people with alcohol problems: a study of the prevalence of sexual abuse and its relationship to drinking behaviour. British Journal of Psychiatry 169(3): 355–60.

Montcreiff J, Farmer R (1998) Sexual abuse and subsequent development of alcohol problems. Alcohol 33(6): 592–601.

Morris R (2001) Gypsies and travellers: new policies, new approaches. Police Research and Management 5(1): 4–49.

Munoz-Baell IM, Ruiz TM (2000) Empowering the deaf: let the deaf be deaf. Journal of Epidemiology and Community Health 54: 40–4.

Rachbeisel J, Scott J, Dixon L (1999) Co-occurring severe mental illness and substance use disorders: a review of recent research. Psychiatric Services 50: 1427–34.

Reeves D, Kokoruwe B, Dobbins J, Newton V (2002) Access to primary care and emergency services for deaf people in the North West. National Primary Care Research and Development Centre, University of Manchester.

Regier DA, Farmer ME, Rae DS, Locke BZ, Keith SJ, Judd LL, Goodwin FK (1990) Co-morbidity of mental disorders with alcohol and other drug abuse: results from the epidemiologic catchment area (ECA) study. Journal of the American Medical Association 264(19): 2511–19.

Rendon ME (1992) Deaf culture and alcohol and substance abuse. Journal of Substance Abuse Treatment 9: 103–10.

RNID (1998) Breaking the sound barrier. London: The Royal National Institute for Deaf People.

Schroedel JG (1984) Analyzing surveys on deaf adults. Implications for survey research on persons with disabilities. Social Sciences and Medicine 19(6): 619–27.

Shope JT, Copeland LA, Maharg R, Dielman TE, Buchart AT (1993) Assessment of adolescent refusal skills in an alcohol misuse prevention study. Health Education Quarterly 20(3): 373–90.

Shubiner H, Tzelepis A, Millberger S, Lockart N, Kruger M, Kelley P, Schoener EP (2000) Prevalence of attention-deficit/hyperactivity disorder among substance abusers. Journal of Clinical Psychiatry 61(4): 244–51.

Singleton E (2001) Psychiatric Morbidity among Adults. London: Office of National Statistics.

Steinberg AG, Sullivan VJ, Loew RC (1998) Cultural and linguistic barriers to mental health service access: the deaf consumer's perspective. American Journal of Psychiatry 155(7): 982–4.

Sullivan P, Brookhouser P, Scanlan J (2000) Maltreatment of deaf and hard of hearing children. In Hindley P and Kitson N (eds) Mental Health and Deafness. London: Whurr, pp. 149–84.

Weaver T, Renton A, Stimson GV, Tyrer P (1999) Severe mental illness and substance misuse co morbidity: research is needed to inform policy and service development. British Medical Journal 318: 137–8.

Westermeyer, J (1995) Cultural aspects of substance abuse and alcoholism: assessment and management. North American Journal of Clinical Psychiatry 18(3): 589–605.

Westermeyer J, Wahmanholm K, Thuras N (2001) Effects of childhood physical abuse on course and severity of substance abuse. American Journal of Addiction 10(2): 101–10.

WHO (2001) World Health Organization Report: Mental Health. http://www.who.int/whr/2001.

CHAPTER 13

Cochlear implants in adults: the role of the psychologist

SALLY AUSTEN

Introduction

This chapter addresses the place of outcome studies in cochlear implantation and the role of the psychologist within these studies. The psychologist's increasing role in candidate selection is illustrated by case studies.

The National Institute for Health (NIH)(1988) suggested that there are few medical interventions that are associated with such variable outcomes as the cochlear implant (CI) and few that have caused such controversy. By 1995 the start of the NIH major recommendations read, 'Cochlear implantation improves communication ability in most adults with severe to profound deafness and frequently leads to positive psychological and social benefits as well.' However, its first recommendation still finished with the statement: 'There is substantial unexplained variability in the performance of implant users of all ages, and implants are not appropriate for all individuals.'

Why people want a cochlear implant

Candidates for implantation have bilaterally profound deafness and are finding hearing aids of little use for speech perception. For many, communication has become difficult, the interactions of everyday life strained and social life is becoming restricted. This may result in feelings of loss, depression, anxiety and isolation and some adults may struggle to maintain their level of functioning at work, college or in the home.

For many people a CI is a solution, at least in part, to these difficulties. The following quotations are all from service users of the Link Centre for Deafened People in Eastbourne UK, (Link Centre for Deafened People, 1996):

Meryl: 'I love it; it has taken away the silence. It isn't like having normal hearing, but it is a sense of sound and I can understand a lot from the information I receive through my implant.'

For partners too, the deafness is a strain and the CI may be part of the solution:

Pat: 'I do not know how Mick would have coped without the implant. I saw him slipping away, becoming quieter and more introspective, and desperately sad and lonely. I think it has saved him in some way.'

However, the CI is not a 'miracle' or 'bionic ear' but a piece of technology that, depending on a number of variables (some that we understand and some that we do not yet understand) may improve speech perception a little, a lot or not at all. Professionals decide whether to implant based on whatever evidence is available. The potential candidate may get only a fraction of this information and, even though able to make an informed choice, may not make an impartial choice.

Bob: 'For me nothing, it seemed, could be worse than the state of total deafness . . . I couldn't get to the operating table fast enough! I don't remember worrying about the outcome at all.'

Role of the psychologist

Given the variable outcomes in this procedure it is unsurprising that researchers are increasingly asking whether psychological factors affect outcome. To this end intelligence, cognitive functioning and personality factors are being investigated as predictors of implant outcome. For example, learning to use an implant is likely to require certain types of cognitive functioning whereas personality may be a predictor for the motivation and active engagement required to cope with the rehabilitation period. However, there is not yet a consensus.

Thus, despite the CI being a fundamentally surgical and audiological procedure, the role of the psychologist is increasing in breadth and significance. However, there have been relatively few papers written about psychological involvement.

Aplin (1993a) commented that few cochlear implant teams around the world have psychologists and recommended that this role increase such that psychologists see all candidates for pre-implant assessment and post-implant follow up.

The role of the psychologist is multifaceted. Pollard (1996) suggested psychological assessment would aid candidate selection, exclusion and readiness, adding that, while psychosocial variables are often considered in the postoperative outcome literature, they are rarely considered in the preoperative candidacy decisions. In the early days of cochlear implantation, Clarke et al. (1977) described two major reasons for carrying out psychological assessment of prospective implantees. First, to help determine whether the patient can adequately cope with all that is required of the procedure and, second to evaluate the results of the surgery. Aplin (1993a) said that the psychologist's role was also to review the patient post implant, to ascertain that no psychological damage has been done to the patient by the implantation, to monitor psychological state and collect long-term data.

The role of the psychologist in candidate selection

The NIH (1995) recommends exclusion on the grounds of severe psychiatric disorders, severe mental retardation and organic brain disorders. However, the definitions of these are not very clear, although people with severe depression or psychosis would probably be excluded or implantation delayed until successful treatment had occurred.

Mental illness

The implant process can be traumatic in itself: the anxiety of the decision-making process; the stress of potentially life threatening surgery; the 5- or 6-week healing process in virtual silence; the intrusive and sometimes meaningless noises of the early switch-on period; possible disappointments of hopes not fulfilled. After implantation, the patient and others will have audiological and psychosocial expectations. A certain level of personal resilience is therefore required to undergo the surgery and complete the rehabilitation in a way that maximizes the outcome of the surgery. Yet this operation is offered to a group of people who are likely to be psychologically compromised by their experience of profound deafness. McKenna, Halam and Hinchcliffe (1991) found that 27% of consecutive referrals to a neuro-otology outpatient clinic for hearing loss had need of psychological help. Fraser (1991) says that all patients should see a psychologist and have an appropriate evaluation to avoid implanting people who are grossly psychologically disturbed, for whom the implant is likely to be a burden to both the patient and the team. McKenna (1991) reports that many CI candidates will be emotionally distressed and that they cannot all be excluded on this basis, but that emotional states can change and that psychological counselling can help.

Pollard (1996) reports that distress at hearing loss is normal but an acute adjustment reaction is not compatible with implant candidacy. At present candidates are rejected if:

- their mental state is so poor it means that they cannot consent;
- the possible deterioration of mental state due to the stress of the operation would not be worth the benefit to hearing;
- that no evidence exists such that CI teams can give the patient a reliable enough prediction of outcome.

Organic brain damage, severe mental retardation and psychotic illnesses may come into this final category, but it may be that implants will be offered to these client groups in the future.

Case study

A 45-year-old profoundly prelingually deafened man presented to an implant team. Knowing he was an unlikely candidate but adamant that his success orally would ensure him a good outcome, he threatened the team with litigation if they did not implant him and promised that he would take responsibility for a poor outcome. The team agreed to implant him, possibly in an attempt to placate him. The outcome unsurprisingly was extremely poor. Hostile allegations of mistreatment followed and the patient demanded that the implant be removed. At this point the team refused to treat the patient further and he presented to a second team, where a clinical psychologist saw him. The psychologist was concerned that the man had a personality disorder with paranoid features. Some of his decisions were not based in reality and some were fuelled by an attraction to chaos. The psychologist concluded that the patient would be unable to give informed consent to having the implant removed without first accepting psychiatric treatment. The patient refused such treatment, still has the implant, which he doesn't use, and is constantly bothered by its presence. Given his difficulties this man probably should not have been implanted. The same issues must be considered whether deciding to implant or remove a CI.

Intelligence and specific cognitive functioning

The relationship between cognitive functioning and outcome of implantation is still in dispute. Clarke et al. (1977) said that one of the major reasons for carrying out psychological assessment of prospective implantees was to determine whether the patient could cope intellectually with all that is required of the procedure. In rehabilitation the patient must be able to understand instructions, describe what is being heard and make detailed comparisons between different signals. This process is rigorous and requires concentration and attention to detail, so Clarke et al. describe it as 'essential' that CI patients 'perform at or above the average level on standardized intelligence tests'.

Knutson et al. (1991) report that IQ measured by the WAIS-R (Weschler Adult Intelligence Scale – Revised) and Raven's Standard Progressive Matrices had been shown not to predict postoperative success and recommends tests of vigilance (for example, the ability to extract information from sequentially arrayed signals and to rapidly process such information) rather than IQ. Despite this, some programs exclude those with a learning disability and some even exclude those with higher borderline intelligence.

There are, to date, still no outcome data concerning adult implantees with more severe learning disabilities. However, it is likely that people with increasing degrees of cognitive impairment will be included in the future. More multiply handicapped people are now surviving and the deaf population is changing. As multiply handicapped people have a higher chance of psychiatric disorder, it will become even more important that psychologists should be involved in CI team assessment and intervention. This group is more likely to use manual communication so psychologists should ideally be able to sign or have access to mental health trained interpreters.

If the relevant radiological components are intact and functioning, the measure of whether individuals should be offered an implant will be:

- Can they or their guardian give consent?
- Can they use rehabilitation so that the implant will be useful?
- Can they maintain use of the implant?
- Will the operation and rehabilitation be too distressing for the possible audiological gains?
- Audiological status apart, do they have the cognitive ability to use speech and hearing (as opposed to not being able to make use of language or to being able to benefit only from a simple sign system such as Makaton)?
- Can they care for the implant?
- Will they be able to attend the numerous appointments?

It would seem that a functional assessment of ability would answer these questions better than a formal IQ test.

Thus, it is generally agreed that a broad understanding of the patients' cognitive abilities will be helpful in the management and rehabilitation of the patient. Aplin (1993b) assesses the reading level of patients so that rehabilitation materials, which often rely on written texts, can be adapted. This is particularly important for adults who were deafened prelingually and who may have an average reading age of below 9 years (Conrad, 1979).

Case study

In this case intelligence was paramount: not to consent to an implant but to refuse one. An 80-year-old man with a mild learning disability presented at an ENT hospital for earwax removal. A keen junior doctor recognized that, audiologically, the patient was a good candidate for an implant and referred him on. Profoundly deafened at the age of 8, he communicated orally using a tiny amount of residual hearing. He had lived in old people's sheltered housing for many years and not only received all the support he needed to help him function independently but, surrounded by other elderly deafened people, was relatively unconcerned by his deafness. By the time he saw a clinical psychologist, the patient had a date set for his implant. The psychologist would not accept 'yes' and 'no' answers requiring the man to repeat back what he had understood at each stage. It soon became apparent that he had no idea as to what he had repeatedly agreed. He was under the impression that he had been referred for a new hearing aid. He had probably said 'yes' inappropriately for a number of reasons: he misunderstood what was being offered, he didn't want to reveal that he hadn't heard or hadn't understood and he was eager to please. When the full story was explained to him in an appropriate manner, he opted for a new hearing aid and some more regular attention to his earwax.

Readiness

As well as intelligence, it is also important to assess the client's readiness for a CI. Pollard (1996) regards readiness as twofold, encompassing motivation and consent.

Motivation

The motives and enthusiasm for the CI will determine willingness to have the operation and the subsequent programming, mapping and training required to maximize its functioning. Knutson et al. (1991) using the Health Opinion Survey showed that medical compliance correlates with audiological outcome. Gantz et al. (1988) found that willingness to comply with the rehabilitation process and a desire for active participation in one's own health care were of benefit to later implant use.

Older teenagers have the lowest usage rate of CIs and this is probably associated with poor motivation as well as psychosocial and identity implications of the implant and its visible body-worn parts. Evans (1989) said that the stigmatizing equipment interferes with the process of crystallizing identity, as teenagers want to conform and identify with peers.

Thus, body image and identity should be considered preoperatively or the patient may not wear the implant, may want it removed or may experience distress. Research to develop a fully implantable device, which will have no visible external parts is under way, but currently patients need to be aware of the external components of a cochlear implant.

A person's motives for having the implant are therefore crucial. It is important to ascertain whether the client is having the implant to please others or hoping for psychological solutions (for example, 'I will be more confident') rather than audiological ones (such as 'I will hear more'). According to McKenna (1991) the nature of the patients' reinforcement will determine whether they are likely to use their implant. For example, if patients are having the implant to impress someone else whom they rarely meet, then wearing the implant will only rarely be reinforcing. Likewise, if they hope the implant will improve their relationships or reduce their isolation and it fails to meet this expectation, the patient is unlikely to continue using it. If there appears a high probability of the patient's expectations being met, then the act of using the device will be reinforced.

Non-users (those having an implant but not attaching the external parts or switching it on) are frequently grouped with persons for whom the device was not audiologically beneficial, even though non-use may not relate to audiological factors. Quittner and Steck (1991) report several non-audiological variables associated with non-use in children. The American Speech and Hearing Association committee report (1986) suggested that as many as 19% of 3M/House single channel implantees could be classified as non-users. By definition, non-users are often lost to follow-up and their motives for non-use not recorded.

Consent

It is fairly obvious that cognitive disability and mental illness can confound the ability to give consent. However, Pollard (1996) says for patients truly to consent to an implant they must have reasonable expectations of it. This should include the patient having knowledge of the device, the surgery and recovery, the mapping and training, expected commitments and appointments, and the possible outcomes. Pollard reports that the psychologist and team should be up to date on all these issues and be able to advise on surgical risks, MRI prohibition and alternatives to implantation. He says that the assessor should verify that the candidate and relevant others have understood and retained this information, just informing the patient is not enough. For informed consent the assessor must also tease out their expectations emotionally, socially, educationally and vocationally. Pollard reports that candidates should really have met successful deafened and culturally Deaf implantees so that they do not base their decision on TV fantasy or extreme publicity.

Consent means choice between the implant and the alternatives. Deafened adults often know little about rehabilitation, technology, their rights and the views about implants of the wider society. For example, people who say they want an implant to be able to speak on the phone should also understand the use of text phones and relay services. People who say that they want an implant to improve their job opportunities should know about their employment rights under the various disability discrimination Acts. People who say they want to be able to hear, need to know they will not necessarily be able to hear speech. Brauer (1993) cautioned against discussions of 'deaf world' versus 'hearing world', as a cochlear implant does not make a deaf person hearing. Pollard says that adults will need at least two sessions with the psychology assessor and that communication should be by writing, if the person does not sign, as the conversation is too important and protracted to do by lip-reading alone.

Few teams have psychologists and those that do most likely leave consent, as Pollard describes it, to the audiological or medical staff. This may be a factor of the dearth of psychologists who reserve their assessment time for the more obviously psychologically vulnerable. Or it may be a result of us, as psychologists, underestimating our own particular skills in assessment and explanation. We may also overestimate these skills in our audiological colleagues, who probably have little training in the psychology of learning and motivation, let alone mental illness. The need for psychologists to be more involved in all aspects of the candidacy assessment is powerfully illustrated by the case studies below. Numerous audiological professionals had seen these clients, and the problem had either not been identified or not been addressed. On each occasion a single meeting with a clinical psychologist made significant progress in identifying the concerns and subsequent meetings or team interventions made significant progress in addressing the problems. As a result of their unique skills, experience, and contribution in this field, it is my opinion that psychologists should see every candidate before and after implantation.

The psychologist will also need to be extremely knowledgeable about the views of cochlear implants within the wider deaf communities, in order to place patients within their own bio-psycho-social context. It is essential that psychologists can reflect on their own beliefs and work to remain impartial in their exploration of this with clients.

Although it is important to check that the patient is not motivated to have an implant to please someone else, it is also important to check that someone else is not pressuring the patient into having an implant.

Case study

A 32-year-old woman from the Middle East, accompanied by her siblings, attended an implant centre. The patient did not speak English and the siblings said she did not sign. The siblings interpreted the assessment procedure and the patient lipread their native spoken language. Suspicions were aroused when the family failed to attend appointments where professional interpreters were guaranteed and when they seemed to change their answers depending on what they thought would ensure an implant. The patient seemed emotionally withdrawn and was referred to a female clinical psychologist. The psychologist used a professional female interpreter and adapted her own British Sign Language into as international form as she could. The patient revealed that she was fluent in her native sign language and had been brought to England against her will to have an implant as the family thought this would increase her chances of marriage. The patient had been living a happy life in her native country, working as a teacher of the Deaf, and she neither wanted to be in England nor to have an implant. To protect the patient from her family's wrath, the family was told that an implant was impossible on audiological grounds and the patient was put in contact with a cultural advocate.

Follow-up and rehabilitation

Audiological follow-up and rehabilitation is considered necessary for both audiological and psychosocial outcomes. Gagne (1992) recommends the use of aural rehabilitation (AR), which involves fitting and adjustment of the speech processing device, training in skills such as speech production, and the provision of information and personal counselling. Hogan (2001) however, recommends that interventions be aimed more directly at psychosocial wellbeing. He promotes psychosocial rehabilitation groups that address assertiveness, communication strategies, and the emotions associated with the clients' deafness and the CI, both of the patients and their partners.

Aplin (1993a) said psychologists should also provide counselling services to patients to review progress, explore benefits, discuss expectations (fulfilled or unfulfilled) and allow space to explore feelings of inadequacy. Aplin conducts psychological reviews 6 months after implant and yearly thereafter, plus others as required.

Outcome studies

Summerfield and Marshall (1995) report that being able to predict outcomes is useful for three reasons:

- individuals could make informed judgments of the benefits they might personally receive from implantation;
- purchasers and providers of health care could identify the patients who would gain most or least from CI;
- following implantation, the CI team could identify those patients who were underperforming relative to expectations and who were therefore candidates for additional rehabilitation.

Success is usually measured by tests of speech perception, but Summerfield and Marshall say that as healthcare decisions are increasingly made based on quality of life (QoL) this is also useful in this arena. Their results show that the more recently deafened, with good lipreading, who retain some usable residual hearing and who are not depressed display better outcomes in performance and QoL. However, QoL was their least accurately predicted outcome measure and therefore not robust enough to make purchasing decisions in this arena.

Psychosocial outcomes

Implanted adults report feeling less isolated generally and more confident in social situations (Tyler and Kelsay, 1990; Aplin, 1993b). On an open-ended questionnaire to elicit the advantages and disadvantages of implantation, 70% of the Tyler and Kelsay's sample reported 'escape from a world of silence' as their main advantage. Knutson et al. (1998) followed up 37 CI users for 54 months after implant and found significant improvements in relation to loneliness, social anxiety and distress. They found that assertiveness and marital satisfaction only improved after long term use of the implant. They conclude that cochlear implantation is associated with long-term psychological benefits but that the association between the audiological benefit and the psychological benefit is not simple. Ramsden et al. (1994) even found that most patients who had relatively poor audiological outcomes, the 'poor performers', were still happy with their results.

Hogan (1997) points out that whereas traditionally efficacy is measured by improvements in speech perception, the psychosocial outcomes are more relevant. He found that post cochlear implant, patients experienced improvements in interpersonal communication skills, social confidence and social anxiety. However, he reported that broader socio-economic gains were not achieved and put this down to the poorer job opportunities for all deaf people.

Psychometric screening measures

Knutson (1988) reported changes on the Beck Depression Inventory (BDI) following implantation, which correlated with measures of audiological ability. It would therefore seem that we need more research on the link between audiological outcome and the various combinations of personality and cognitive measures. However, Clark et al. (1977) found that there was no impairment or improvement in cognitive or neuropsychological functions nor were there significant changes in personality dimensions pre- and post- implant. Others found likewise and as a result stopped including these parameters in their pre- and post- measures (McKenna, 1991; Crary et al., 1982). McKenna was concerned that not only did the conventional psychometrics not seem able to predict patients' benefits, but that the tests did not lend themselves to use with deaf populations. As a result he uses a less formal clinical interview to gather data and suggests that tests of emotional distress would be more useful than tests of personality.

Aplin (1993a, 1993b) continues to use a battery of cognitive and personality assessments on every implant candidate and is concerned that, by not doing so, there will be a paucity of longitudinal data. Most current research has a relatively short follow-up time but we need to know how the patient will fare in the long-term future. This has particularly been the case with IQ level. The results showing that IQ level does not correlate with outcome have resulted in a tendency to dismiss the use of IQ testing pre-implant, and yet adults with global learning disabilities have been excluded from implantation. The lack of significance of IQ may change if a wider range of scores were included from the start. Similarly, McKenna (1991) believes that by including only candidates with normal personality profiles in implant programs, the question of whether people with deviant personality profiles are in fact poor CI users, remains unanswered.

Although the IQ itself may not presently be considered useful in predicting outcome, more detailed cognitive assessment is. Aplin (1993b) says that intellectual functioning data with particular emphasis placed on recall, information processing and attention to detail, are useful. Knutson et al. (1991) hypothesized that making sense of the sounds and learning to use the implant requires attentional cognitive processing skills. This highlighted that the ability to extract information from sequentially arrayed signals and to rapidly process that information was related to CI outcome. Knutson thought such information would be useful, not to exclude candidates, but to advise about outcomes and therefore more informed consent.

Conclusion

More psychologists are required to work in CI teams, to continue and expand the role. Psychologists – particularly clinical psychologists – have unique skills and experience, which should be applied to all aspects of the CI assessment, rehabilitation and research.

The psychologist should take a lead role in assessing whether the client can consent to the implant and should advise the team of issues indicating exclusion or postponement.

The link between psychological factors and the outcome of surgery (either audiological or psychosocial) is still unclear. Further research is required particularly with reference to the long-term collection of data and the widening of breadth and size of samples. However, there is also a need for some policing of the methodology of these studies, as much of the present research is sponsored by the CI companies and many of the studies only use the more successful implant users as subjects. Very little research or even discussion looks at those with poorer outcomes or those that go on to become non-users.

The role of the psychologist within the CI team is both challenging and rewarding. In order to remain objective, the psychologist should understand the issues important to the wider deaf communities as well as the procedures involved in implantation and habilitation.

References

Aplin DY (1993a) Psychological assessment of multi-channel cochlear implant patients. Journal of Laryngology and Otology 107: 298–304.

Aplin DY (1993b) Psychological evaluation of adults in a cochlear implant program. American Annals of the Deaf 138(5): 415–9.

American Speech and Hearing Association (1986) Report of the Ad Hoc Committee on Cochlear Implants. Rockville MD: ASHA, pp. 29–49.

Brauer BA (1993) Leap of faith. Hearing Health (June/July): 1–4.

Clarke GM, O'Loughlin BJ, Rickards FW, Tong YC, Williams AJ (1977) The clinical assessment of cochlear implant patients. Journal of Laryngology and Otology 91(8): 697–708.

Conrad R (1979) The reading ability of deaf school leavers. British Journal of Educational Psychology 47: 138–48.

Crary WG, Berliner KI, Wexler M, Miller LW (1982) Psychometric studies and clinical interviews with cochlear implant patients. Annals of Otology, Rhinology and Laryngology (Supp) 91: 55–8.

Evans JW (1989) Thoughts on the psychosocial implications of cochlear implantation in children. In Owens E, Kessler DK (eds) Cochlear Implantation in Young Deaf Children. Boston MA: College-Hill Press and Little, Brown, pp. 307–14.

Fraser G (1991) The cochlear implant team. In Cooper H (ed.) Cochlear Implants: A Practical Guide. London: Whurr, pp. 84–91.

Gagne JP (1992) Ancillary aural rehabilitation services for adult cochlear implant recipients: a review and analysis of the literature. Journal of Speech-Language Pathology and Audiology 16(2): 121–8.

Gantz BJ, Tyler RS, Knutson JF, Woodworth G, Abbas P, McCabe BF, Hinrichs J, Tye-Murray N, Lansing C, Kuk F, Brown C (1988) Evaluation of five different cochlear implant designs: audiologic assessment and predictors of performance. Laryngoscope 98: 1100–6.

Hogan A (1997) Implant outcomes: towards a mixed methodology for evaluating the efficacy of adult cochlear implant programmes. Disability and Rehabilitation 19(6): 235–43.

Hogan A (2001) Hearing Rehabilitation For Deafened Adults: A Psychosocial Approach. London: Whurr.

Knutson JF (1988) Psychological variables in the use of cochlear implants: predicting success and measuring change. Presented at NIH Consensus Development Conference, Washington DC, 2–4 May.

Knutson JF, Hinrichs JV, Tyler RS, Gantz BJ, Schartz HA, Woodworth G (1991) Psychological predictors of audiological outcomes of multichannel cochlear implants: preliminary findings. Annals of Otololgy, Rhinology and Laryngology 100: 817–22.

Knutson JF, Murray KT, Husare KS, Westerhouse K, Woodworth G, Gantz BJ, Tyler RS (1998) Psychological change over 54 months of cochlear implant use. Ear and Hearing 19(3):191–201.

Link Centre for Deafened People (1996) Cochlear implants in deafened adults. Advanced Bionics. Eastbourne: Link Centre for Deafened People.

McKenna L (1991) The assessment of psychological variables in cochlear implant patients. In Cooper H (ed.) (1991) Cochlear Implants: A Practical Guide. London: Whurr, pp. 125–45.

McKenna L, Hallam RS, Hinchcliffe R (1991) The prevalence of psychological disturbance in neurotology outpatients. Clinical Otolaryngology and Allied Sciences 16(5): 452–6.

National Institute of Health (1988) Cochlear Implant 7(2). Washington DC: US Government Printing Office.

National Institute of Health (1995) Cochlear implants in adults and children. National Institute of Health Consensus Statements 13(2): 1–30. Washington DC: US Government Printing Office.

Pollard RQ Jr (1996) Conceptualizing and conducting preoperative psychological assessments of cochlear implant candidates. Journal of Deaf Studies and Deaf Education 1(1): 16–28.

Quittner AL, Steck, JT (1991) Predictors of cochlear implant use in children. American Journal of Otology 12 (Supplement): 89–94.

Ramsden R, Aplin Y, Boyd P, Giles E (1994) The poor performers – what can they teach us? In Hochmair-Desoyer IJ, Hochmair ES (eds) (1994) Advances in Cochlear Implants. Wein: Manz, pp. 369–73.

Summerfield AQ, Marshall DH (1995) Preoperative predictors of outcomes from cochlear implantation in adults: performance and quality of life. Annals of Otology, Rhinology, and Laryngology Supplement 166: 105–8.

Tyler RS, Kelsay DK (1990) Advantages and disadvantages reported by some better cochlear implant patients. American Journal of Otology 11(4): 282–9.

CHAPTER 14

The causes of schizophrenia and its implications for Deaf people

ALISON GRAY AND MARGARET DU FEU

Introduction

Research about schizophrenia in hearing people has established predisposing, precipitating and perpetuating factors for the illness. This chapter will highlight which of these factors impact more strongly on Deaf people. However, there are few robust community studies looking at the incidence and prevalence of psychoses in Deaf people in the UK. The paucity of research directly with Deaf people makes much of this comment speculative and inferential. Although it is recognized that research on hearing people may not be directly transferable to Deaf people, we believe this is the best evidence currently available. The evidence suggests that both the incidence and prevalence of schizophrenia may be higher in the Deaf population than in a comparable hearing group.

The term Deaf will be used to refer to those whose preferred language is British Sign Language and who identify with the Deaf community; those who identify more with the English using hearing culture will be referred to as deaf.

Schizophrenia

Schizophrenia is a severe and enduring mental illness. It is a psychotic illness, meaning that, when acutely unwell, sufferers are out of touch with reality. They will experience hallucinations – for example, hearing voices when there is no one in the room, seeing peoples' faces distort (for instance, into devils) and as a result of these experiences they may develop delusions (beliefs based on inadequate evidence). There are several causes of psychosis other than schizophrenia, including manic depression, medical illnesses and the use of some drugs. Brief psychotic symptoms are not uncommon in the general population. A first diagnosis is usually an inclusive term such as 'psychotic illness' and only later the diagnosis of schizophrenia become clear. Schizophrenic illness can vary in severity between people: about one third of people who have a schizophrenic breakdown recover and do not become ill again; another third recover well and then relapse; the final third never really recover from the first breakdown. The longer it is before adequate treatment is instituted and the more frequently someone relapses, the worse the outcome.

The vulnerability to the illness is lifelong, but many people do recover from schizophrenia, some with no further problems and some with ongoing symptoms. Follow-up studies show that 62% of people who had been severely ill had fully recovered over 20 years (Harding, 1987). Some of these people still took medication or had symptoms at times, but were functioning in society without difficulties. People who have been unwell with many symptoms have gone on to train as professionals.

Schizophrenia most commonly develops in young people, in the later teenage years and early twenties. It is rare before puberty and tends to begin later in women than men. This illness interferes with people at a significant period of their lives, when careers are being determined and adult relationships formed.

Schizophrenia is a clinical diagnosis. There is no blood test or X-ray that proves the presence of schizophrenia; instead such tests demonstrate the absence of other illnesses that can cause similar symptoms (such as brain tumours). The diagnosis is made on a typical set of positive or negative symptoms and signs: positive symptoms include:

- voices talking about or directly to the person, or commenting on the persons' actions (for example, 'now he's having a bath');
- the sensation of thoughts being put into or removed from one's mind;
- the feeling that others can read one's thoughts;
- the sensation that an external force controls one's feelings, bodily experiences or actions;
- a sudden delusion, which arises fully formed (for example 'he looked at the traffic light and knew he was a space alien').

Negative symptoms include social withdrawal (a common early sign of psychosis), apathy, lack of emotional response and reduced amounts of speech.

The other group of abnormalities in schizophrenia are abnormalities in the patients' communication, referred to as 'thought disorder'. Often schizophrenics jump from subject to subject without obvious links, and are preoccupied with odd themes, making them difficult to understand. Positive symptoms and thought disorder are more likely to respond to medication; negative symptoms are more difficult to treat. All symptoms tend to become worse if there are repeated episodes of illness.

Stress vulnerability model

Schizophrenia has many causes. For the full illness to develop there must be 'multiple hits' – both a genetic predisposition and a number of social or environmental factors present. The stress-vulnerability model (Zubin and Spring, 1977) argues that many people have a biological vulnerability to psychosis, but that it is life experiences that determine who will develop the illness (Gispen-de Wied and Jansen, 2002). If psychosis were caused purely biologically there would be nothing an individual could do to prevent occurrence or relapse of the illness. The stress vulnerability model argues that by looking at stressors, altering lifestyle and improving psychological coping mechanisms one can decrease the risk of relapse – see Birchwood, Spencer and McGovern (2000) for a summary of the evidence and practical applications.

Deafness and mental health

Deaf people are *people* first and foremost, with similar problems to hearing people. Some will also have the added dimensions of physical problems related to the cause of deafness, poor access to services due to communication difference or difficulty, or language deprivation. Ninety per cent of Deaf children have hearing parents and, to encourage them to speak, some parents may have been advised not to sign to them. There is no evidence that this strategy promotes speech, in fact, in cases of profound prelingual deafness this can result in language deprivation for the child. This potentially results in adults of normal IQ having restricted communication skills. In one project nearly 20% of deaf young people with a normal IQ score were unable to complete an interview in either speech or sign language (Gregory, Bishop and Sheldon, 1995). This inevitably decreases educational opportunities leading to lower paid jobs and long-term relative poverty. Deaf people are often excluded from hearing society and services.

Deafness and schizophrenia

The precise prevalence of schizophrenia in Deaf people is difficult to establish as little research has been done in the area. However, schizophrenia in Deaf people seems to present in a very similar way to that in hearing people. The voices that hearing people experience may be experienced as people signing to the patient, or they may believe that they are acquiring hearing (Du Feu and McKenna, 1999).

Deaf people and diagnosis

The general practitioner should be the first point of assessment for mental health problems (Department of Health, 1999), yet most Deaf service users in the UK receive a poor service from primary care and many avoid appointments because they cannot understand the GP (Bruce, McKennell and Walker, 1991). Few GPs or mental health professionals have experience of Deaf people, their language, culture, or their mental health. Most GP surgeries and community mental health teams do not have a minicom and struggle to access suitable interpreters. Thus, there is a need for greater investment in Deaf awareness training, communication technologies and in interpreter training to bring equity of access to Deaf patients and maximize the chance of accurate and timely diagnosis.

There are currently three specialist multidisciplinary mental health services for Deaf people in the UK at which assessment may take place if: the Deaf service is known to the referrer; the resident health authority agrees to fund the assessment; the patient lives within travelling distance of the Deaf service; the Deaf service has the skills relevant to the patient's particular clinical difficulties. The Deaf patient may also be assessed by a mainstream (hearing) service using an interpreter. Accessing either the specialist or mainstream route is likely to involve delays, which result in late diagnosis. Communication may make diagnosis complicated even by specialist Deaf mental health teams, with odd behaviour as a result of psychosis often being blamed on the deafness. If diagnosis is delayed then treatment is also delayed.

Communication difficulties can make diagnosis particularly difficult in deaf people. Subtle changes in behaviour in the early stages of illness may be missed or masked by deafness. Thought disorder, which compromises language fluency, is difficult to establish if the individual's communication is limited and normal baseline functioning is unclear. Some Deaf people have limited life experiences such that it is difficult for them to determine fact from fantasy – for example, Deaf teenagers may be unsure if space aliens are objectively real or not and hence may seem deluded when they are just misinformed.

Use of interpreters

Interviewing via interpreters will always distort interaction to some degree. Farroq and Fear (2003) found that people express more psychotic content when interviewed in their first language. Thus, studies using interpreters are likely to give falsely low rates of psychosis. Given that many Deaf people will be interviewed using sign language interpreters, it is likely that psychosis may therefore go undiagnosed in some Deaf people.

The pool of sign language interpreters who are skilled in mental health work is small. However, using friends and family as interpreters is rarely appropriate as they may try to conceal difficulties or normalize the language. Horror stories abound of hearing children interpreting for Deaf parents, and it is recognized that this is unacceptable (except in dire emergencies) in the case of other language groups (Farooq and Fear, 2003). The ideal situation is to have mental health professionals whose first language is BSL. However, this would have major implications for professional training, access to which is currently limited in the UK. In the US, the Americans with Disabilities Act of 1990 has improved access for Deaf people to training courses leading to a body of qualified Deaf professionals. Trained Deaf relay interpreters may improve accuracy of assessment.

Comordibity

Comorbidity of substance misuse complicates diagnosis. Psychosis resulting from amphetamines and cannabis use recovers rapidly, but for some, drugs precipitate a psychosis that remains and acts in the long term as schizophrenia. To further complicate diagnosis, illicit drugs and alcohol may be used to self-medicate early symptoms of psychosis, such as difficulty sleeping. The presence of substance abuse or alcohol dependence makes treatment of the psychosis more difficult and less likely to succeed. Deaf people seem to have similar levels of alcohol abuse to hearing people, but less access to information and services (Austen and Checinski, 2002).

Factors that lead to higher prevalence of schizophrenia and psychotic illnesses

Factors that lead to a higher prevalence of severe and enduring mental illness in the general population will be discussed and their relevance to people with pre-lingual or very early deafness considered.

Psychiatric illness factors

There is a genetic predisposition towards developing a psychotic illness and the lifetime incidence of schizophrenia is 1% in the general population. If an individual has one parent with schizophrenia the incidence goes up to 13%, and if both parents are affected the rate is nearly 50%, regardless of whether the person is brought up by the affected parent or not (thus, disturbed environment cannot be solely to blame). Researchers have tried to find a single gene responsible for schizophrenia, but it is now generally accepted that there are a number of susceptibility genes. However, genes alone cannot be responsible for incidence of schizophrenia, otherwise, in cases where both parents were affected, the prevalence rate would be nearer 100%.

Neurological risk for both deafness and schizophrenia

Schizophrenia most commonly begins in late adolescence. Young people who develop schizophrenia at a younger age tend to have more severe illness and a poorer long-term outcome. Imaging techniques have shown a number of abnormalities in the brains of people with schizophrenia that suggest abnormalities in the developing nervous system. These changes are found at the very start of schizophrenia and do not worsen as the disease progresses (Sawa and Kamiya, 2003). These consistently include an increase in the size of the ventricles, fluid-filled spaces inside the brain. The brain shows small nerve cells but none of the repair processes that would suggest ongoing neurodegeneration. All these factors suggest damage to the brain early in development. Some authors have suggested that this damage is due to a viral infection during gestation (Sawa and Kamiya, 2003).

Deafness can also be caused by a variety of insults to the brain in early development, for example, rubella, mumps, prematurity and low birth weight. It is known that people with brain damage have a greatly increased risk of psychiatric illness in general (Graham and Rutter, 1968) and, although this has not been adequately investigated, we would predict therefore that D/deaf people would have an increased rate of schizophrenia.

Genetic conditions causing deafness and a potential mental health difficulty

Some genetic problems that cause deafness can also cause psychosis. For example, MELAS is a syndrome of mitochondrial myopathy, encephalopathy, lactic acidosis and stroke-like episodes, which usually results in early death. MELAS is caused by genetic abnormalities in the mitochondria and is associated with multiple problems including hearing loss and psychotic illness (Damian et al., 1995).

Usher's syndrome is a recessive genetic condition with three subtypes. It causes early profound deafness and retinitis pigmentosa, which causes tunnel vision and blindness. As well as the psychological problems caused by adjusting to becoming a deaf-blind person there is some, albeit scant, evidence for increased rates of psychosis (Hallgren, 1959).

Social factors

People with severe mental health problems are generally feared and looked down on. A MIND survey 'Not just sticks and stones' (Read and Baker, 1996) of people with a mental illness, identified problems accessing health, justice, education and housing services.

Stigma

Stigma is a barrier to people accessing services. The negative image of mental illness makes people reluctant to recognize a mental health problem in themselves or their loved ones. Once a diagnosis is made stigma can lead to difficulties engaging with the service, poor compliance with treatment and correspondingly poor outcomes. Internalised stigma can lower people's self esteem and lead to them taking up an unnecessary sick role (Gray, 2002). People who are Deaf experience much discrimination and lack of understanding (Higgins, 1980). Those who go on to develop a major mental illness are in double jeopardy, often unable to fit in with the Deaf community due to illness and odd behaviour, but unable to access the (hearing) mental-health service user movement due to communication difficulties. Some services have supported the development of Deaf service user groups although the small size of the Deaf community can create problems of confidentiality.

General psychiatric services

The British government has recognized the poor services received by many people who have severe and enduring mental illnesses. In the National Service Framework (NSF) (Department of Health, 1999) a shift in emphasis was proposed to concentrate services on those with the most severe illnesses. This has led to the development of early intervention teams to work with people in the first 2 years of psychotic illness, home treatment teams as an alternative to hospital admission and assertive outreach (AOT) to focus on those who find it difficult to engage with services. Early intervention has the aim of decreasing the length of time someone is ill before they receive treatment, referred to as the duration of untreated psychosis (DUP). The aim is to provide rapid effective and user-friendly treatment as soon as psychosis is identified, because longer DUPs are linked with worse overall outcome (Linszen et al., 1998). It is hypothesized that the relative difficulty in diagnosing Deaf people will lead to an increase in average DUP and that this will create an increase in the proportion of Deaf people having a chronic mental health problem.

Home treatment and crisis intervention teams aim to manage a mental health crisis without admission to hospital, visiting several times a day for short periods when necessary. For such services to be accessible to Deaf people, sign language interpreters would need to be available at short notice, an unlikely feat given the present shortage of interpreters in most parts of the UK.

Assertive outreach was developed in the US as a response to needs in city areas (Drake, 1998). Assertive Outreach teams have a high staff to patient ratio and work intensively with a small number of 'difficult' clients. This paradigm relies on a large local population to ensure that the services are focusing only on those who need such intensive support. A number of assertive outreach services have been developed for people of particular ethnic groups: this model has been used for the Deaf community in London. However, Deaf people do not tend to live in geographically close communities so it is hard to see how assertive outreach to Deaf people can be provided outside large urban conurbations.

Local community

Certain features of the local community and social environment can lead to a higher than usual prevalence of schizophrenia – for example areas with low social capital (McKenzie, Whitley and Weich, 2002). Social capital is a measure of the 'glue' that binds communities together. Low social capital is reflected in crime and vandalism and the inability of the community to improve things. Communities are not necessarily geographical and people can belong to several such communities. For example, there is an inverse correlation between social capital and incidence of psychosis in South London (Boydell, Van Os, McKenzie, 2001), meaning that the more deprived your home area the more likely you are to develop schizophrenia. In this study the effect of growing up in an urban, low social capital area remained even when people moved to areas of higher social capital before becoming ill (Van Os and Sham, 2002). Research on social capital is at an early stage and Deaf communities have not been widely studied.

It has long been accepted that migrants have a higher rate of schizophrenia than those of the same racial group in the host country; it is not clear whether this is due to differential migration (of those who were becoming ill) or the stress of being in a new country. Certainly having experienced racist abuse or assault (Karlsen and Nazroo, 2002) and being a member of a small minority community (Boydell, Van Os, McKenzie, 2001) are both linked to higher rates of schizophrenia. This may in part explain the high rates of diagnosis of psychosis in young black men. Living in an area with many people from your minority community is protective.

Deaf children are likely to come from all socio-economic backgrounds but often have very few deaf peers in the locality; they may experience discrimination and difficulties fitting in, similar to a black child in a predominantly white area. Deaf people regularly experience discrimination (RNID, 1998) and may, as a community, feel powerless to improve things.

Social role

Poverty, unemployment and low educational achievement are all linked with increased rates of mental disorders (Fryers, Melzer and Jenkins, 2003). Having a valued social role (for example, paid or voluntary work or being a member of a Church community) promotes recovery from psychosis (Boardman et al., 2003), while promoting employment decreases the need for mental health support in people with severe and enduring mental illness (Bond et al., 1997).

Young people in the early stages of psychosis report smaller social networks compared to those without mental illness (Macdonald, Hayes and Baglioni, 2000). Whether this social isolation causes the illness or reflects a developing illness, is not clear. In people with established schizophrenia those with good social support were more likely to be in work and have good self care independent of their level of illness (Evert et al., 2003).

People who are Deaf may have considerable difficulties in obtaining appropriate employment and on average have low educational achievement (Conrad, 1979). They are also more likely to be socially isolated than hearing people. Most Deaf people are born into hearing families and even those who had a strong peer group at Deaf school are likely to have returned to their hometown and become socially and linguistically isolated once more. Therefore, it is hypothesized that Deaf people will have a worse social outcome for psychoses compared to hearing people with a similar severity of illness.

Victimization

It has long been reported that victimization experiences increase the long-term risk of developing psychosis. The British National Survey of Psychiatric morbidity, a very large general population survey in the UK, demonstrated that having experienced sexual or physical abuse was strongly associated with a diagnosis of psychotic illness (Bebbington et al., in preparation). Deaf and hard-of-hearing children (along with children with other forms of disability) are more vulnerable to neglect and emotional, physical and sexual abuse (Brookhouser and Scanlan, 2000).

Interpersonal and intrafamilial factors.

Living in a family with a lot of critical and demanding interactions, known as high expressed emotion (EE), is likely to lead to a relapse of schizophrenia (Vaughn and Leff, 1976). Behavioural family therapy works with families to help them improve their style of interactions and reduce levels of EE. Expressed emotion was studied with white Western families, but in African American families high EE is perceived as a sign of caring and concern and linked with less relapse and better outcomes (Rosenfarb and Bellack, 2003). Hearing parents of Deaf children are reported to be more directive, controlling and intrusive than either Deaf parents of Deaf children or hearing parents of hearing children (Schlesinger and Meadow, 1972). The interaction styles of families having a psychotically ill Deaf member have not been formally investigated. Anecdotally, such families often have high levels of expressed emotion, but whether this is experienced as positive or negative by the Deaf service user has not been investigated.

Separation from family of origin

Even without the experience of abuse, being separated from your parents is a traumatic experience and along with other factors can predispose to later schizophrenia. Early separation from parents is very frequent in those African-Caribbean people in the UK who later go on to develop schizophrenia (Mallet et al, 2002). In the middle of the last century many deaf children, some as young as 3 years old, were reportedly sent away to deaf schools and had little contact with their family for months at a time. Most of the deaf schools had oral policies, but many deaf children learned sign language from their peers. Institutional care and having lived in a children's home were also associated with higher rates of psychosis in the British National Survey of Psychiatric morbidity (Bebbington et al., in preparation).

Recovery

We have considered the social, physical and psychological factors, which contribute to a greater risk of developing schizophrenia, or higher risk of experiencing ongoing difficulties. Now we consider factors working in the opposite direction, towards recovery from the illness.

Since the late 1980s work has been published on the possibility of recovery from severe psychosis, for example *www.mhrecovery.com*. The term 'recovery' is used to mean a recovery of wholeness, self-esteem and valued social roles whether or not the person still has some symptoms or still takes medication. Recovery is a long journey of rebuilding, of coming to terms with what has happened, with an ongoing vulnerability to illness and need for medication.

In trying to be realistic, not to raise false hopes, or not put too much pressure on the patient, services have often been guilty of undermining the possibility of recovery and limiting people's lives unnecessarily.

Coping with diagnosis

Most people who develop schizophrenia are very distressed about its implications. On receiving a psychiatric diagnosis people feel disbelief, shame, terror, isolation, grief, and anger (O'Donoghue, 1994). Social rejection causes loss of self-esteem, diminished self-efficacy and lack of self-confidence, which lead to social withdrawal and secrecy (Holmes and River, 1998). Internalizing other people's negative attitudes may lead to the service user giving up trying and accepting a very poor quality of life as normal and appropriate. A similar process is active in some profoundly Deaf people who may already have lower self-esteem and who may become discouraged by communication difficulties and withdraw from mainstream society.

Positive coping strategies such as collecting information on the problem, talking things through with friends, contacting support groups and accessing professional care are often more difficult for Deaf people due to their communication and literacy problems (Mentality, 2003). Adjustment to diagnosis and treatment compliance may be made more difficult by a lack of adequate comprehensible explanation about treatments: for example, none of the UK major drug companies produce patient information as a BSL video. Likewise the Deaf community tends to have limited knowledge about mental health (Connolly, in preparation). Those who are language deprived may find it difficult to express their concerns and to understand the information being given to them about their illness, and one would predict these individuals would need extra help to come to terms with their illness and psychotic experiences.

Spiritual factors

Many service users describe their recovery in spiritual terms (Deegan, 1996). Anyone who has been through a psychosis will need to make sense of it. 'Why me?' 'What does this mean for my future?' 'What is my purpose in life?' These are spiritual questions. They are not the direct concern of medically based services, but mental health workers can acknowledge these concerns and encourage people to find the right spiritual support for them (Nolan and Crawford, 1997). Spirituality is much broader than organized religion and can be found through nature, yoga, and creativity as well as through prayer and communal worship. Many service users find belonging to a faith community helpful and supportive (Health Education Authority, 1999).

All service users, deaf or hearing, should be able to access peer support groups, spiritual support, and faith communities as well as active rehabilitation services to help them fulfil their potential.

Insight

People who lack insight into their schizophrenia and deny that they have any problems may develop 'revolving door syndrome' (Davis, 1975). This describes someone who comes into hospital very unwell, takes the medication, recovers, goes home, stops taking the medication and is readmitted soon after. Trying to find a compromise such that the individual does not have to take on the whole medical/illness model seems most successful. For example, agreeing, 'when the neighbours start bothering you and you're not sleeping so well, is the time to take more tablets' can be effective in preventing relapse and eventually lead to some degree of insight. This slow and patient work is particularly undertaken by assertive outreach teams and as previously discussed, outside of London; Deaf people rarely have access to this form of service.

Factors likely to complicate recovery

As discussed earlier, comorbidity of substance misuse problems with schizophrenia can complicate recovery. Likewise, the continued presence of some of the causal factors such as victimization, social isolation, lack of social role and so on may affect progress. Personality disorder is also thought to negatively affect recovery.

Personality disorders

People who have a personality disorder along with their psychotic illness are more difficult to treat. At one time clinicians identified a specific deaf personality disorder 'surdophrenia'. Basilier, writing in 1964, emphasized impulsiveness and aggressive behaviour in his description of disturbed deaf young men. The term 'surdophrenia' is now not generally used; the concept of adjustment disorder is usually found to be more helpful. These behaviours are not unique to Deaf people and can be found in hearing people brought up in institutions, and in those with organic brain disorders (Kitson and Thacker, 2002).

The frequency of certain personality disorders are increased by experiences of severe abuse and neglect in childhood. Given the increased incidence of abuse of Deaf people one would expect this to lead to proportionately more Deaf adults with damaged personalities. A survey of the patient population of the National Deaf Mental Health service in Birmingham, UK (Appleford, 2003) demonstrated that there was a much higher rate of personality disorder diagnoses in their ward patients when compared with those in a hearing service.

Discusssion

There is a lack of accurate data on the incidence of severe mental health problems in the Deaf community and future research needs to collect accurate epidemiology to enable appropriate levels of funding and services to work with this socially excluded group.

It has been demonstrated, however, that there are many factors active in Deaf people and their environment that would tend to predict a higher incidence and prevalence of psychotic illnesses in this group. As well as neurological and genetic risks, Deaf people experience poorer job prospects, higher unemployment, relative poverty, and social isolation that are all associated with more psychotic illnesses.

Some of these factors will be modified by the changes in social and educational practice towards bilingualism and away from purely oral techniques with the aim of age-appropriate language development. Intensive signing input for hearing families with a Deaf member would benefit both the family and wider society.

Diagnosis of Deaf people can be difficult and comorbid substance abuse, personality difficulties, and language deprivation would tend to increase the demand on specialist Deaf psychiatric services and require a higher level of resources than a hearing service with similar numbers and demographics.

Once ill, Deaf people find it harder to access skilled health care. The National Institute of Clinical Excellence guidelines state that early intervention and assertive outreach services should be accessible by all members of the community (NICE, 2002) but are presently only available, in part, to Deaf people in London.

Mental health promotion resources, which aid recovery, are generally not available in sign-language forms, despite being available in other minority languages, and self-help groups are difficult to access without an interpreter. A shortage of sign language interpreters with mental health experience and a dearth of qualified Deaf mental health professionals contribute to the inequality of access for Deaf people to mental health services.

References

Appleford J (2003) Clinical activity within a specialist mental health service for deaf people: comparison with a general psychiatric service. Psychiatric Bulletin 27: 375–7.

Austen S, Checinski K (2002) Addictive behaviour and deafness. In Hindley P and Kitson N (eds) (2002) Mental Health and Deafness. London: Whurr, pp. 253–81.

Basilier T (1964) Surdophrenia: the psychic consequences of congenital or early acquired deafness. Acta Psychiatrica Scandinavica 40: 362–71.

Bebbington P, Bhugra D, Brugha T, Singleton P, Farrell M, Jenkins R, Lewis G, Melzer H (In preparation) Psychosis, Victimization and Childhood Disadvantage. Evidence from the Second British National Survey of Psychiatric Morbidity.

Birchwood M, Spencer E, McGovern D (2000) Schizophrenia: early warning signs. Advances in Psychiatric Treatment 6: 93–101.

Boardman J, Grove B, Perkins R, Shepherd G (2003) Work and employment for people with psychiatric disabilities. British Journal of Psychiatry 182: 467–8.

Bond GR, Drake RE, Mueser KT, Becker DR (1997) An update on supported employment for people with severe mental illness. Psychiatric Services 48(3): 335–46.

Boydell J, Van Os J, McKenzie K (2001) Incidence of schizophrenia in ethnic minorities in London: ecological study into interactions with environment. British Medical Journal 323: 1336.

Brookhouser P, Scanlan J (2000) Maltreatment of deaf and hard of hearing children. In Hindley P, Kitson N (eds) Mental Health and Deafness. London: Whurr Publishers Ltd, pp.149–84.

Bruce I, McKennell A, Walker E (1991) Blind and Partially Sighted Adults in Britain: the RNIB Survey. Vol. 1. London: HMSO.

Connolly C (in preparation) Unpublished doctoral thesis. Attitudes of Deaf People to Mental Health and Translating/Validating the 'Clinical Outcomes in Routine Evaluation – Outcome Measurement' for Deaf People. Birmingham University, England.

Conrad R (1979) The Deaf Schoolchild. London: Harper & Row.

Damian MS, Seibel P, Reichmann H, Schachenmayr W, Laube H, Bachmann G, Wassill KH, Dorndorf W (1995) Clinical spectrum of the MELAS mutation in a large pedigree. Acta Neurologica Scandinavica 92(5): 409–15.

Davis JM (1975) Overview: maintenance therapy in psychiatry: I Schizophrenia. American Journal of Psychiatry 132(12): 1237–45.

Deegan P (1996) Recovery and the Conspiracy of Hope. www.bu.edu/resilience/examples/recovery-conspiracyofhope.txt. Accessed 28/4/04.

Department of Health (1999) http://www.doh.gov.uk/nsf/mentalhealth.htm (accessed 10 December 2003).

Drake RE (1998) A brief history, current status, and future place of assertive community treatment. America Journal of Orthopsychiatry 68(2): 172–75.

Du Feu M, McKennell (1999) Prelingually profoundly deaf schizophrenic patients who hear voices: a phenomenological analysis. Acta Psychiatrica Scandinavica 99(6): 453–9.

Evert H, Harvey C, Trauer T, Herrman H (2003)(The relationship between social networks and occupational and self-care functioning in people with psychosis. Social Psychiatry and Psychiatric Epidemiology 38(4): 180–8.

Farooq S, Fear C (2003) Working through interpreters. Advances in Psychiatric Treatment 9: 104–9.

Fryers T, Melzer D, Jenkins R (2003) Social inequalities and the common mental disorders: a systematic review of the evidence. Social Psychiatry and Psychiatric Epidemiology 38(5): 229–37.

Gispen-de Wied CC, Jansen LM (2002) The stress-vulnerability hypothesis in psychotic disorders: focus on the stress response systems. Current Psychiatry Report 4(3): 166–70.

Graham P, Rutter M (1968) Organic brain dysfunction and child psychiatric disorder. British Medical Journal 3: 695–700.

Gray AJ (2002) Stigma in psychiatry. Journal of the Royal Society of Medicine 95: 72–6.

Gregory S, Bishop J, Sheldon L (1995) Deaf Young People and Their Families. Developing Understanding. Cambridge: Cambridge University Press.

Hallgren B (1959) Retinits pigmentosa combined with congenital deafness with vesitbulocerebellar ataxia and mental abnormality in a proportion of cases: a clinical and genetico-statistical study. Acta Psychiatrica Scandanavica 34(138): 1–97.

Harding CM (1987) American Journal of Psychiatry 144 (6): 718–35.

Health Education Authority (1999) Promoting Mental Health: The Role of Faith Communities – Jewish and Christian Perspectives. London: HEA.

Higgins PC (1980) Outsiders in a Hearing World – A Sociology of Deafness. Beverley Hills CA: Sage Publications.

Holmes EP, River LP (1998) Individual strategies for coping with the stigma of severe mental illness. Cognitive and Behavioural Practice 5: 231–9.

Karlsen S, Nazroo JY (2002) Relation between racial discrimination, social class, and health among ethnic minority groups. American Journal of Public Health 92(4): 624–31.

Kitson N, Thacker (2002) Adult psychiatry. In Hindley P, Kitson N (eds) (2002) Mental Health and Deafness. London: Whurr, pp. 75–98.

Linszen D, Lenior M, De Haan L, Dingemans P, Gersons B (1998) Early intervention, untreated psychosis and the course of early schizophrenia. British Journal of Psychiatry 172(33): 84–9.

Macdonald EM, Hayes RL, Baglioni AJ Jr (2000) The quantity and quality of the social networks of young people with early psychosis compared with closely matched controls. Schizophrenia Research 46(1): 25–30.

Mallett R, Ieff J, Bhugra D, Pang D, Zhao JH (2002) Social environment, ethnicity and schizophrenia. A case-control study. Social Psychiatry Psychiatric Epidemiology 37(7): 329–35.

McKenzie K, Whitley R, Weich S (2002) Social capital and mental health. British Journal of Psychiatry 181: 280–3.

Mentality (2003) www.mentality.org.uk/services/positive.htm. Accessed 28/4/04.

National Institute for Clinical Excellence (2002) Schizophrenia: Core Interventions in the Treatment and Management of Schizophrenia in Primary and Secondary Care. Clinical Guideline 1, December. London: NICE.

Nolan P, Crawford P (1997) Towards a rhetoric of spirituality in mental health care. Journal of Advanced Nursing 26: 289–94.

O'Donoghue D (1994) Breaking down barriers. The stigma of mental illness: a user's point of view. In Sayce L (ed.) (2000) From Psychiatric Patient to Citizen. London: Macmillan Press.

Read J, Baker S (1996) Not Just Sticks and Stones: a Survey of the Stigma, Taboos and Discrimination Experienced by People with Mental Health Problems. London: Mind.

RNID (1998) Breaking the Sound Barrier. London: The Royal National Institute for Deaf People.

Rosenfarb IS, Bellack AS (2003) Relative's Negative Affect and the Course of Schizophrenia in African-American Patients. Presented at 'Schizophrenia Not Just Biological' conference, London.

Sawa A, Kamiya A (2003) Elucidating the pathogenesis of schizophrenia. British Medical Journal 327: 632–3.

Schlesinger HP, Meadow KP (1972) Development of maturity in deaf children. Exceptional Children Feb: 461–7.

Vaughn C, Leff J (1976) The influence of family life and social factors on the course of psychiatric illness. A comparison of schizophrenic and depressed neurotic patients. British Journal of Psychiatry 129: 2125–37.

Van Os J, Sham P (2002) Gene-environment interactions. In Murray RM, Jones PB (eds) The Epidemiology of Schizophrenia. Cambridge: Cambridge University Press.

Zubin J, Spring B (1977) Vulnerability – a new view of schizophrenia. Journal of Abnormal Psychology 86: 103–26.

CHAPTER 15

At-risk deaf parents and their children

ELIZABETH STONE CHARLSON

Introduction

This chapter reports on a research study of Child Protective Service records involving the abuse of children by deaf parents. The purpose of this study was not to determine whether deaf parents are more or less likely to abuse their children than hearing parents; rather, this chapter illustrates the potential risk factors for deaf parents and the consequences for children who are victims of physical, sexual, and emotional abuse, exploitation and neglect. Certainly, deafness alone does not make a parent likely to abuse, although deaf parents and their children face complex challenges that extend beyond identity issues and communication modalities. Parents who are culturally deaf, deafened, or oral-educated deaf people are referred to with the small 'd'. 'Deaf' is used throughout this chapter to refer to the community of deaf people who use sign language to communicate and associate with great frequency with other deaf people.

The question is often raised how parents who differ linguistically and culturally from their children fare. In the case of parents who are deaf, most have children who can hear (Preston, 1996). Such families may initially call to mind refugee or immigrant families where parents have arrived in a new country, unfamiliar with the language, schooling, and cultural ways of the new land. Their children easily learn the language and ways of the 'new country', which may have far-reaching implications for the immigrant parents. It seems as though the parents and children are forging different paths and it is the children who must pave the way for the immigrant parents (Singleton and Tittle, 2000). For parents who are deaf, raising children who can hear can feel like the new territory of immigrants. Many deaf parents attended residential schools, away from their biological families, used a language foreign to the larger community, and had limited opportunities to integrate into mainstream society. The

222

children of these parents will fare well if their parents are resourceful and resilient, have had good parenting models themselves, and can rely on formal or informal social support systems for guidance in raising children (Maestas y Moores, 1981; Rea, Bonvillian, and Richards, 1988, Rienzi, 1990). Pollard and Rendon (1999) state that deaf/hearing issues per se are seldom attributable to family dysfunction, rather normal family relationships depend on the family's general mental health. Pollard and Rendon also note that for competent deaf parents, 'deafness might present an occasional challenge, but it is not a tragedy or insurmountable problem in living or in parenting . . .'

A great support network for parents is affiliation with a Deaf community. Deaf communities are formed through marriage to other deaf people, membership in Deaf clubs, organizations or religious groups, and affiliations with schools for Deaf children. Deaf communities share in the use of sign language and act as a means of bonding and protection against the negative experiences of the 'hearing world'. Preston (1994) states, 'cultural deafness is not just about hearing loss. Being culturally Deaf is interdependent on the individuals' identification with the group and the group's evaluation and acceptance of the individual.' Without this acceptance, deaf parents may be without a community to support their parenting role. Participation in a socially supportive network is believed to lessen the likelihood of child maltreatment (Barth, 1991).

In an earlier study by Charlson (1989) on hearing adolescents with deaf parents, many teens were no longer living with their biological parents who had been unable to care for their children during the challenging teenage years, and had frequently sent the children to live with grandparents or other relatives. Deaf parents with cognitive or psychological impairments and overwhelming social stressors may not have the resources to provide for the care and safety of their children, regardless of whether they have deaf or hearing children.

At the Center on Deafness, San Francisco, California (a research, training, and mental health centre) we had been struck by the problems of deaf parents who abuse or neglect their children and the characteristics of both hearing and deaf children of deaf parents who have experienced abuse or neglect. Frequently, families are court-ordered to the clinic for professional evaluation of the likelihood of family reunification after a child has been made a dependent of the court. The problems and issues with which the clients at the clinic presented differed greatly from those described in the literature of the past several decades. Those earlier studies concerned with similar clinical populations of deaf parents and their hearing children, focused on the issues surrounding the communication and cultural differences of deaf parents and their hearing children (see Charlson, 1989). The cases seen at the Center on Deafness, San Francisco, were often horrific and the psychological and physical damage to children often beyond comprehension. The parenting needs were overwhelming. Additionally, therapists and caseworkers were faced with a lack of appropriate community resources for deaf parents and their children. The future of these families was uncertain.

Research study

A study was undertaken to explore those deaf parent families and their children in the most serious of crisis situations – where the children had been temporarily or permanently removed from the parents' home due to severe abuse or neglect. Readers should be reminded that the Deaf community is heterogeneous and, like any community, stressors experienced by some of its members do not reflect upon the community as a whole. The purpose of the study was to examine the following:

- What are the characteristics of families with deaf parents where there is abuse and neglect? Are they similar to families with hearing parents where there is abuse and neglect of children?
- What happens to children as a result of abuse and neglect?
- What is the range of services available to parents and children?
- How do the characteristics of at-risk deaf parent families compare to deaf parent families who successfully raise children?

In other words, how are deaf parent families at-risk different than hearing parents at-risk, and how might a community best respond?

Deaf parents with hearing children

To date, there are no published demographic reports on deaf parents whose children are at risk of abuse or neglect. During the 1970s and 1980s, a small number of clinical studies described the social and emotional impact that parental deafness can have on hearing children (Robinson and Weathers, 1974; Bene, 1977; Halbreich, 1979; Taska and Rhoads, 1981; Dent, 1982; Frankenberg, Sloman and Perry, 1985; Wagenheim, 1985). Generally, these children were impaired by their parents' lack of insight into their children's psychological needs and either themselves or their parents had sought psychotherapy. The parents had limited communication and cognitive skills and thus were unable to mediate the world for their children satisfactorily, although they were noted as having great concern and regard for their children. In addition to social-emotional problems, children were often described as having delayed speech development and having mild learning disabilities. The parents in these families were typically married to deaf spouses, worked at low paying jobs, and had stable home lives.

Children who parent

The hearing children of deaf parents are often depicted as 'parentified'. Role reversal often occurs when parents are limited by any kind of disability or are not fluent in the language of the majority of the community. Deaf parents who need sign language interpretation to have access to the world around them may have understandably become dependent on their hearing children. Interview and survey data of children of deaf parents conducted by Bunde (1979) and Preston (1996) describe the heavy responsibilities put on these children by their parents. Preston describes interpreting, whether it was sporadic or incessant, as the 'seminal aspect of being the hearing child of deaf parents'. Today, however, advanced technology has enabled deaf parents to rely on sources other than their children for communication access. Free or low-cost telecommunications devices (TDDs), state-run telephone relay services, television sub-titles, electronic mail and the Internet have relieved many contemporary children from the responsibilities carried by earlier generations of children of deaf parents.

Other research studies indicated that hearing children of deaf parents tended toward more emotional problems, anxiety, and motor excess than a matched group of children of hearing parents (Sanders, 1984). Another study found that hearing adolescent children of deaf parents living in intact homes appear to have significant personal and/or school problems but these students scored similarly to hearing teenagers on assessment of self-concept and social understanding (Charlson, 1989). A 1975 study by Tendler of hearing children of deaf psychiatric patients found that the children had poor analytic functioning, impulse control and reality judgment.

Abuse

Cycles of abuse

Children who themselves have been abused are known to be at risk of growing up to abuse their own children (Heineman, 1998). Parents with disabilities are more likely to have been abused as children and therefore might be at greater risk for abusing and neglecting their children than non-disabled parents (Sullivan and Knutson, 2000). It has been estimated that the sexual abuse among deaf children is about 50% (Sullivan, Vernon, and Scanlan, 1987) and large-scale abuse of children has been reported at several residential schools for the deaf (Sullivan, Brookhouser and Scanlan, 2000). We know that even to this day, many hearing parents cannot communicate with their deaf children, and that leaves deaf parents with poor developmental experiences and inadequate models of parenting and family life. Pollard and Rendon (1999) state that many deaf parents from a clinical population, or those who seek treatment, have themselves been neglected, have inadequate education, and have histories of poor family communication. These parents describe fears of incompetence in raising their children. As 90% of the children of deaf parents can hear, from Pollard and Rendon's clinical experience, the inability of some parents to identify with their children or to feel competent in raising a child that is different from themselves may cause old childhood memories of powerlessness to resurface and be played out with their own children.

Risk factors of child abuse

Other risk factors of parental abuse of children are low economic status coupled with low social status (Webster-Stratton, 1985), lack of social supports (Avison, Turner, Noh, 1986), history of sexual abuse, absence of mother's father during mother's childhood, previous history of psychiatric illness, low educational achievement and teen motherhood (Sidebotham and Golding, 2001). Coohey and Braun (1997) also found through their research of hearing adults that mothers most likely to physically abuse their children had early exposure to aggression from their own mothers and experienced domestic violence as adults. Deaf adults are traditionally under- or unemployed and may be isolated communicatively from hearing family members and neighbours, so that the development of social networks for support and information in child-rearing may be absent for many deaf parents. It has been estimated, for example, that between the ages of 20 and 24 years, the national unemployment rates for deaf adults are two-and-a-half times greater than for the same age group and deaf women's employment is even lower than that of deaf men (MacLeod-Gallinge, 1992).

California research

In order to describe the characteristics of deaf parents and their children at risk, seven Child Protective Services (CPS) agencies within the State of California in the United States were contacted. The purpose of the study was explained and agencies were requested to provide us with all cases from 1985 to 1990 involving deaf parents and their children. Specifically, we requested cases that had reached the dependency stage. In other words, at sometime within the previous 5 years, the court had taken jurisdiction over one or all the children within a family. Most often, dependency means that the child or children are removed from the home and placed in emergency shelter, in foster care, or with relatives for a brief to extended period of time. If the children are unable to return to the parents, adoption, long-term foster care or guardianship might be established. In some instances, the courts may take jurisdiction but return the child to the parents' home with on-going court supervision.

Of the seven counties contacted, all indicated that they had no system for identifying families through a computer search of records and that their agency had never kept any statistics on deaf parent families they had been in contact with. Although child disability is often coded for the CPS computer systems, parental disability typically is not. As a result, CPS supervisors had to question social workers personally to generate a list of cases. This method resulted in two counties being unable to identify any cases. Although social workers knew such cases existed, they could not recall the families' names. Another county could only identify one case that had recently been opened. Therefore, the cases reported in this study do not represent a random sample. Moreover, they may be indicative of more severe, notorious, or unusual cases that social workers could still remember. The large majority of the cases examined were currently 'open' cases at the time of review. In all, the study covered five counties in California involving forty-seven families with a total of one hundred and twenty children (79% hearing and 11% deaf, the remaining unknown).

After each county identified cases, the juvenile court in that county was petitioned for access to the records. In all counties permission was granted and the principal investigator and two research associates read each case file thoroughly and recorded information onto a form designed for that purpose. Data extracted from the case files included basic demographic information on the parents (and in most cases those individuals in the role of parents, such as mother's boyfriend); children's history of abuse or neglect; the services provided to the families by CPS; the allegations made of the parents under the Welfare and Institutions Code Section 300; children's ages, developmental history, and hearing status; the mental health status of the parents, and parental histories of substance abuse; child abuse and domestic violence. Information in the files varied by county, but typically included a family history taken by a social worker, psychological evaluations, copies of child abuse/neglect reporting forms, police reports, court reports, and financial information. While we were able to collect an enormous amount of data on each family, many files were incomplete in some areas, particularly on the backgrounds of adult males involved in the cases. In more than 60% of the cases, the families' primary social worker reviewed our notes for accuracy. A minor amount of missing data (usually updates not yet recorded in the files) were added to our form, but generally the social workers confirmed our accuracy.

All data were then transferred to a second coding form containing 252 data points. The principal investigator and a third research associate coded all 47 cases separately and compared coding on all cases. Any errors in coding were corrected.

To further contrast at-risk deaf parent families from functional families, eight intact families of deaf parents with hearing adolescent children were interviewed as part of this study. The children in these families had never been under jurisdiction of Child Protective Services. Each family was given the Conflicts Tactics Scale (CTS), which measures the self-reported amount of violence in the home. The CTS is a frequently used measure of child maltreatment (Straus et al, 1998). The CTS confirmed that these families were not 'at-risk' of child maltreatment or family violence. In contrast to the families where there is abuse and neglect, we found that non-abusive families were part of the Deaf community (involved in clubs and activities that kept them in close contact with other Deaf people who used American Sign Language); had warm feelings toward their own parents whether they were deaf or hearing; had a long employment history; did not have drug or substance abuse problems, and did not experience abuse or domestic violence as a child. These parents reported that they used friends, popular literature, and their own parents as resources for the typical challenges that parents encounter.

Research findings

Generally, it is our sense that the profile of deaf parents involved in abuse and neglect cases looks very different from the descriptions of deaf parent families found in the previous clinical literature that emphasized communication difficulties and occasionally speech, developmental, or learning delays. These parents were not just culturally or linguistically different from their children and fighting to navigate a hearing culture. The 47 families in our study more closely resembled current profiles of abusive hearing parents as described earlier in this paper and well-documented elsewhere. The cyclical nature of abuse and the role of environmental and societal stressors that lead hearing parents to abuse were also apparent in at-risk deaf parents.

Mothers

The deaf mothers were cited as the perpetrators of abuse or neglect in 52% of the allegations. Their average age at the time of birth of their first child was 21:9 years. Many mothers had oral skills sufficient for communication and/or had graduated from mainstream high school programmes. Thirty-six per cent of the mothers in this study were abused themselves during early childhood and at least 75% were victims of domestic or spousal violence. Almost all of the mothers were unemployed and on public assistance. Fifty-six per cent of the mothers had a reported drug history, mostly of cocaine and alcohol abuse. The true figure is probably higher, as many cases did not report mothers' drug/substance use. Most of the mothers were not currently married and most had never married. The majority of the mothers lived isolated, transient lives. As a group they appear to be victims themselves of all society's worst ills. Many relied on hearing family members but had little contact with other deaf people, although 66% of the mothers were American Sign Language (ASL) users and 19% used both voice and sign to communicate.

Fathers

Far less is known of the fathers in this study. Mothers tended toward multiple partners who were the suspected perpetrators of abuse or neglect in 39% of the allegations. Of mothers' most recent male companion, at least one-third were hearing (many were unable to sign and only able to grossly communicate with their deaf partners) and almost half had either abandoned the family or were incarcerated during the time of children's dependency. Forty per cent of the mother's current partners were unemployed. While mothers are more likely to be perpetrators of abuse, mothers' partners who are not the biological parents of the children are frequently cited as perpetrators. This phenomenon has also been noted in studies of hearing families (Margolin, 1992).

Children

Profiles of children identified in our study also depicted more severe problems than reported in previous clinical studies. One hundred and twenty children were identified in the 47 families studied and, within these families, 82% had been reported as abused or neglected. Seventy-nine per cent of the children were hearing, 11% deaf, and 10% had unknown hearing status. All but one deaf child in the study was a reported victim. For these families with a deaf child, the expectation that communication and identification between parent and child would be more 'normal' did not offer protection. Seventeen per cent of the children who were hearing (plus three additional children currently under evaluation) had been placed in special education programmes or early developmental enrichment programmes because of language delays, emotional disturbance, behavioural disturbance, academic delays, or general developmental/motor delay. An additional 23% of the children had identified delays or disturbances, but were not receiving specialized educational services. Fifty one children in all were identified as having one or a combination of behavioural, developmental, and/or emotional problems; drug abuse, motor delays, academic delays, or language delays. In all families, the children were placed out of the home for either a short-term or long-term period. Most children had several placements, bouncing from foster care, back to parents, to relatives, and back again. Several children had made suicide attempts and a few had begun abuse of younger children.

It is impossible to determine conclusively the outcome for the children studied (as many cases are ongoing, closed and then reopened, or appear again in other jurisdictions) but our analysis does indicate that most children had several placements. Fifty seven per cent of the children studied were placed with grandparents or other relatives at some period during their court dependency. The difficulty of reparenting grandchildren who have been emotionally and physically traumatized must be overwhelming. Presumably many of these grandparents had failed to parent effectively or protect their own deaf children from either institutional or familial abuse. There is no evidence that these grandparents *can* successfully guide their grandchildren in stable, non-abusive homes. Children are frequently reunified with their parents, but often only temporarily until another instance of abuse or neglect is reported. Forty five per cent of the family case files contained three to nine allegation reports.

Services

Although the study took place in large urban counties, few families with a deaf parent received more than short-term individual or family therapy. Other services provided to parents included interpreter services, transportation services (such as bus vouchers) to travel to and from appointments, and alcohol and drug treatment. In most programmes, communication was geared toward hearing individuals even though most mothers in our study communicated in American Sign Language or 'home signs'. In our sample, an interpreter was usually available for intervention programmes, but the content in many cases remained inaccessible for the parents (for example, extensive reliance on reading material or references to unfamiliar hearing cultural media such as TV shows or movies). Deafness often prohibited parents from using intervention programmes to gain the kind of social support that hearing parents might gain from such contacts. In substance abuse treatment programmes in particular, the bonding and support amongst deaf clients is an essential component of the recovery process. Programmes that use only sign language inter-preters and do not have signing staff are often unsuccessful in their treatment approaches (Guthmann and Blozis, 2001). Only seven families were provided with parenting classes focusing on the needs of deaf fami-lies. Treatment for children consisted most often of short-term therapy, referrals for special education or early child development programs. Twenty eight of the 47 families received psychotherapeutic services for the children, and 27 families received psychotherapy for the parents. Yet, only one family of the 47 was supported with practical services such as in-home independent living skills, nutrition instruction, services of a public health nurse, housing assistance, or respite care. While the availability of psychotherapy to deaf parents and their children should be a component of reunification services, parents who are drug addicted or who are lin-guistically impaired may see limited results from such insight-oriented psychotherapy, especially if services are short term. Only seven families received parenting classes where other deaf parents were present. Parenting classes that are directed at hearing participants may do little to alleviate the social isolation that many of these abusive and neglectful deaf parents experience and may not be appropriate for the special needs of these parents who may be linguistically or cognitively impaired.

Conclusions

It is not the purpose of this study to state if deaf parents are more or less abusive than hearing parents. Our data, however, can be compared pro-portionately to available statistics of the general population within the communities we studied in relation to ethnic diversity and types of abuse reported. While all our cases were drawn from California, the state's 1990 reporting/allegation rate (California Consortium for the Prevention of Child Abuse, 1990) matches very closely the rate reported in our sample, sup-porting the notion that at-risk deaf families have a similar profile to hearing families. In relation to ethnic diversity, while the numbers of Caucasian and Hispanic families identified in this study were fairly consistent with pro-portions of diversity within the five counties studied, African-American families were over-represented and Asian families unrepresented. This study also closely replicated findings of a study of 206 children from hear-ing families conducted in Massachusetts (Jellinek et al., 1992), which identified similar psychological and substance issues for mothers, as well as poverty, and the overwhelmingly absence of data on fathers.

Generally, it is our sense that the profile of deaf parents involved in abuse and neglect cases, which are serious enough to warrant the courts taking jurisdiction over all or some of the children in these families, looks remarkably similar to profiles of at-risk hearing parents. This differs from previously reported clinical studies of deaf parents whose children were experiencing mental health problems, or from interview studies that focused on difficulties around identity and communication (Preston, 1994). Our data suggests that higher percentages than might be expected, of deaf women whose children are at risk, are involved in relationships with hearing men. Frequently, these men are unable to communicate in the mothers' primary language, and the nature of the relationships is usually transient and violent. The data also indicates that a high percentage of mothers themselves were abused as children, are victims of domestic violence, are likely to be substance abusers, and are overwhelmingly poor and unemployed. There were no indications that these families were part of a Deaf community. Abusive behaviours and drug-addiction would create an insurmountable barrier to access to this supportive community.

Again, while these descriptors look fairly similar to that of hearing abusive parents, we know that access to services for deaf parents is severely limited and usually does not take into consideration their linguistic, cognitive, or social support needs. The families at greatest risk represent a multitude of problems, with deafness being just one component of focus. Effective interventions must take into account poverty, family involvement in substance abuse, domestic violence, and the needs of single mothers. Care must be taken to work with children, as the next cycle of abuse is already emerging within this population.

It is not easy to confront the severity of problems of deaf parents 'at risk', but it is essential that the mental health and deaf education community address this segment of the population. Efforts to increase early parent–child communication, provide adequate job preparation and training, and have accessible mental health, substance abuse, and violence prevention programmes, may make some impact. These families fall between the Deaf and hearing worlds, and the gap can have tragic consequences.

References

Avison W, Turner R, Noh S (1986) Screening for problem parenting: preliminary evidence on a promising instrument. Child Abuse and Neglect 10: 157–70.

Barth RP (1991) An experimental evaluation of in-home child abuse prevention services. Child Abuse and Neglect 15(4): 363–75.

Bene A (1977) The influence of deaf and dumb parents on a child's development. Psychoanalytic Study of the Child 32: 175–94.

Bunde L (1979) Deaf Parents – Hearing Children: Toward a Greater Understanding of the Unique Aspects, Needs, and Problems Relative to the Communication Factors caused by Deafness. Washington DC: Registry of Interpreters for the Deaf.

California Consortium for the Prevention of Child Abuse (1990) Child Abuse Incidents in California 1980-1989. Sacramento CA: California Consortium for the Prevention of Child Abuse.

Charlson E (1989) Social Cognition and Self-concept of Hearing Adolescents with Deaf Parents. Unpublished doctoral dissertation, University of California, Berkeley and San Francisco State University.

Coohey C, Braun N (1997) Toward an integrated framework for understanding child physical abuse. Child Abuse and Neglect 21:1081–94.

Dent K (1982) Two daughters of a deaf mute mother: implications for ego and cognitive development. Journal of the American Academy of Psychoanalysis 10: 427–41.

Frankenburg FR, Sloman L, Perry A (1985) Issues in the therapy of hearing children with deaf parents. Canadian Journal of Psychiatry 30(2): 98–102.

Guthmann D, Blozis S (2001) Unique issues faced by deaf individuals entering substance abuse treatment and following discharge. American Annals of the Deaf 146: 294–303.

Halbreich U (1979) Influence of deaf-mute parents on the character of their offspring. Acuta Psychiatria Scandinava 59: 129–38.

Heineman T (1998) The Abused Child: Psychodynamic Understanding and Treatment. New York NY: Guilford Press.

Jellinek MS, Murphy JM, Poitrast F, Quinn D, Bishop SJ, Goshko M (1992) Serious child mistreatment in Massachusetts: the course of 206 children through the courts. Child Abuse and Neglect 16(2): 179–85.

MacLeod-Gallinge J (1992) The career status of deaf women: a comparative look. American Annals of the Deaf 137: 315–25.

Maestas y Moores M (1981) A descriptive study of communication modes and pragmatic functions used by three prelinguistic, profoundly deaf mothers with their infants one to six months of age in their homes. Dissertation Abstracts International (4) 7-A: 3049-3050.

Margolin L (1992) Child abuse by mothers' boyfriends: why the over-representation? Child Abuse and Neglect 16: 541–51.

Pollard R, Rendon M (1999) Mixed deaf-hearing families: maximizing benefits and minimizing risks. Journal of Deaf Studies and Deaf Education 4: 156–61.

Preston P (1994) Mother Father Deaf: Living Between Sound and Silence. Cambridge MA: Harvard University Press.

Preston P (1996) Chameleon voices: interpreting for deaf parents. Social Science and Medicine 42: 1681–90.

Rea C, Bonvillian J, Richards H (1988) Mother-infant interactive behaviors: the impact of maternal deafness. American Annals of the Deaf 133: 317–24.

Rienzi B (1990) Influence and adaptability in families with deaf parents and hearing children. American Annals of the Deaf 135: 402–8.

Robinson L, Weathers O (1974) Family therapy of deaf parents and hearing children: a new dimension in psychotherapeutic intervention. American Annals of the Deaf 119: 325–30.

Sanders M (1984) An Examination of the Academic Achievement and Social/emotional Adjustment of Normally Hearing Children Reared by Deaf Parents. Unpublished doctoral dissertation, University of Tennessee.

Sidebotham P, Golding J (2001) Child maltreatment in the 'children of the nineties': a longitudinal study of parental risk factors. Journal of Child Abuse and Neglect 25: 1177–200.

Singleton J, Tittle M (2000) Deaf parents and their hearing children. Journal of Deaf Studies and Deaf Education 5: 221–36.

Straus M., Hamby S, Finkelhor D, Moore D, Runyan D (1998) Identification of child maltreatment with the parent–child Conflict Tactics Scales: development with psychometric data for a national sample of American parents. Child Abuse and Neglect 22: 249–70.

Sullivan P, Brookhouse P, Scanlan M (2000) Maltreatment of deaf and hard of hearing children. In Hindley P, Kitson N (eds) (2000) Mental Health and Deafness. London: Whurr, pp. 149–84.

Sullivan PM, Knutson JF (2000) Maltreatment and disabilities: a population-based epidemiological study. Child Abuse and Neglect 24(10): 1257–73.

Sullivan P, Vernon M, Scanlan J (1987) Sexual abuse of the deaf youth. American Annals of the Deaf 132: 256–62.

Taska R, Rhoads J (1981) Psychodynamic issues in a hearing woman raised by deaf parents. The Psychiatric Forum 10: 11–16.

Tendler R (1975) Maternal Correlates of Differentiation in Hearing Children of the Deaf. Unpublished doctoral dissertation, Yeshiva University.

Wagenheim H (1985) Aspects of the analysis of an adult son of deaf-mute parents. Journal of the American Psychoanalytic Association 33: 413–35.

Webster-Stratton C (1985) Comparison of abusive and non-abusive families with conduct-disordered children. American Journal of Orthorpsychiatry 55: 59–69.

CHAPTER 16

Paediatric cochlear implantation

EMMA SANDS AND SUSAN CROCKER

Introduction

In addition to representing a significant advancement in technology and medical fields, cochlear implantation has generated considerable interest surrounding the ethical issues and choices associated with the procedure. This has been particularly pertinent over the past 20 years when children first became recipients of the device.

Whether a child receives a cochlear implant or not is a complex decision made by the family and the assessment team. Throughout, the chapter will emphasize the influence of families' experience (for example, coping), expectations and beliefs relating to both the child's deafness and cochlear implantation itself, which are themselves subject to personal and sociocultural influences. The impact of these factors on families' decisions regarding implantation, aspects of outcome following implantation and degree of parental satisfaction, highlights the importance for services to be aware of their complex inter-play though assessment, surgery and habilitation.

This chapter will follow the child and parents' journey from diagnosis through the pre-implant assessment and decision making, to surgery and (re)habilitation.

Psychological perspectives; pre-implantation

Traditionally, research into childhood disability, non-specific to deafness, has tended to focus on the adjustment of the index child. More recently studies have looked at the child's social environment and the family's accommodation to disability, which in turn may affect the adjustment of the child. Recognition of the influential role of families has led to an increase in research investigating the relationship between family factors (for example, response to diagnosis, coping) and outcome following cochlear implantation.

Parental reaction to diagnosis

Parents' own experience of deafness, and whether they had any suspicion of the hearing impairment, can influence their initial reaction to diagnosis and subsequent response to a cochlear implant.

It is widely thought that hearing parents react by grieving with the news of their child's deafness, both in terms of their emotional and behavioural responses. The Transitional Model helps us to have a structure for understanding this (Luterman, 1979; Moses, 1985). The initial affective state is typically defined as a period of shock, characterized by the subjective experience of numbness. Many parents participating in a qualitative, retrospective study commented that their unfamiliarity with deafness, both within their own families and in the wider society, contributed to their initial shock (Christiansen and Leigh, 2002). The second stage of recognition, characterized by a multitude of intense feelings, defines the period when parents begin to recognize the severity and permanence of their child's deafness. Christiansen and Leigh (2002) found that parents described their emotional experience in terms of frustration, disappointment, despair, anger, helplessness, confusion and guilt. The parents also commented that they felt these emotional responses were justified given their pre-existing assumptions and expectations about their children and their future. The etiology of the child's hearing loss and the context surrounding the diagnosis may influence parents' emotional response. For example, if the child is deafened following traumatic illness or injury, parents may describe feeling relieved at the outcome compared to the possibility of death or surviving with health concerns they perceive to be more serious (Christiansen and Leigh, 2002).

Parents in the subsequent stage of denial may know their child is deaf at a cognitive level but are unable to recognize the permanence or implications of this and may therefore persevere with searching for a cure. In the final stage of acknowledgement and constructive action parents are more able to discuss the deafness, assess the reality of the situation, assimilate necessary information and make decisions regarding intervention.

Thus, it is easy to see how the impact of parents' reactions to deafness affects their decisions surrounding cochlear implantation. The following section will discuss the application of a coping paradigm in this respect and the implications for cochlear implant services.

Application of a coping paradigm

Parents' appraisal of their child's deafness, or the meaning they attach to this event, has the potential for causing stress. The applied transitional model proposes that whether parents perceive the deafness as desirable or undesirable, disruptive, controllable or important, has a direct effect on the mourning process (Kampfe, 1989). This model also suggests that individual or situational variables, such as parents' own experiences, personal resources, social support availability and the nature of the deafness or circumstances surrounding the diagnosis, moderate the relationship between parents' perception of the deafness and their reaction.

The stress-coping model (Folkman, Scjaefer and Lazarus, 1979) emphasizes the importance of appraisal and proposes that when an event is perceived to be stressful, people attempt to minimize the impact of stress through coping behaviours. Coping is conceptualized as an ongoing process consisting of a series of appraisals and responses to the stressful event. Thus, the coping strategies employed influence outcome. When the transitional model is applied to parental reaction to the child's deafness, the ultimate outcome is achieving and maintaining the constructive action stage of the mourning process. According to Folkman, Scjaefer and Lazarus (1979) coping strategies either regulate emotion and adjust the person–environment relationship, or are focused on active problem solving. Parents implementing emotion-focused coping may seek out other parents of deaf children to validate their feelings, while those using problem-focused coping may be more likely to request literature and enquire about opportunities and resources for their child (Fehrer-Prout, 1996).

Implications of a coping paradigm for cochlear implant teams

Parents of deaf children make various decisions for their child (for example, about the auditory device, communication mode, educational placement), and both the type of option selected and the approach taken by parents towards these decisions can be conceptualized within a coping paradigm. Cochlear implantation is one possible option and is also a prime example of an intervention and approach to deafness, which carries various beliefs and assumptions at an individual and societal level. It is therefore important that cochlear implant teams assess families for their position in the grieving process, their coping strategies for managing with a deaf child and their beliefs and assumptions about deafness and cochlear implants.

Assessment

In most centres, the assessment for a cochlear implant involves a multidisciplinary team. For psychologists in teams assessing a child and family's ability to consent to a cochlear implant, understanding a child's learning abilities and possible additional difficulties – as well as parental emotions (for example, coping, grieving) – seem to be their predominant role.

Expectations of parents

A key element for assessment is the expectations families have for cochlear implants and these in turn are likely to be influenced by their response to the child's deafness and their coping style (Downs et al., 1986; Kampfe et al., 1993). Cochlear implantation is an intervention surrounded by expectations, with implications for both the pre-implantation, decision-making stage and parental satisfaction and outcome after implantation.

It is argued that realistic parental expectations optimize outcome and ensure they have a clear understanding of the benefits and limitations of this and alternative options to make an informed choice on behalf of their child (Kampfe et al., 1993; Vernon, 1994). Parents in the early recognition stage might be seeking a cochlear implant without having adjusted to the meaning and implications of having a deaf child in their family. Due to the experience of strong emotions, parents may not be able to focus on information regarding the potential outcome and limitations of the intervention. Parents in denial might be seeking an implant as a miracle cure to restore their child's hearing to normal, while parents in the constructive action stage are more likely to recognize the possibility for an implant to provide additional auditory input rather than offer a complete or immediate cure. Parents in this final phase of the process may also be interested in exploring a variety of communication options and thinking about identity issues for children in both deaf and hearing communities.

Implications for teams

As hearing parents may not have had much exposure to implanted children, opportunities for their expectations to be confirmed or rejected are limited. Thus, parents need to be introduced to a range of potential outcomes through the assimilation of objective information, video material and contact with other parents (who regard the implant as negative as well as positive). It may also be helpful for parents to consider alternative methods of communication and to meet families who elected not to proceed with implantation for their child. Parents with a desire for a hearing child may be more likely to maintain stronger expectations for implantation, further indicating the need for families to be supported appropriately, according to their position in the grieving process. Finally, expectations are strengthened when other members of the family or social network share similar expectations.

Implications for parental satisfaction

Ensuring the parents have realistic expectations before embarking on cochlear implantation for their child is critically important, as expectations are thought to influence outcome. Performance indicators post-implantation that match parents' expectations, are likely to result in feelings of satisfaction, even if the positive changes are not large or immediate (Perold, 2001). Satisfaction, in turn, positively reinforces parents' compliance with the habilitation programme. Conversely, parents who experience a discrepancy between their expectations and the reality post-implantation may feel disappointed with the outcome. It has been suggested that inappropriately high expectations increase the likelihood that implant use will be discontinued due to inadequate parental support and poor compliance (Kampfe et al., 1993), while expectations that are too low may limit the child's development due to insufficient parental encouragement and commitment towards progress (Tye-Murray, 1993).

Expectations and parental anxiety

Parental expectations are not static, but are thought to fluctuate at significant milestones in the child's life and developmental progression with a cochlear implant. In an interview study, mothers were found to re-experience aspects of the grieving process at times of stress or disappointment and their expectations regarding implantation were subsequently influenced by varying degrees of hope or knowledge (Perold, 2001). During the pre-implant assessment stage, knowledge-based expectations were found to dominate and maternal anxiety was low. The switch-on period, after surgery, was characterized by increased anxiety and, consequently, mothers tended to rely less on their knowledge and more on hope-based expectations. This association was particularly evident with increasing disparity between mothers' pre-existing expectations and outcomes following switch-on of the device. When the children started responding to new sounds, anxiety decreased and knowledge-based expectations once again dominated. The non-appearance of meaningful speech, however, gave rise to increased anxiety and the potential for mothers to doubt their implant decision. Together these findings suggest that teams have a role in ensuring that parental anxiety is addressed by providing accurate information and opportunities for asking questions, thereby encouraging increased reliance on knowledge rather than on potential unrealistic hopes for outcome.

Consent from parent/child

Consent issues are very pertinent to elective surgery. From legal information, it is possible to understand where we stand in relation to children and young people (Mental Health Act Code of Practice, 1999). Where a child is under the age of 16, whether or not a child has an implant (operation) is ultimately the parent's decision. However, if the child or young person is deemed competent to provide consent then their view has to be taken into consideration. Where views differ, the primary obligation is to consider the child's best interests. For very young children, consent cannot be sought, however, understanding their current relationship to a number of factors needs to be taken into account alongside parental views. Some of these factors are explored later in this chapter and are as follows:

- motivation to wear hearing aids;
- interest in using any residual hearing;
- ability to cope with change;
- response to medical/audiological intervention;
- response to coming to the centre for multiple assessment visits;
- additional difficulties;
- predicted ability to use the information that the implant will potentially supply.

For older children (over age 6) an estimation of their self-esteem, self-image, confidence, culture (BSL/Oral), peer group and their understanding about implants also need to be taken into account. When children consistently express that they do not want an implant, then a team should not proceed.

Developmental assessment

Understanding how a child thinks and feels is important, not only in relation to decision making for or against implantation, but also to predict rate of development with an implant and to think about needs in relation to re/habilitation. This will have an effect on both parental expectations and the amount and type of multidisciplinary team input required of each individual child.

Play

Play assessment is useful for all children pre-adolescence, but especially for younger children where a more formal cognitive assessment is not possible due to age or behaviour, or if the child has significant additional difficulties. Play can also augment any formal assessment and is useful in a number of ways. Specifically, it enables one

- to see the range of toys that are explored – for example, just concrete toys (construction, puzzles) or a mix of mediums (drawing, cause and effect, puzzles, dolls, tea set);
- to look at specific skills – for example, colour matching, grouping of categories of toys, naming of items and so forth;

- to look at emotional development, drawing is the best medium as well as play assessment;
- to see how a child is playing with the toys – for example, exploratory, relational, self-pretend, decentred-pretend, symbolic or imaginative play;
- to look at a child's concentration, attention and problem-solving skills;
- to see how a child will let the assessor or parent/sibling join them in play, ability to take turns, adapt their play or include other people's ideas.

Communication

Alongside the play assessment, communication can be assessed in relation to both pre-verbal and informal verbal/signed skills – for example, who a child goes to when showing pleasure, or for needs (drink, toilet, hurt). Looking at children's relationships with parents and siblings will be informative for thinking about attachment and also whether there may be any underlying disorder of communication. Ideally a speech and language therapist will formally assess a child's language skills.

Cognition

Most psychologists on cochlear implant teams administer a basic cognitive assessment to all candidates, as the child's cognitive profile is useful in identifying areas of difficulty and providing additional information regarding the possible expected outcome following implantation. Most commonly used assessment tools are the Leiter-R, a non-verbal assessment battery (Roid and Miller, 1997) and the Snijders-Ooman Nonverbal Intelligence Test (Snijders, Tellegen and Laros, 1989). Non-verbal measures are used to assess ability that is not related to language skills.

Additional difficulties

Related to a child's communication, learning and play we can see that many children who are assessed for a cochlear implant have additional difficulties. This is not surprising as the literature states that deafness is associated with additional difficulties in approximately 25% to 40% of cases (Rawlings and Gentile, 1970; Schein and Delk, 1974; Flathouse, 1979).

In an as yet unpublished study looking at all children assessed over an 18-month period at a paediatric cochlear implant centre, it was felt that 40% had complex needs (Hare and Crocker, in preparation). There has been thought in the past that children with significant social communication or learning needs would not be implanted, but this seems to vary from team to team. Complexity is always assessed on an individual basis looking at the likely benefits to communication and auditory awareness versus the possible negative effects, such as surgery, parental and child stress, amount of habilitation required and whether a child can be programmed audiologically.

Behaviour

Assessment of the child's behaviour may also guide teams and indicate whether behavioural intervention might be required, prior to surgery to optimize progress. Observation and discussion in a clinical setting, together with standardized questionnaires, are useful assessment techniques in this regard. It is important, however, that the behaviour rating scale selected provides clinically relevant information and has good face validity, and that these measures are developed specifically for use with deaf children. A widely used measure among child mental health services, and often used by cochlear implant teams, is the Child Behaviour Checklist (CBCL) rated by parents (Achenbach and Edelbrock, 1991). This is not specifically designed for a deaf population, however the availability of two standardized versions of the CBCL for children aged 2 to 3 years and 4 to 18 years makes this measure a popular choice. A study investigating the detection of behavioural and emotional problems among deaf children compared the utility of the CBCL with a parent checklist developed specifically for the young deaf population. Both scales were found to have a high degree of agreement on problem severity (Vostanis et al., 1997), and the authors concluded that the sound psychometric properties of the CBCL allow for a closer estimate of clinical cases.

Parental motivation

Whether children wear their hearing devices is an important measure in most cases of both the child's motivation for listening and the parents persistence with encouraging the child to wear the device. But device wearing can be much more than this. If children wear their hearing aids before implantation then it is a good predictor that they will wear a cochlear implant (Knutson et al., 1997). This not only reflects whether children can pick up on any sounds but also whether they will tolerate wearing a hearing device.

Assessing the families' willingness and ability to be actively involved in (re)habilitation is an important part of the assessment for suitability for an implant, and indeed hearing-aid use has been identified as a key indicator in predicting families' participation in this process (Downs et al., 1986). Hearing-aid use itself may indicate parents' level of acceptance of their children's deafness, further highlighting the importance of including these issues in a comprehensive assessment for a cochlear implant.

Motivation has been found to be the best predictor for a successful outcome. In the case of a young child the motivation needs to stem from the parents and those associated with the child, whereas with an adolescent, this needs primarily to be internal (Knutson et al., 1997).

Adolescent cochlear implant candidates

There are many issues pertinent for adolescents that may influence their implant use, such as consent, their own expectations, or issues relating to their identity and self-image. The authors also identified the need to consider the attitudinal culture towards cochlear implants of the child/young person's educational environment, as this may impact on implant use.

Motivation

When adolescents are referred for assessment, teams need to be mindful of the unique issues that are pertinent for this group and tailor the assessment accordingly. It is essential that the adolescent's own reasons for investigating or pursuing this option are identified and it has been recommended that the young person has the opportunity to discuss this initially alone with the team member (Downs et al., 1986). It is possible that the adolescent may hold expectations that are unrealistic and different from those of their parents. It is also important that young people are presented with all the relevant information appropriately so they have an adequate understanding of implantation and the various alternative options, to enable them to take an active role in the decision-making process together with their family and the team.

Informed consent

How teams address the issue of informed consent, and prepare adolescents preoperatively, differs depending on the age and developmental level of the young person. The application of a developmental framework in preparing adolescents for surgery and hospitalization generally has been described (Busen, 2001) and is useful in understanding the issues specific for cochlear implantation. Understanding the adolescents' cognitive and psychosocial functioning is crucial for teams to be able to provide information and reassurance in a meaningful and useful way.

Development and self-image

Cognitive development in adolescence is characterized by the transition from concrete operational thought to formal operational thought (the ability to think logically and use deductive and abstract reasoning) (Piaget, 1952). Between 11 and 14 years of age, teenagers have a limited capacity to anticipate future events and therefore find it difficult to reflect in an abstract way on the potential benefits of implantation. At this age, it may be helpful to involve other teenage implant users in providing information, to assist the candidate in viewing potential outcome more concretely. By 15 to 17 years adolescents are more able to understand the consequences of events, although conformity with the peer group is of primary importance with issues of body image particularly salient. At this stage adolescents are often sensitive to any aspect of their physical appearance that contributes to them feeling different from their peers, indicating that the young person's feelings about wearing the external device needs to be explored pre-operatively. If this is perceived by the user to be conspicuous it may result in feelings of difference and social isolation (Evans, 1989).

Identity

Associated with the issue of self-image is that of individual identity and it may be helpful to talk with the young people about their own culture and social network, as this may indicate possible influences and pressures impinging on them. Thus, from the adolescent's perspective, the risks of surgery and expectations from rehabilitation may be less important than other psychosocial needs, such as physical appearance or potential disruption to school routines or social activities.

A study using the young people themselves as participants found that deaf adolescents, with and without cochlear implants, held similar beliefs about their identity in relation to hearing/deaf culture (Wald and Knutson, 2000). Both groups responded to statements reflecting a balanced view of hearing and deaf culture, indicating a high degree of bicultural identity. The authors suggest on the basis of these findings that adolescents with cochlear implants are able to develop a social identity that embraces both hearing and deaf cultures, rather than feeling they are not firmly affiliated with either group.

Preventing non-use

Christiansen and Leigh (2002) reported that a main theme of interview among a group of adolescent and young adult implantees was that the role they had in deciding about implantation initially influenced whether they continued using the device. Interestingly, the users who reported that they were too young to participate in the initial decision-making process were generally satisfied with their implant. Based on studies of adolescent users and non-users, practical ideals for involving adolescents in the decision-making process have been described (Chute, 1993). These ideas included the following components:

- training (individuals are encouraged to wear a vibrotactile device, to help them realize the commitment aspect of rehabilitation and for them to experience wearing an external device);
- education (encompassing all aspects of cochlear implant performance and surgery);
- expectations assessment;
- networking (meeting other implanted teenagers);
- supportive counselling (ongoing during assessment and post-implantation).

Decision making: familial and professional considerations

Cochlear implant teams have a role in guiding families through the decision-making process. The complexity surrounding this phase is apparent due to the elective nature of the surgical intervention and the uncertainty regarding the precise degree of predictive benefit that a cochlear implant may provide. In a retrospective interview study parents reported that the primary motivating factor for proceeding with implantation was their desire for their child to function as a 'normal', hearing person (Kluwin and Stewart, 2000). Other key factors identified were the parents' own frustration with their child's communication and the influence of significant family members or the child's teacher. The first two of these factors again highlight the relationship between parents' experience and assumptions about having a deaf child and their reasons for selecting implantation.

The results of Kluwin and Stewart's (2000) study indicated two further types of decision-making sequence related to the primary source of information about cochlear implants. Firstly, parents who initially learned about implantation from medical professionals and continued to use this contact as their exclusive information source rated communication difficulties or their desire for a hearing child as the highest motivating factor to proceed. Parents who learned about cochlear implants via their own sources, such as the Internet or from other parents, tended to be more active in seeking out information, and hence the opinion of others was found to have the greatest influence. The results tentatively suggest that information presented in a medical setting may carry the assumption that deafness is curable. Teams therefore need to be mindful of parents' position in the grieving process and present information accordingly. The beliefs that families hold about each option may need to be assessed before guiding them through a problem-solving process that involves carefully considering the benefits and limitations or risks of each option. Some families may ultimately decide that the potential benefits of implantation do not outweigh the associated risks or commitment required, choosing instead to pursue an alternative auditory device and communication mode.

Throughout the assessment, cochlear implant teams are also continuously assessing and making decisions from audiological, medical, educational, speech and language and psychological perspectives. The themes highlighted in this discussion have addressed issues of coping, parental expectations, adjustment to deafness, development and consent, forming an important part of the assessment. While teams do not only use this understanding to inform a pass-fail decision about the child's suitability as a cochlear implant candidate, it can often suggest further recommendations for assessment and intervention prior to proceeding with surgery. Thus, the one goal of assessment is to establish a baseline to allow the prediction and implementation of successful implant use (Downs et al., 1986).

Assessment measures

To assist teams in decision making, questionnaires may be used in conjunction with clinical interviews. Measures assessing expectations may be particularly helpful in guiding teams about whether further information or counselling is required. They may be completed directly by an adolescent candidate – for example, House Ear Institute Cochlear Implant Questionnaire (House, 1980) – or by parents – for example, Kampfe-Harrison Modified House Ear Institute Cochlear Implant Questionnaire (Kampfe et al., 1993).

Once the overall assessment is finalized, teams may complete a summary scale together, for example, Child Implant Profile (ChIP) (Hellman et al., 1991). This will indicate their level of concern for the key aspects of the multidisciplinary assessment, incorporating the psychosocial elements. At this point, the team and the family ultimately discuss the plan for proceeding with implantation.

Preparation for surgery and habilitation

All children and parents require preparation for surgery at differing levels, dependent on specific factors, for example, parents' or child's previous response to hospitalization, medical procedures, child's ability to cope with change (Lynch, Craddock and Crocker, 1999). Also specific difficulties may have been uncovered, such as a child's or parent's needle phobia, or a child's fear of gas. Generally a team will offer a package to support this preparation, which would include:

- parental information about the stay in hospital e.g. what to bring, what to expect;
- child and sibling information about what will happen in hospital e.g. in the style of a colouring book;
- video showing the surgery (if parent's desire) and the size of the bandage on the child's head after surgery;
- a hospital visit with the whole family to see where the child will be having the operation;
- additional sessions with a psychologist (if required) to work through specific issues such as needle phobia;
- meeting with other families to discuss all aspects of the operation and habilitation procedures.

After surgery the children and families will need similar preparation for the habilitation process. Helping children and families to feel informed, in control and to have ownership of the new device (at their own pace and according to their developmental needs) will aid outcome (Peterson and Shigatomi, 1981).

Psychological perspectives: after implantation

Psychosocial outcome

There is a wealth of research into the physical consequences following a cochlear implant such as speech discrimination and language improvements, however, research investigating the psychosocial consequences of cochlear implantation for the child and family is limited. While there is some evidence for the effectiveness of interventions addressing parental adjustment to coping with a deaf child, as previously outlined, there are fewer outcome studies investigating parental stress and psychological adjustment following paediatric cochlear implantation. Indeed, the available evidence does not support the hypothesis that a cochlear implant reduces parental stress and emotional difficulty (Quittner, Thompson, Steck and Rouiller, 1991). Caution is needed in interpreting these results due to the small sample size, however they highlight the importance of parents receiving continued support in the post-implantation phase. The child's behaviour is a further factor identified in this discussion as forming an important part of the assessment, which may be used to provide some indication of future implant use (Knutson et al., 2000a).

Some of the studies investigating psychosocial outcome have focused on aspects of the child's social functioning and social relationships following cochlear implantation. A longitudinal study employing both quantitative and qualitative methodology to explore peer relationships, reported that 68% of parents indicated an improvement post-implantation, in how their child interacted with other children. The parents tended to attribute this to their child's greater social extroversion (Bat-Chava and Deignan, 2001). The findings from this study also indicated a significant relationship between the quality of peer relationships and the child's oral communication ability, post-implantation. A study looking specifically at sibling relationships found no difference between cochlear implant and hearing aid users in the quality of their relationships with siblings (Bat-Chava and Martin, 2002), although this study did not compare the quality of sibling relationships before and after implantation. One longitudinal study investigating the relationship between audiological benefit and psychological change reported no evidence of any detrimental effects of cochlear implantation on children's psychological well being (Knutson et al., 2000b).

Quality of life

Many of the studies described so far have used parental report to assess change following implantation and there are few studies documenting children's own perceptions of benefit or problems associated with implantation. One retrospective study that did measure quality of life changes perceived by the cochlear implant recipients and their parents, found that both groups reported substantial benefits and few problems following implantation (Chmiel, Sutton and Jenkins, 2000). Parents and children in this study rated the perceived benefit and problems of the cochlear implant for each of the specified areas. Clearly, quality of life questionnaires are valuable as clinical tools to evaluate the benefit of cochlear implantation but further research is needed to develop and standardize such measures.

Conclusion

The role of the clinical psychologist in paediatric cochlear implant teams is certainly multifaceted. As illustrated throughout this chapter, the psychologist plays an important part in assessing a child's suitability for an implant and helping the family through the decision-making process, involving the child/adolescent in this process in an age-appropriate manner. The psychologist must tailor the assessment and presentation of information in preparing the child for surgery and habilitation according to both their age and developmental level. However, a comprehensive assessment also considers the complex interplay of personal and socio-cultural factors influencing each family's own approach towards assessment and cochlear implantation. Psychologists draw upon their knowledge of child development and theoretical models of stress and coping during assessment. However, with additional longitudinal research investigating the psychosocial outcomes for the child and family following implantation, the assessment process may be further enhanced with subsequent improvements in satisfaction and device use. A further direction for future work in this field to aid assessment and optimize outcome, is the development of assessment tools and evaluation measures for deaf paediatric populations, to enable more research into psychological domains to be completed.

References

Achenbach TM, Edelbrock C (1991) Manual for the Child Behavior Checklist. Burlington VT: University of Vermont.

Bat-Chava Y, Deignan E (2001) Peer relationships of children with cochlear implants. Journal of Deaf Studies and Deaf Education 6: 186–99.

Bat-Chava Y, Martin D (2002) Sibling relationships of deaf children: The impact of child and family characteristics. Rehabilitation Psychology 47(1): 73–91.

Busen NH (2001) Perioperative preparation of the adolescent surgical patient: a review. AORN Journal 73(2): 337–41.

Chmiel R, Sutton L, Jenkins H (2000) Quality of life in children with cochlear implants. Annals of Otology, Rhinology and Laryngology 185(supplement): 103–5.

Christiansen JBL, Leigh IW (2002) Cochlear implants in children: Ethics and Choices. Washington DC: Gallaudet University Press.

Chute P (1993) Cochlear implants in adolescents. Cochlear Implants 48: 210–15.

Downs MP, Campos CT, Firemark R, Martin E, Myres W (1986) Psychosocial issues surrounding children receiving cochlear implants. Seminars in Hearing 7(4): 383–405.

Evans JW (1989) Thoughts on the psychosocial implications of cochlear implantation in children. In E Kessler (ed.) Cochlear Implants in Young Deaf Children. Boston MA: College-Hill Publications.

Fehrer-Prout T (1996) Stress and coping in families with deaf children. Journal of Deaf Studies and Deaf Education 1(3): 155–66.

Flathouse VE (1979) Multihandicapped deaf children and public law 94-142. Exceptional Children 45: 560–65.

Folkman S, Scjaefer C, Lazarus R (1979) Cognitive processes as mediators of stress and coping. In Warburton V (ed.) Human Stress and Cognition. New York: John Wiley.

Hare J, Crocker SR (In preparation) Profiling the complex needs of children referred to a paediatric cochlear implant centre. RNTNE Paediatric Cochlear Implant Team.

Hellman SA, Chute PM, Kretschmer ME, Nevins SC, Pariser LC, Thurston LC (1991) The development of a children's implant profile. American Annals of the Deaf 136: 77–81.

House WF (1980) Cochlear implant questionnaire, cochlear implant clinical trials manual. Los Angeles CA: House Ear Institute.

Kampfe CM (1989) Parental reaction to a child's hearing impairment. American Annals of the Deaf 134: 255–9.

Kampfe CM, Harrison M, Oettinger T, Ludington J, McDonald-Bell C, Pillsbury HC (1993) Parental expectations as a factor in evaluating children for the multi-channel cochlear implant. American Annals of the Deaf 138(3): 297–303.

Kluwin TN, Stewart DA (2000) Cochlear implants for younger children: a preliminary description of the parental decision process and outcomes. American Annals of the Deaf 145(1): 26–32.

Knutson JF, Boyd BC, Goldman M, Sullivan PM (1997) Psychological characteristics of child cochlear implant candidates and children with hearing impairment. Ear Hear 18(5): 355–63.

Knutson JF, Ehlers SL, Wald RL, Tyler RS (2000a). Psychological predictors of paediatric cochlear implant use and benefit Annals of Otology, Rhinology and Laryngology 185(Supplement): 100–3.

Knutson JF, Wald RL, Ehlers SL, Tyler RS (2000b). Psychological consequences of pediatric cochlear implant use. Annals of Otology, Rhinology and Laryngology 185(Supplement): 103–5.

Luterman D (1979) Counselling parents of hearing-impaired children. Boston MA: Little, Brown & Co.

Lynch C, Craddock LC, Crocker SR (1999) Developing a child-centred approach for paediatric audiologists: a model in the context of cochlear implant programming. The Ear 1: 10–16.

Mental Health Act Code of Practice (1999) Department of Health, Health Service Circular 050: LAC (99) 11.

Moses KL (1985) Infant deafness and parental grief: Psychosocial early intervention. in T Powell, S Friel-Patti, D Henderson (ed.) Education of the hearing impaired child. San Diego CA: College Hill Press.

Perold JL (2001) An investigation into the expectations of mothers of children with cochlear implants Cochlear Implants International 2(1): 39–58.

Peterson L, Shigatomi C (1981) The use of techniques to minimise anxiety in hospitalised children. Behaviour Therapy 12: 1–14.

Piaget J (1952) The Origins of Intelligence in Children. New York: International Universities Press.

Quittner AL, Thompson Steck J, Rouiller RL (1991) Cochlear implants in children: a study of parental stress and adjustment. The American Journal of Otology, 12(Supplement): 95–104.

Rawlings B, Gentile A (1970) Additional handicapping conditions, age at onset of hearing loss and other characteristics of hearing-impaired students. Washington DC: Office of demographic studies, Gallaudet University.

Roid GH, Miller LJ (1997) Leiter International Performance Scale-Revised. Wood Dale IL: Stoelting Co.

Schein JD, Delk MT Jr (1974) The deaf population of the United States. Silver Spring MD: National Association of the Deaf.

Snijders JTH, Tellegen PJ, Laros JA (1989) Snijers-Ooman Non-verbal Intelligence Test SON-R 51/2-17. Manual and Research report. Groningen: Wolters-Noordhoff.

Tye-Murray N (1993) Aural rehabilitation and patient management. In RS Tyler (ed) Cochlear Implants: Audiological foundations. San Diego: Singular.

Vernon MA (1994) Issues in the use of cochlear implants with prelingually deaf children American Annals of the Deaf 139(5): 485–91.

Vostanis P, Hayes M, Feu MD, Warren J (1997) Detection of behavioural and emotional problems in deaf children and adolescents: comparison of two rating scales. Child Care Health and Development 23(3): 233–46.

Wald RL, Knutson JF (2000) Deaf cultural identity of adolescents with and without cochlear implants. Annals of Otology, Rhinology and Laryngology 185(Supplement): 87–9.

CHAPTER 17

Deafness and additional difficulties

SUSAN CROCKER AND LINDSEY EDWARDS

Overview of chapter

This chapter will focus on the deaf or hearing-impaired child. In this chapter we will use the term 'additional difficulties' to mean an additional impairment, disability or handicap alongside deafness. We will also use the term 'deafness' to mean all forms and levels of hearing impairment.

The chapter is divided up into three main parts:

- the definition of 'additional difficulties' for this population;
- the types of additional difficulties;
- the psychological and other factors associated with concomitant impairments.

Definition of deafness and additional difficulties

It is necessary to begin this chapter with a brief discussion of the terms 'disability', 'impairment' and 'handicap' in order that we understand what we are looking at and trying to explore in the following pages. The well-established 1980 World Health Organization (WHO) definition of the three concepts reads:

> impairment is any loss or abnormality of psychological, or anatomical structure. Disability refers to any restriction or lack of ability to perform an activity in the manner or within the range considered normal for a human being. Handicap refers to the disadvantages for an individual resulting from an impairment or a disability, that limit or prevent the fulfilment of a role that is normal . . . for that individual. (WHO, 1980).

We use the term 'additional difficulties' to refer to all three categories.

Another definition of 'additional difficulties' comes from Gallaudet University: 'Additional handicapping condition is defined as any physical, mental, emotional, or behavioural disorder that significantly adds to the complexity of educating a hearing-impaired student' (Gentile and McCarthy, 1973). In relation to the above definition, we will also look at the medical needs of children associated with additional difficulties. In this chapter we will not be focusing on the educational needs of children per se, rather we will look at children's psychological needs in all aspects of life.

Prevalence

Historically, it seems to have been difficult to generate prevalence figures for this population. One factor may be that due to the children's communication needs, additional difficulties have sometimes been ignored. Extreme behavioural difficulties, for example, may have been put down to a child being deaf rather than having difficulties additional to the deafness. Tools to measure accompanying disabilities in a valid manner have not always been reliable, and psychologists with an understanding of deafness and appropriate communication skills remain in short supply.

Another difficulty with the prevalence literature is that children with deafness and additional difficulties may be classified in several disability categories. However, attempts have been made to look at incidence figures. In 1971–2 the Office of Education in the UK estimated that there were 40,000 multihandicapped children. In 1972 10,000 of these were reported to be hearing impaired (Flathouse, 1979), the largest category being deaf-learning disabled. A similar report from the US (Craig and Craig, 1981), found that the largest group consisted of deaf-blind students, followed by deaf learning-disabled, then deaf children with emotional/behavioural difficulties.

Other studies reveal estimates of how many deaf students will require additional assistance in an educational setting (not including language interpretation). Rawlings and Gentile (1970) state that this figure is one in every four students, whereas Schein and Delk (1974) regard this to be four in 10 students. Flathouse (1979) gives a general figure of between one-quarter and one-third of all deaf students having additional difficulties. Hogan (2000) researched deaf children's self-reports of disability. His findings show that 23% reported additional 'physical difficulties', 20% rated themselves as having 'sensory disabilities', 19% 'learning' and 'attentional' difficulties and 26% having other areas of need, for example epilepsy.

Overall, the literature suggests that one-third of deaf children are likely to have additional difficulties, so it is important that we assess children thoroughly before intervening.

Additional difficulties: genetic causes of deafness

Due to the problems in describing the additional difficulties associated with deafness, a variety of terms are used to classify the additional difficulties. For example, some studies report difficulties in 'independence', 'mobility', and 'mental deficits', whereas others refer to 'mental retardation', 'autism spectrum disorder', 'neuropsychiatric disorder' and 'visual abnormalities'. However, for each of the main aetiologies of sensori-neural hearing loss we will endeavour to consider as wide a range of additional difficulties as possible.

The children to whom we refer have deafness either as part of an identifiable syndrome of medical anomalies, or have deafness which is not linked to a specific syndrome, but due to chromosomal anomalies. Rehm and Morton (1999) report that approximately 70% of deafness is non-syndromic, and these children do not generally exhibit difficulties in addition to the primary clinical finding of hearing loss. However, this leaves the remaining 30% or so whose etiology of deafness is one of more than 400 possible syndromes. The most common of these include Alport syndrome, Jervell and Lange-Nielsen syndrome, Pendred syndrome, Stickler syndrome, Usher syndrome, Klippel Feil syndrome and Waardenberg syndrome. The associated medical anomalies include nephritis, cardiac defects, retinitis pigmentosa and thyroid disorder. Rehm and Morton (1999) report that 77% of the syndromic cases are autosomal recessive, 22% are autosomal dominant and 1% are X-linked. Up to 50% of the non-syndromic recessive deafness is caused by mutations in the GJB2 gene, which encodes the connexin 26 protein.

As already stated, where deafness occurs as an isolated 'medical' problem in an individual, and is not part of a syndrome with multiple medical anomalies, additional difficulties such as intellectual disabilities are much less common. However, it is important to be aware that in any individual, with or without a syndromal etiology of deafness, additional difficulties can co-exist coincidentally, in the same way as a person with arthritis may have learning difficulties, without the two being linked in any way. Similarly, it is important to keep in mind the possibility that just because a recognized pattern of additional difficulties has not been documented in a particular syndrome or genetic disorder, it does not mean that those difficulties will not occur. At present, only gross developmental delay or significant behavioural and learning difficulties tend to be reported in the literature, but it is probably safe to assume that more subtle difficulties also exist, but are overshadowed by the primary diagnoses for the individual.

Having said this, there are a number of syndromes where additional difficulties, particularly involving impaired global development or intellectual disabilities, are well documented. Retarded intellectual development in CHARGE syndrome has been reported by several authors (see, for example, Grimm, Thomas and White, 1997; Tellier et al., 2000). Waardenburg syndrome has been associated with cognitive and motor developmental delays and other neurological abnormalities to varying degrees (see DeSaxe, Kromberg and Jenkins, 1984; Kawabata et al., 1987). Similarly, Alport syndrome, which results in sensorineural deafness, visual problems and systemic disease, has been associated with developmental delay and difficulties in 'social integration' (McCarthy and Maino, 2000). Visual and audiological abnormalities are central to Usher syndrome, which in addition to mild developmental delay in some cases, has also been associated with depression or bipolar affective disorder at higher rates than in the general population (Tamayo et al., 1996).

Additional difficulties: deafness caused by insult or injury

In this section, the etiologies of deafness are divided into those that are congenital, and those that can occur at any time during the individual's lifespan.

Congenital causes of deafness

Congenital causes of deafness, which are non-hereditary, include intrauterine rubella infection, prematurity, intrauterine cytomegalovirus (CMV) infection, hypoxia, hyperbilirubinemia and untreated toxoplasmosis. This section will focus on the first three of these.

There is considerable variability in the degree of hearing loss between individuals, and some causes are associated with progressive hearing impairment. However, a significant proportion of individuals experience difficulties in addition to their deafness. Das (1996) reports that over a 10-year period 339 children were born in Greater Manchester, UK with an average bilateral hearing-impairment of 30 dB HL or greater. In these children the etiology was rubella infection in 18 (5.3%), CMV infection in 10 (2.9%) and perinatal problems in 26 (7.7%). Additional difficulties, described as predominantly developmental delay or visual impairment were found in 44%, 80% and 60% respectively. Williamson et al. (1982) reported that 53% of 17 children with symptomatic congenital CMV were 'performing in the retarded range', and developmental verbal dyspraxia had been diagnosed in at least 2 of the children.

Maternal rubella infection during pregnancy results in a high proportion of babies with disabilities, including auditory, visual and learning disabilities. Kelly et al. (1993) surveyed 238 children aged four to 21 years attending a residential school for the deaf, and found that those children with acquired deafness (including rubella infection and meningitis) were significantly more likely to experience attention deficits compared with their peers whose deafness was hereditary.

Severe prematurity has also been associated with a wide range of consequent disabilities. Rikards et al. (1987) describe a group of 60 extremely low birth-weight infants, who were assessed aged 5 years or more. Twenty-six per cent were found to have some degree of disability. Only one child was deaf but around 50% were noted to have behaviour problems (so this child had one chance in two of also having behaviour problems). In a more recent study, Monset-Couchard, De Bethmann and Kastler (2002) report the neurodevelopmental outcome of 151 extremely low birth weight babies. In this group 2% had cerebral palsy, 15% had other motor difficulties, 8% were severely delayed in the early years and 28% evidenced some degree of cognitive difficulties by age 14 years. Seven children (5%) had permanent hearing loss, and 31% displayed language delay and 42% behavioural disturbances. In addition to reporting rates of difficulties in their review of studies of prematurity, Msall and Tremont (2002) also describe the functional impact of prematurity. In their sample, rates of functional limitation in pre-schoolers were up to 27% for motor difficulties, 30% for self-care and 22% for communication difficulties. In the school-age group rates of functional disabilities exceeded 50%, and adolescent activity limitation was found in up to 32% of cases. The extent of co-morbidity of additional difficulties in this group is not clear, although Lorenz (2001) notes that approximately half of disabled survivors of prematurity have more than one major disability.

Acquired causes of deafness

There are a number of causes of deafness which occur as a result of insult or injury to the brain or auditory system at some time after birth, for example from bacterial meningitis, head trauma, noise, leukaemia and ototoxic medication. Thankfully all but the first of these are very rare. Despite the introduction of vaccinations against certain of the bacteria responsible for meningitis, and therefore a reduction in the number of cases of deafness caused by meningitis, there remains a significant number of children who develop sensorineural deafness following infection each year. Almuneef et al. (1998) reviewed 70 children who had bacterial meningitis over an 11-year period, and report that 14% had hearing loss, 10% experienced seizures of some description, 9% were diagnosed with developmental delay and 30% with a motor deficit. They do not report the overlap in prevalence between these additional difficulties. Thomas (1992) also examined the outcome of cases of paediatric bacterial meningitis from an 11-year period. Sensorineural hearing loss was identified in 6 of 71 children (9%), which was bilateral and severe in 4 (6%). Other difficulties included learning difficulties (13%), motor problems (7%) speech delay (7%), hyperactivity (4%), blindness (3%), hydrocephalus (3%) and recurrent seizures (3%). Again, it is not clear to what extent these additional difficulties may co-exist in any one individual, but it is probably safe to assume that in many children more than one is apparent.

Associated difficulties: functional

In our clinical work, we see many deaf children with additional difficulties. For some the additional difficulty is obvious – for example, the child comes with microcephaly or a recognized syndrome. For others, we slowly come to realize that children's difficulties cannot all be explained by their deafness. These children may have additional specific learning or language needs, praxis difficulties or behavioural/emotional difficulties. For children with concomitant difficulties, the associated needs can be great.

Motor development (praxis)

Children need the ability to take in, process and integrate sensation from movement and the environment. They need to use that information to plan and organize their behaviour and physical skills in order to master everyday activities. These include play, learning, self-care, self-regulation, motor and sensory skills, social and interaction skills, and sense of self. Deaf children with additional physical difficulties will obviously find the planning and execution of these skills more taxing.

It is also important to note that a deaf child's physical milestones may be delayed due to balance difficulties (for instance, if a child has absent semi-circular canals), which is not necessarily an indication of an overall developmental delay. With deaf children with additional difficulties, in order to give informed diagnosis and support, a clear understanding of development in all areas is important.

Communication

There is much written in the literature about mental health outcomes for deaf children with poor communication skills (Sinkkonen, 1994). Coupled with learning disabilities or other additional difficulties, this increases risk factors (Carvill, 2001). If communication development is very late, we know from the literature that this affects intellectual, language and social development, as well as emotional learning (Sachs, 1990). As most deaf children are born to hearing parents, the initial communication mode is oral. Even if a family takes on BSL while the child is still very young, the child and parents are learning the language at the same time, which is different from hearing children of hearing parents or deaf children with deaf parents. We are aware that, in this situation, hearing parents learning BSL tend to use language in a functional way initially, with much more limited emotional and conversational aspects of language (Schlesinger and Meadows, 1972). This will have implications for all areas of development as a chid will most likely have an impaired ability for mental representations and hypothesizing (theory of mind is discussed later in this chapter).

Language disorder

Language disorders can present themselves within the domains of expressive, receptive or as mixed disorders. A language disorder includes difficulties with speech processing and production (phonology), understanding word meaning (semantics), and poor grammatical knowledge or sentence use (syntactic or morphological). Difficulties are also seen in the integration of language and context (decoding meaning) and understanding intended meaning (social communication and pragmatics) (Bishop, 1999). In some children there can be a disorder of the speech system (production). These difficulties with language therefore spill out into the social spheres and affect peer relationships.

Deaf children with a concomitant language disorder (for example semantic-pragmatic disorder) will often, not surprisingly, present with behavioural difficulties. They may find it difficult to behave appropriately in unpredictable situations, for example, social situations with peers, as they are not able to read the social cues easily and thus decode meaning that is not explicitly shared. As young children, they may hit out (possibly as an attempt to interact) or withdraw (maybe preferring to play on their own) (Fujiki, 1999). Thus, understanding the rules of social communication will be difficult, as seen in the learning of turn taking in toddlers.

Assessment and diagnosis of language disorders is particularly difficult in hearing-impaired children, as language delays resulting from the deafness may 'mask' difficulties that in a hearing child would be categorized as specific language disorders. A few standardized assessment batteries do present some data, usually on a small sample, for hearing-impaired children, but this assumes that it has been possible to administer the tests in the first place: many deaf children do not have the verbal language or literacy skills needed to understand and follow the instructions, or respond verbally. Although it is sometimes possible to use sign language for both the administration and response mode, this typically makes the test very difficult to score, and more particularly, difficult to interpret the results. Hence assessment frequently falls into the qualitative domain, with some supporting evidence from standardized tests.

Autism and theory of mind (ToM)

Deafness and autism has been highlighted by Jure et al. (1991). Since both diagnoses affect communication, their co-existence is likely to have severe consequences. In all cases of autism, whether as part of a dual diagnosis or not, an inability to master theory of mind (ToM) underpins the diagnosis alongside the triad of difficulties. An assessment to know whether learning difficulties are also present is essential. Meeting the needs of children affected by deafness and autism will take a lot of expertise. Profiling all of their needs and not just the deafness is paramount. Sometimes the deafness is not the primary disability and thus it may be necessary to consider an appropriate educational placement to reflect this.

In many cases, autism may be detected late in a deaf child (Jure et al., 1991), as the behavioural problems are put down to communication difficulties attributable to the hearing loss. Similarly styles of behaviour, for example rigidity and desire for routine can be misinterpreted as features of autism rather than a hearing-impaired child's need to understand the world and to feel in control of what is happening. Thus specialist knowledge about both language delay and social communication disorders need to be understood in relation to deafness, before a diagnosis of autism can be made.

There has been an increasing amount of research in recent years looking at ToM in deaf children not affected by autism. Theory of mind is often seen as related to an ability to hold shared attention with another person (to the same object or event) and understand metarepresentations (Baron-Cohen and Swettenham, 1996). Metarepresentation is the ability to use mental representations of hypothetical events, often seen in children emerging through symbolic play. Theory of mind, therefore, is the ability to put oneself in the position of another, to be able to see a situation from the other's perspective. It is generally felt that these skills emerge in the preschool years, predominantly through interaction, where a child can learn about mental states and how these relate to behaviour (Peterson and Siegal, 1995).

With deaf children raised in a spoken language environment, a delay in the development of theory of mind is more often present. A number of studies confirm that the performance level of deaf children is significantly below that of hearing peers. In a study by Russel et al. (1998) many children failed 'false belief' questions. False belief is an understanding that how people behave depends on what they believe (even if that belief is false). Deaf children's performance rose after the age of 13, with the performance of the 8-to-12 year olds being no better than the 4-to-7 year group. Only 14% of the deaf 4-to-12 year olds passed the test compared to 85% of 3-to-5-year-old hearing children. There was still a high failure rate in the 13-to-16 year group, with 40% not completing the task successfully. These findings have recently been replicated (Peterson, 2002). It was found that having ToM was not dependent on cognitive ability (Baron-Cohen, Leslie and Frith 1985), emotional disturbance or specific expressive language disorder (Leslie and Frith, 1988). What is interesting to note is that with deaf children from deaf parents, the pass rate of false belief tasks was consistent with the outcome of the hearing children. Therefore, this group did not have a delay in this area (Peterson and Siegal, 1995) indicating that language is the underlying need to pass ToM tests.

A deficit in ToM is not exclusive to autism but is indicative of poor language development and communication opportunities, and thus the ability to understand that people think and feel differently to themselves, which has consequences for behaviour and actions. Not having this ability in the pre-school years is debilitating for deaf children, and it's consequences potentially far reaching for relationships, emotional development and the potential to live independently as adults.

Learning

The association between developmental delay or intellectual disability and deafness is an important one to remember as the combination results in the individual being more vulnerable to developing behavioural problems and psychiatric illness (Carvill, 2001). In addition, hearing impairment frequently impedes learning through its impact on language and communication, leading to an increase in the level of intellectual disability, which in turn reduces the individual's ability to cognitively process auditory information, setting up a vicious circle.

Learning problems in children may be specific or global in nature. With global difficulties, there is a spectrum of severity from mild to profound. Also a learning disability can be primary or secondary in nature. It is important to assess whether a child's learning needs are global (whether they affect all aspects of the child's learning) or specific (for example in dyslexia, dyspraxia or central auditory processing) as this may affect their intervention and education placement options.

When testing a deaf child's cognition, it is advisable to use a nonverbal tool as a global assessment of learning, to show how a child is functioning without language being a confounding variable. By defining whether a learning need is specific or global, appropriate intervention can be put into place and a child's learning potential achieved more easily.

Many deaf children will not have a primary learning difficulty – their non-verbal cognition will be average. They may, however, have secondary learning needs due to their style of communication being different from those around them. The same child in an environment where everyone uses the same communication mode will not have any secondary learning needs. By not fully understanding the relationship between a primary and secondary learning disability, we do not allow children to gain in confidence and esteem, due to the expectations of those around them. Children with a primary global learning disability and deafness are not well represented in the deaf literature (Bowe, 1988).

Attention

Assessments of attention are also sometimes used with deaf children. They form an important part of a diagnosis of attention deficit hyperactivity disorder (Samar, Parasnis and Berent, 1998) and can be useful in differentiating problems with executive function from memory or attention difficulties. There are a number of questionnaire measures that may be used with hearing-impaired children, which require relatively little modification to render them appropriate for this population. Typically there are versions that can be completed by the parent/caregiver and teacher, and this allows comparison of behaviour in different contexts and environments. As noted previously, Kelly et al, (1993) found that children with an acquired sensorineural hearing loss were at greater risk for attention problems than their hearing peers. However, there was no difference between the children with congenital hearing loss and the normative data. When assessing a child with suspected attention problems it is important to consider how being deaf may affect behavioural manifestations of attention problems, for example, impulsivity may be due to the social and psychological consequences of being deaf in a hearing world, rather than primary disability, and thus decisions regarding an appropriate education placement may need to reflect this.

Associated difficulties: psychological

When working with children, much of the psychological work is carried out with the system involved in the child's care. Children will sometimes have time to think about their needs on their own, but mainly organizations, parents and other carers are engaged to think about changing the environment and their understanding of a child, to bring about changes with the child. Supporting the system to carry out intervention programmes and to respond to new information, or ways of thinking, is a very important but at times lengthy and difficult process. Thoughts about how to change and move forward need to be embraced with sensitivity, with the understanding that all situations are unique.

Emotional

The disability literature is well referenced with regard to the emotional development of children. Often this links to particular subgroups of children and does not look at concomitant difficulties. In the deafness field, emotional aspects of a child's development are outlined by a number of authors (for example, Leigh et al., 1989) and mainly relate to the early attachment difficulties or due to the effects of not hearing and/or poor communication. Hindley (in Hindley and Kitson, 2000) suggested that the prevalence of psychiatric disorder is two to five times higher in deaf children than in control groups. These difficulties seem to be relating to anxiety and behaviour disorders (Roberts and Hindley, 1999), with emotional problems, or difficulties relating to low self esteem and depression occurring alongside conduct disorders (Hindley and Kitson, 2001). However, little is written about the emotional development of children with deafness and additional difficulties.

Behavioural

Although not often documented for specific syndromes, in the deaf population as a whole, behaviour and personality disorders are generally considered more prevalent than in the general population (Hindley, in Hindley and Kitson, 2000). However, estimation is made more difficult by inadequacies in communication, test administration, validity of measures and inappropriate norms. Many problem behaviours linked with deafness may not be anything to do with the deafness per se, but rather a consequence of the interaction of the individual with their environment.

It is well known that deaf children may have behaviour difficulties reported in their early years, often associated with late language acquisition. Frequently we see children of 2 or 3 years old, who do not have good language models. With these children, reported areas of need are often around toilet training, sleep difficulties, feeding problems, adherence to routines and temper tantrums. Advice to families about parenting a deaf child is useful and often enables parents to understand that difficult behaviour is frequently a form of communication.

Deaf children with limited language skills respond positively to routine and predictability in their environment so that they can make sense of what is going on and feel safe. This is a normal developmental need and will reduce as children are able to express themselves, understand what is happening and question their environment through language. Deaf children without additional difficulties in their learning or language should be showing a desire to communicate and be eager to learn even without a structured language available to them. For some children, we slowly realize that they do not desire to communicate and act upon their environment. These children may have additional difficulties that require careful assessment. As with all behavioural interventions, a complete and thorough assessment to reveal any underlying cause is essential. A child displaying aggressive behaviour, for example, could be due to poor parenting, emotional difficulties, learning difficulties, social and communication difficulties or language needs to name but a few.

Self-esteem

Hindley and Kitson (2001) suggest that deaf children are at risk of developing mental health difficulties due to being deaf in a hearing orientated society. This is thought to be due to:

* poor self image and identity as a deaf person, and
* not being a part of 'deaf culture'.

Establishing good self image, identity and links with deaf culture are thus seen to protect against poor mental health (Yetman, 2002). Deaf students in this study, who used hearing peers for social comparison, had lower self-esteem, whereas those students who compared themselves to deaf peers had higher esteem across a number of domains.

Self-esteem in children with disabilities is rarely discussed, and almost no literature has been found relating to how deaf children with additional difficulties see themselves or what their self-attributes are. It is clearly going to be difficult to obtain this information from children who do not have a good language system to portray their thoughts and feelings. Nevertheless, the use of art or play therapy might be a way to assess and work with a deaf child with identity and esteem problems and who has multiple disabilities.

Associated difficulties: social

Children with deafness and additional difficulties, such as learning disabilities, often do not have the chance to interact in Deaf cultural networks. As their deafness is not acknowledged, they are generally absorbed into the learning disabilities services with little attention to their cultural deafness needs (Carvill, 2001).

Parenting

Many studies of deaf children with hearing parents focus on differences in parent–child interactions (Gregory, 1976). This relates to a parent's acceptance of deafness and to their acceptance of other modes of communication. Parental feelings (shock, anxiety, anger, depression, guilt, resentment, vulnerability, denial and overprotection) are often discussed in relation to how they relate to the changes ahead of them once their child is diagnosed as deaf (Luterman, 1987). This response will have a significant effect on a parent's ability to cope and successfully parent the child, as in any other situation of disability or upheaval. Alongside the shock of parenting a child in need of interventions from a multi-disciplinary team (for example, health and education professionals), a family may also need to adjust to significant communication needs, and possibly co-morbid additional difficulties.

Many parents do not have a shared language with their deaf child. This means that deaf children cannot learn to understand other people through communication (Greenberg in Hindley and Kitson, 2000), thus increasing communication through behaviour or by withdrawing. This will make parenting a deaf child increasingly difficult.

Communication needs and additional difficulties aside, is there anything different in parenting a deaf child? The recent report produced by the National Deaf Children's Society (2003) supported by the Department of Health, outlined that there are aspects of parenting a deaf child that are the same and aspects that are different, compared to parenting a hearing child. This needs assessment study of 1,300 parents of deaf children highlighted particular needs for hearing parents: expert input from professionals who know about deafness and learning what to do with regards to education, communication and so on. The report highlighted that having a deaf child affects the whole family, for example, siblings, where a family lives, relationships outside of the home, and internal changes to the parent, for example in assertiveness.

One finding was that deaf parents appraised communication, developmental and parenting tasks as being much easier than hearing parents of deaf children. They also saw professional support as far less important.

Hearing parents of deaf children with additional disabilities rated parenting tasks as significantly more difficult than for the other parents in the study and gave high importance to professional support.

Siblings

The Children Act (HMSO, 1991) states: 'the needs of brothers and sisters should not be overlooked and they should be provided for as part of a package of services for the child with a disability.' A higher incidence of emotional behavioural problems in siblings of deaf and hearing-impaired children has been identified (Dunn and McGuire, 1992). In a study of 14 hearing female adolescents with younger deaf siblings, it was found that the siblings had poorer identity and self worth than their peers with hearing siblings (Israelite, 1986).

As with all siblings with a brother or sister with a disability, there is the need to consider children's attribution concerning the cause of disability (Senapati and Hayes, 1988) as this may have an impact on their understanding of their own future. For example, some children with an older deaf sibling might believe that they themselves will become deaf, or that deafness is caused by an illness or infection. Thus, an absence of communication leaves children feeling confused about a sibling's condition (Wasserman, 1983).

Issues of responsibility, guilt, anger, resentment, anxiety about the future and high parental expectations have all been cited as experiences of siblings (Badger, 1988). However, this is not always the case, as many siblings are well adjusted, responsible and mature (Blatcher, 1984). For some, the experience of having a deaf child in the family positively affects their compassion and life choices. It has been noted however, that siblings with younger deaf brothers or sisters have more home responsibilities, less independence and decreased social activities (Schwirian, 1976). Thus, it is vital for any service to consider sibling issues as part of any assessment and intervention given to families.

Summary

Many deaf and hearing-impaired children have difficulties in addition to their deafness. These difficulties can take many different forms, from a mild case of a specific learning difficulty such as dyspraxia, to highly complex multiple handicaps involving physical disabilities, learning difficulties and behaviour problems, for example. In this chapter we have aimed to provide the reader with a flavour of the additional difficulties that hearing-impaired children may experience. We have given some indication of the ways in which the additional difficulties may interact with each other and the hearing-impairment, resulting in highly complex clinical presentations. Thorough assessment is emphasized as the cornerstone of appropriate, effective intervention or management for these children. The presence of additional difficulties for hearing-impaired children has potentially profound consequences for their social and emotional development throughout their life. Psychological input is therefore an essential component of the multi-disciplinary, multi-agency approach to the care of these children.

References

Almuneef M, Memish Z, Khan Y, Kagallwala A, Alshaalan M (1998) Childhood bacterial meningitis in Saudi Arabia. Journal of Infection 36: 157-160.

Badger A (1988) The brothers and sisters group. A group for siblings of children with physical disabilities. Groupwork 3: 262–8.

Baron-Cohen S, Leslie AM, Frith U (1985) Does the autistic child have theory of mind? Cognition: 21: 37–46.

Baron-Cohen S, Swettenham J (1996) The relationship between SAM and TOMM: two hypotheses. In Carruthers P, Smith PK (eds) Theories of Theories of Mind. Cambridge: Cambridge University Press, pp. 158–68.

Bishop DUM (1999) Uncommon Understanding. Development and Disorders of Language Comprehension in Children. Hove: Psychology Press.

Blacher J (1984) Severely Handicapped Young Children and their Families: Research in Review. Orlando FL: Academic Press.

Bowe F (1988) Toward Equality: Education of the Deaf (Report on the Commission on the Education of the Deaf). Washington DC: US Government Printing Office.

Carvill S (2001) Sensory impairments, intellectual disability and psychiatry. Journal of Intellectual Disability Research 45(6): 467–83.

Craig W, Craig H (1981) Directory of educational programmes and services. American Annals of the Deaf 126: 190–206.

Das VK (1996) Aetiology of bilateral sensorineural hearing impairment in children: a 10 year study. Archives of Disease in Childhood 74: 8–12.

De Saxe M, Kromberg JG, Jenkins T (1984) Waardenburg syndrome in South Africa. Part 1. An evaluation of the clinical findings in 11 families. South African Medical Journal 66: 256–61.

Dunn J, McGuire S (1992) Sibling and peer relationships in childhood. Journal of Child Psychology and Psychiatry 33: 67-105.

Flathouse VE (1979) Multihandicapped deaf children and public law 94-142. Exceptional Children 45: 560–5.

Fujiki M, Brinton, B, Morgan, M, Hart CH (1999) Withdrawn sociable behaviour of children with language disorder. Language Speech and Hearing Services in Schools, 30: 183–95.

Gentile A, McCarthy B (1973) Additional handicapping conditions among hearing-impaired students, United States: 1971–72. Washington DC: Office of Demographic Studies, Gallaudet University.

Greenberg MT (2000) Educational Interventions: Prevention and Promotion of Competence. In Hindley P, Kitson N (eds) Mental Health and Deafness. London: Whurr.

Gregory S (1976) The Deaf Child and his Family. New York: Halsted Press.

Grimm SE 3rd, Thomas GP, White MJ (1997) CHARGE syndrome: review of literature and report of case Coloboma, heart disease, atresia of choanae, retarded mental development, genital hypoplasia, ear abnormalities-deafness. ASDC Journal of Dentistry for Children 64: 218–21.

Hindley P, Kitson N (2000) Mental Health and Deafness. London: Whurr.

Hindley P, Kitson N (2001) Deafness and Mental Health. In Graham J, Martin M (eds), Ballantyne's Deafness. 6 edn. London: Whurr.

HMSO (1991) The Children Act Guidance and Regulations. Vol. 6. London.

Hogan A (2000) The well-being of students with disabilities. Presentation given at the Royal National Throat Nose and Ear Hospital, London.

Israelite NK (1986) Hearing-impaired children and the psychological functioning of their normal hearing siblings. Volta Review 88: 47–54.

Jure R, Rapin I, Tuchman R F (1991) Hearing-impaired children. Developmental Medicine and Child Neurology 33: 1062–72.

Kawabata E, Ohba N, Nakamura A, Izumo S, Osame M (1987) Waardenburg syndrome: a variant with neurological involvement. Ophthalmic Paediatric Genetics 8: 165–70.

Kelly DP, Kelly BJ, Jones ML, Moulton NJ, Verhulst SJ, Bell SA (1993) Attention deficits in children and adolescents with hearing loss: a survey. American Journal of Disabled Children 147: 737–41.

Leigh IW, Robins C J, Welkowitz J, Bond RN (1989) Toward greater understanding of depression in deaf individuals. American Annals of the Deaf 134: 249–54.

Leslie AM, Firth U (1988) Autistic children's understanding of seeing, knowing and believing. British Journal of Developmental Psychology 6: 315–24.

Lorenz JM (2001) The outcome of extreme prematurity. Seminars in Perinatology 25: 348–59.

Luterman D (1987) Deafness in the Family. Boston MA: Little, Brown.

McCarthy PA, Maino DM (2000) Alport syndrome: a review. Clinical Eye and Vision Care 12(3–4): 139–50.

Monset-Couchard M, De Bethmann O, Kastler B (2002) Mid- and long-term outcome of 166 premature infants weighing less than 1,000 g at birth, all small for gestational age. Biological Neonate 81: 244–54.

Msall ME, Tremont MR (2002) Measuring functional outcomes after prematurity: Developmental impact of very low birth weight and extremely low birth weight status on childhood disability. Mental Retardation and Developmental Disabilities Research and Review 8: 258–72.

National Deaf Children's Society (2003) Parenting and Deaf Children: Report on the Needs Assessment Study Undertaken as Part of the NDCS Parent's Toolkit Development Project. London: NDCS.

Peterson CC, Siegal M (1995) Deafness and theory of mind. Journal of Child Psychology and Psychiatry 36(3): 458–74.

Peterson CC (2002) Drawing insight from pictures: The development of concepts of false belief in children with deafness, normal hearing, and autism. Child Development 73 (5): 1442–59.

Rawlings B, Gentile A. (1970) Additional Handicapping Conditions, Age at Onset of Hearing Loss and Other Characteristics of Hearing-impaired Students. Washington DC: Office of Demographic Studies, Gallaudet University.

Rehm HL, Morton CC (1999) A new age in the genetics of deafness. Genetics in Medicine 1(6): 295–302.

Rikards AL, Ford GW, Kitchen WH, Doyle LW, Lissenden JV, Keith O (1987) Extremely-low-birthweight infants: neurological, psychological, growth and health status beyond five years of age. Medical Journal of Australia 147: 476–81.

Roberts C, Hindley P (1999) Practitioner Review: the assessment and treatment of deaf children with psychiatric disorder. Journal of Child Psychology and Psychiatry 40(2): 151–67.

Russell PA, Hosie CD, Gray CD, Scott C, Hunter N (1998) The development of theory of mind in deaf children. Journal of Child Psychology and Psychiatry 39(6): 903–10.

Samar VJ, Parasnis I, Berent GP (1998) Learning disabilities, attention deficit disorders and deafness. In Marschark M, Clark MD (eds) Psychological Perspectives on Deafness. Vol. 2. Hillsdale NJ: Erlbaum.

Schein JD, Delk MT Jr (1974) The Deaf Population of the United States. Silver Spring MD: National Association of the Deaf.

Schlesinger HP, Meadows KP (1972) Development of maturity in deaf children. Exceptional Children (February): 461–7.

Schwirian P (1976) Effects of the presence of a hearing-impaired preschool child in the family on behaviour patterns of older 'normal' siblings. American Annals of the Deaf 121: 373–80.

Senapati R, Hayes A (1988) Sibling relationships of handicapped children: a review of conceptual and methodological issues. International Journal of Behavioural Development 11: 89–115.

Sinkkonen J (1994) Hearing Impairment, Communication and Personality Development. Department of Child Psychiatry, University of Helsinki, Helsinki.

Tamayo ML, Maldonado C, Plaza SL, Alvira GM, Tamayo GE, Zambrano M, Frias JL, Bernal JE (1996) Neuroradiology and clinical aspects of Usher syndrome. Clinical Genetics 50: 126–32.

Tellier AL, Amiel J, Delezoide AL, Audollent S, Auge J, Esnault D, Encha-Razavi F, Munnich A, Lyonnet S, Vekemans M, Attie-Bitach T (2000) Expression of the PAX2 gene in human embryos and exclusion in the CHARGE syndrome. American Journal of Medical Genetics 93: 85–8.

Thomas DG (1992) Outcome of paediatric bacterial meningitis 1979–1989. Medical Journal of Australia 157: 519–20.

Wasserman R (1983) Identifying the counselling needs of the siblings of mentally retarded children. Personnel and Guidance Journal 61: 622–7.

Williamson WD, Desmond MM, LaFevers N, Taber LH, Catlin FI, Weaver TG (1982) Symptomatic congenital cytomegalovirus. Disorders of language, learning, and hearing. American Journal of Diseases of Children 136: 902–5.

World Health Organization (1980) International Classification of Impairments, Disabilities and Handicaps. Geneva: WHO.

Yetman MM (2002) Peer relations and self esteem among deaf children in a mainstream school environment. Dissertation Abstracts International: Section B: the Sciences and Engineering. Vol. 62 (12-B), 5984, US: University Microfilms International.

PART 4
NEW DEVELOPMENTS IN
PSYCHOLOGY AND DEAFNESS

CHAPTER 18

Suggestibility and related concepts: implications for clinical and forensic practice with Deaf people

SUE O'ROURKE AND NIGEL BEAIL

Introduction

The concept of vulnerability in the criminal justice system relates primarily to the reliability of certain kinds of witness. Prominent cases of 'miscarriages of justice' have led to the study of the psychological processes involved in interrogation, giving evidence and confessing to crimes. This work is relevant to the situation of Deaf people within the criminal justice system and also has implications for psychological processes that need to be considered when interviewing Deaf people in other situations, for example within the field of forensic mental health.

Suggestibility

Gudjonsson and Clark (1986) define interrogative suggestibility as 'the extent to which, within a closed social interaction, people come to accept messages communicated during formal questioning, as the result of which their subsequent behavioural response is affected.'

This relates primarily to 'leading' questions – that is, questions that contain premises, which may or may not be well founded.

Gudjonsson (1992) also outlines a second distinct type of suggestibility relating to a 'shift' in response, which results from criticism or negative feedback: being told overtly that a response is wrong, or by implication. In the latter the question is repeated, denoting that the interrogator does not accept the first response.

Concepts related to suggestibility are *acquiescence* – the tendency to answer questions in the affirmative, regardless of content – and *compliance*, which is the tendency to go along with the propositions or requests for instrumental gain, without internal acceptance of this. The latter is in contrast with suggestibility where personal acceptance of the proposition offered during questioning is present (Gudjonsson, 1992).

Evidence indicates a weak correlation between acquiescence and suggestibility, and a moderate correlation between suggestibility and compliance (Gudjonsson, 1992).

The Gudjonsson Suggestibility Scales (GSS) were developed as a means of assessing suggestibility in individual forensic cases (Gudjonsson, 1992). The GSS procedure requires the individual to listen to a short passage, presented as a test of verbal memory, followed by free recall. Twenty questions relating to the passage are then presented, 15 of which are leading. The extent to which the individual is 'led' produces a score 'yield 1'. The examiner then firmly states that the questions will be repeated because errors have been made (even if they have not). The 20 questions are repeated, giving a 'yield 2' score and a 'shift' score relating to responses which are altered as a result of negative feedback. Yield 1 and shift are combined to produce a total suggestibility score. Other scores can be obtained for delayed recall and for confabulation on either immediate or delayed recall – confabulation being the extent to which additional items not present in the original story are inserted to fill gaps in memory.

Studies have indicated the robust psychometric properties of these scales (e.g. Merckelbach et al., 1998). Factor analysis confirms the existence of two types of interrogative suggestibility – yield and shift (Gudjonsson, 1984). Test–retest reliability indicates the stability of suggestibility within an individual, across time when measured under similar conditions (Gudjonsson, 1987). Richardson and Smith (1993) present data indicating high inter-rater reliability. These studies have confirmed the psychometric robustness of the measures on both community and forensic populations (Gudjonsson, 1992).

Factors affecting suggestibility

The individual may be more or less suggestible, according to factors relating to him or herself, or alternatively factors relating to the interrogation situation. The age of the individual may render him/her more suggestible. A consistent finding is that intelligence, as measured by standardized psychometric tests, produces a negative correlation between IQ and suggestibility – but only within the below-average range: those with a lower IQ being more suggestible than those with a higher IQ (Gudjonsson, 1990). Suggestibility has been shown to correlate negatively with memory (Gudjonsson, 1988a), self-esteem and assertiveness (Singh and Gudjonsson, 1984) and positively with anxiety (Gudjonsson, 1988b). This not only indicates the types of individuals who are likely to be more suggestible, but also implies that certain characteristics of the interrogation situations or methods of questioning (designed to increase anxiety and reduce confidence and self-esteem) are likely to increase suggestibility (Gudjonsson, 1992). Situational factors, which may increase suggestibility, include the nature of instructions given prior to and during questioning and the effect of the experimenter/interrogator (Gudjonsson and Hilton 1989).

Suggestibility and deafness

Why then should Deaf people be a vulnerable group, in terms of suggestibility? It is proposed that Deaf people are likely to be vulnerable on two counts. The first relates to the position of a Deaf person in the interview situation and the second relates to the nature of BSL and how this affects the interview process.

Cognition

In the past, it has been assumed that Deaf individuals are incompetent – both in the general sense and relating to the criminal justice system. Assumptions of incompetence may be reflected in frequent requests for assessments of fitness to plead in the case of Deaf defendants (Young, Monteiro and Ridgeway, 2000). In a comprehensive meta-analysis of psychometric assessments of Deaf people, Braden (1994) illustrated that non-verbal measures of IQ are reliable and valid indicators of intellectual ability in Deaf individuals. Whereas a slight skewing to the lower end may be observed (due to some etiologies of deafness being coincidental with some etiologies of learning disability), by and large IQ, as measured by non-verbal means, is normally distributed with a mean of 100, as for hearing norms (Braden, 1994).

In contrast, verbal measures, even when translated into sign language, produce mean scores approximately one standard deviation below the mean for non-verbal tests (Braden, 1994). This illustrates the extent to which verbal IQ reflects acquired knowledge (via written/spoken English) and is thus taken as a measure of the deprivation of knowledge and information suffered by Deaf people generally. This finding suggests not that Deaf people are vulnerable to suggestibility by virtue of low IQ but that they may be vulnerable due to lack of knowledge. In other words, an average Deaf person, given the experiences and opportunities that a person is likely to have missed, is likely to be disadvantaged relative to a hearing person of the same intellectual capacity. Not only the fact of this disadvantage, but an awareness of it may lead to low self-esteem, increased uncertainty and stress, leading to greater potential for suggestibility.

Although there is no reason to suppose that Deaf people have poorer memories in terms of recall of information, encoding information may be difficult if relying on lip-reading or other unreliable means of receiving information. Thus, when it comes to recall and questioning, the likelihood of uncertainty is increased.

Culture

Studies in cross-cultural research illustrate how the cultural distance between interviewer and interviewee can affect feelings of disempowerment and alter responses (Paniagua, 2001). Gudjonsson and Lister's (1984) study supports this in relation to suggestibility. They found that the larger the perceived distance between the self and the experimenter, in terms of competence, power and control, the more suggestible the participants. When a Deaf person is questioned by a hearing person, the Deaf person is likely to feel disadvantaged, based on the position of Deaf people in a hearing world (Higgins, 1980). He or she is likely to experience anxiety as a result of this perceived power imbalance, just by virtue of the Deaf/hearing interaction, thus increasing vulnerability. It can be argued that this effect would be reduced in proportion to the degree of 'Deaf awareness' of the hearing interviewer – for example, a totally naïve unaware interviewer would produce heightened anxiety whereas a signing hearing interviewer would be least anxiety provoking.

Epidemiological studies of psychological difficulties show that Deaf people have more difficulties coping with the problems in day-to-day life (Denmark, 1985). Given the difficulties accessing information through appropriate means, it is reasonable to suppose that many Deaf individuals are likely to lack the range of coping strategies available to hearing adults in a stressful situation. This again, may render them vulnerable to suggestibility.

Communication

In the UK, the Police and Criminal Evidence Act (PACE) dictates that Deaf people within the criminal justice system should be provided with a registered qualified BSL interpreter. Police officers, lawyers, judges and jurors often labour under the illusion that BSL is a word-for-sign encoding of English. In employing an interpreter the format of the question may be changed to a more 'Deaf-friendly' version. The problem is, that in doing the latter, the psychological effect is ignored – the question may become more 'leading'. This is likely to be the direction of distortion, since native BSL users tend to use closed, rather than open, questions that are more likely to be leading when based on an uninformed premise. A study by Brennan and Brown (1997) showed that interpreters frequently did just this in a court setting – they turned an open question into a closed question. They give examples of open-ended questions being interpreted into multiple-choice type questions or yes/no answers. Although their study addressed linguistic unreliability rather than psychological impact of this distortion, the possibility of leading the witness is evident from the examples they give.

Finally, Deaf people are frequently in a position of not understanding or half-understanding. The strategy of 'best-guessing', based on limited information, may be one that Deaf people frequently employ – a little like latching onto a few recognizable words in a foreign language and trying to piece it together to make sense. Positive or negative feedback, in the form of other's reactions, may then help to ascertain if this 'best guess' was correct. It would seem that a lifelong experience of doing this when faced with uncertainty may make Deaf individuals more likely to yield to leading questions, as this involves picking up clues to the 'right answer' contained in the question. In addition, they may be particularly likely to shift their responses as a result of negative feedback.

Research evidence

To date, there has been only one study addressing suggestibility and Deafness (O'Rourke and Beail in preparation). The study investigated whether Deaf people are vulnerable to interrogative suggestibility using the Gudjonsson methodology described above. The main hypothesis was that Deaf people are more suggestible than hearing people of similar intellectual ability for reasons discussed. The study was designed to be linguistically and culturally appropriate for Deaf people by conducting the assessment in BSL: the Gudjonsson story was presented in BSL, as were the questions. Results in this study indicated that, using this methodology, Deaf people were not more suggestible than their hearing counterparts. It is purported that, in fact, this study demonstrates conditions under which Deaf people are *not* vulnerable to leading questions and negative feedback. It is therefore interesting to consider why this might be the case and if, under other conditions, different results may have been produced.

As already stated, the previous research has demonstrated the effect of the setting and personal style of the interrogator on the extent of suggestibility (Gudjonsson and Hilton, 1989; Gudjonsson, 1995). Also, issues of assertiveness, self-esteem, control and anxiety have been shown to be important factors related to suggestibility (Gudjonsson and Lister, 1984; Gudjonsson, 1988b). It may be that the conditions of the assessment in this study were such as to promote self-esteem and reduce anxiety by communicating in BSL, thus reducing the sociocultural distance between assessor and assessee. This would echo findings in relation to other cultural minorities when undergoing psychometric assessment (Paniagua, 2001), although the issue of socio-cultural distance has not been addressed specifically as it relates to suggestibility. Gudjonsson (1992) emphasizes the importance of formality in the assessment. It is the contention here that by communicating directly in BSL the perceived power imbalance is reduced, which may impact on suggestibility.

British Sign Language translation

Detailed consideration of the process of translating the GSS can shed light on how linguistic features can be leading in BSL where the equivalent in English is not so. It can be argued that, because the assessment does not rely on the particular words used, the procedure lends itself to interpretation into BSL. However, certain items of content seemed to be more leading in BSL than in English, owing to their visual nature. Facial expression and body language, crucial grammatical features of BSL, often provide more detailed information than the equivalent English words. For example, in signing, 'One Tuesday morning in July the couple were leaving the house to go to work', it is easy to convey, in BSL, by the manner of their walking and facial expression, the type of day it was. This later relates to the question: 'Was the weather wet or dry when the accident happened?' This illustrates how BSL can add-in information unintentionally and become leading. This is particularly the case when using terms that have no general form in BSL but can only be expressed in context. For example the sign for 'grab' cannot be expressed without reference to that which is being grabbed. So, in the GSS, the leading question 'Did John grab the boy's arm or shoulder?' (the answer is neither, he catches hold of the bike) the hand shape used in the original for catching hold of a bike, can easily be very similar to catching hold of someone's shoulders – thus leading the person to a particular response to the question.

A further issue in questioning is the use of implied either/or questions. In the English version 'Did the couple have a dog or a cat?' intonation can be used to infer that the respondent should choose one or the other. In BSL, this is achieved by the addition of the sign 'which?' The choice in BSL is: 'Did the couple have a dog or a cat?' (implies 'or nothing', requiring a yes/no response) or 'Did the couple have a dog or a cat, which?' (implies that they had one or the other and requires a choice). It is clear how the first example is less likely to lead, while the second is more leading.

These observations of the detail of the GSS lead to concerns about the reliability and equivalence of interrogation when it is interpreted from

English to BSL or vice versa. It would appear that reliability in general can be improved, and the potential for a suggestible response minimized, only when these linguistic factors are appreciated and video recordings of BSL interpretation is widely used to investigate what is 'added in' in the process of interpretation.

On closer examination, the fact that Deaf people were not more suggestible than their hearing peers under these conditions is unsurprising. However, it would be highly unusual for Deaf people to be interviewed directly in BSL within the criminal justice system. In addition, the events or incident about which they are being questioned are equally unlikely to have been as accessible in BSL. In the O'Rourke and Beail study, the passage was signed just 5–10 minutes prior to questioning. In reality, it is likely that Deaf people find themselves involved in incidents that they only half understand, about which they are interviewed some time later by high-status hearing people using a BSL interpreter. It could be argued that a more ecologically valid approach, aimed at mirroring this process, would have produced very different results.

Implications of suggestibility for clinical practice

The study described above (O'Rourke and Beail, in preparation) illustrates the conditions under which Deaf people are not more suggestible than their hearing peers. Although it may have demonstrated the viability of using the Gudjonsson methodology for assessment, it also raises the question of whether a more ecologically valid measure is required: one that reflects the naturalistic experiences of Deaf people.

The criminal justice system

If Deaf people are unreliable witnesses it would seem that this could be accounted for by many factors. It may be that difficulties occur at the 'input' stage, where information is misunderstood, or only partly understood because of problems of accessibility. Alternatively, difficulties may arise at the 'output' stage, as a result of questioning that is inaccessible or leading. What is clear is that we are only just beginning to think about suggestibility in relation to Deaf people and that the potential for unreliability in the criminal justice system is enormous. Most people involved at the time are unable to understand both English and BSL and therefore are not in a position to even be aware of the dangers inherent in questioning a Deaf individual.

Forensic mental health

Within the criminal justice system and also in a forensic mental health setting individuals are frequently in a position of wanting to 'look good' for
understandable reasons. The defendant wants to make a good impression
in court; the forensic patient may want to earn the approval of his or her
clinical team as a means of hastening discharge. In assessment and review
this may manifest itself in the desire the pick up clues to the 'right
answer'. In this case, the way BSL tends to be used, particularly when
interviewing a person with minimal language skills, may result in highly
suggestible responses. British Sign Language, in everyday use, tends to
use closed rather than open questions. For example, whereas in English
we might say 'Did you buy any furniture?' in BSL this would translate as
'You bought what? Table, chair, wardrobe?' In this example the difficulty
is that BSL does not tend to use collective nouns. In other situations this
is not the case, but nevertheless a naturalistic use of BSL would still tend
towards this way of structuring questions. For example, 'How do you
feel?' may become 'You feel happy? Sad? Angry?' This is not to say that BSL
does not have the facility for asking the more general question in this
example – merely that Deaf people tend to use this closed, multiple
choice type of questioning.

This can be likened to the popular game show *Who Wants to be a
Millionaire?* (thanks to Brenda Smith, Senior Sign Language Interpreter
and Advisor, for this observation). In the show contestants are asked general knowledge questions of increasing difficulty and, in order to increase
the chance of success, given four possible answers. They also have 'life-
lines' to use when in difficulty. These are '50:50' – two wrong answers are
removed, thus increasing their chance of a right answer; 'ask the audience' – the contestant asks the audience to respond to the question and
has the opportunity to take the majority view; and 'phone a friend' – the
contestant phones a friend and asks that person to answer the question.
At times it would appear that the way BSL is structured gives clues as to
the right answer and in a situation where the patient is suggestible can
create the possibility of leading where English would not. A brief example
from a ward round illustrates the point:

Hearing professional: Last week you said you felt like raping nurse X. How
do you feel now?

Interpreter: Last week you say you want rape X. You feel now what?

Patient: fine *(responding to the latter half of the question only, about how
he feels now)*.

Hearing professional: No, how do you feel about what you said last week?

Interpreter: No, last week you say you want rape X . You feel what? Happy? Sad? Angry? Feel bad? (Guilty?) *(interpreter offers multiple choice answers).*

Patient: Sad? Bad? *(Patient goes 50:50, guessing that he is not supposed to be happy or angry.)* What do you think Steve? *(Unsure of his response he 'phones a friend' – a Deaf professional.)* Am I right? *(Looking round to the rest of the clinical team – he 'asks the audience'.)*

This example shows how the change in style of the question via the interpreting process, entirely in keeping with common usage of BSL, changes the interaction, limiting the range of possible responses and leading the respondent to the 'correct' answer. Of great importance is the fact that the hearing professional, unless fluent in BSL, is not aware of this process unless the way in which his question has been altered is explicitly explained.

Other factors within a forensic setting may also lead to a tendency towards suggestibility in Deaf patients. The power imbalance between the hearing professional and patient is exaggerated by the individual's incarceration. In specialist Deaf services this is acknowledged and addressed by the presence of Deaf co-workers who, as well as having a role in clarifying communication, also reduce the perceived distance between interviewer and patient.

Many Deaf patients in a forensic setting have limited facility in BSL, regardless of whether or not they have a learning disability. The tendency towards structuring BSL in a leading fashion, liable to add to problems of suggestibility, is observed to increase as linguistic competence decreases.

Therapy

Within forensic practice the implications of suggestibility are that responses to offence related questions might be rendered unreliable, impacting on risk assessment. In other settings issues of suggestibility, acquiescence and compliance may interfere with the individual's ability to engage with and benefit from the therapeutic process. Clinicians will be familiar with the Deaf patient 'nodding' in response to questions, particularly to 'do you understand?' for fear of looking stupid and wishing to be seen as competent. Although this acquiescent style tends to be fairly obvious, more subtle is the effect of suggestibility in therapy, as the patient desperately searches for clues to the 'correct' response. In therapy it is common to repeat a question or reflect back a patient's response, in order to seek clarification or elaboration. If individuals are suggestible, this may be a cue for them to shift their response, the implication of the therapist's repetition or reflection being that the first response was 'wrong'.

The issue of suggestibility in relation to clinical work is not addressed in the literature. However, when working with Deaf patients there are theoretical reasons why this may need to be considered as a 'therapy interfering behaviour'. The clinician needs to be aware of these issues, particularly if using an interpreter, rather than communicating directly in BSL. Taking this into account then becomes a matter of being explicit about the way in which BSL may be more leading than English and having a dialogue with the interpreter about the best way to manage this in relation to a particular patient's communication needs. The relationship between therapist and patient impacts on suggestibility and indicates the need to consider co-working with a Deaf professional. Finally, explicitly dealing with the individual's anxiety and tackling the issue of 'right and wrong' answers in therapy may be a necessary first stage of the therapeutic process, in building the relationship and coming to a shared model of working therapeutically.

Conclusion

Suggestibility has been investigated primarily within the criminal justice system and little work has been carried out in relation to Deaf people. Although Deaf people are not necessarily more suggestible (O'Rourke and Beail, in preparation), there are strong theoretical reasons why, in many circumstances, they may be. This relates to the power relationship between Deaf and hearing people, issues of self-esteem and anxiety and, crucially, to the nature of BSL, which previously has not been considered. It is argued that issues of suggestibility are also of significance when working with Deaf patients in clinical settings and that this particularly needs to be taken into account in therapy.

References

Braden JP (1994) Deafness, Deprivation and IQ. New York: Plenum Press.
Brennan M, Brown K (1997) Equality Before the Law. Deaf People's Access to Justice. Durham: University of Durham, Deaf Services Research Unit.
Denmark JC (1985) A study of 250 patients referred to a department of psychiatry for the deaf. British Journal of Psychiatry 140: 282–6.
Gudjonsson G (1984) A new scale of interrogative suggestibility. Personality and Individual Differences 5(3): 303–14.
Gudjonsson G (1987) The relationship between memory and suggestibility. Social Behaviour 2: 29–33.
Gudjonsson G (1988a) The relationship of intelligence and memory to interrogative suggestibility. British Journal of Clinical Psychology 27: 185–198.

Gudjonsson G (1988b) Interrogative suggestibility: it's relationship with assertiveness, social-evaluative anxiety, state anxiety and method of coping. British Journal of Clinical Psychology 27: 159–66.

Gudjonsson G (1990) The relationship of intellectual skills to suggestibility, compliance and acquiescence. Personality and Individual Differences 3: 227–31.

Gudjonsson G (1992) The Psychology of Interrogations, Confessions and Testimony. Chichester: Wiley.

Gudjonsson G (1995) Interrogative suggestibility: does the setting where subjects are tested make a difference to the scores on the GSS1 and GSS2? Personality and Individual Differences 18(6): 789–90.

Gudjonsson G, Clark NK (1986) Suggestibility in police interrogation: a social psychological model. Social Behaviour 1: 38–104.

Gudjonsson G, Hilton M (1989) The effect of instructional manipulation on interrogative suggestibility. Social Behaviour 4: 189–93.

Gudjonsson G, Lister S (1984) Interrogative suggestibility and its relationship with self-esteem and control. Journal of the Forensic Science Society 24: 99–110.

Higgins PC (1980) Outsiders in a Hearing World. A Sociology of Deafness. Beverley Hills CA: Sage.

Merckelbach H, Peters M, Wessel I, Van Koppen PJ (1998) The Gudjonsson Suggestibility Scale (GSS): further data on its reliability, validity and metacognition correlates. Social Behaviour and Personality 26: 203–10.

O'Rourke SH, Beail N (in preparation) Interrogative suggestibility and deafness: a preliminary study.

Paniagua (2001) Diagnosis in a Multicultural Context: A Casebook for Mental Health Professionals. London: Sage.

Richardson G, Smith P (1993) The inter-rater reliability of the Gudjonsson Suggestibility Scale. Personality and Individual Differences: 14(1) 251–3.

Singh KK, Gudjonsson GH (1984) Interrogative suggestibility, delayed memory and self-concept. Personality and Individual Differences 5: 203–9.

Young A, Monteiro B, Ridgeway S (2000) Deaf people with mental health needs in the criminal justice system: a review of the UK literature. Journal of Forensic Psychiatry 11(3): 556–70.

Chapter 19

Stroke in users of BSL: investigating sign language impairments*

Jane Marshall, Joanna Atkinson, Alice Thacker and Bencie Woll

Introduction

This chapter is based on the work of the Deaf Stroke Project, which was funded by the Wellcome Trust to investigate sign language disorders arising from neurological damage. Following an introduction to stroke and aphasia, the chapter will discuss the development of language tests and describe some of the measures created by the project. We then present two case studies showing different patterns of impairment on these (and other) measures. Finally, we consider service provision and make recommendations for the future.

Stroke and aphasia

Strokes, or cerebral vascular accidents (CVA), affect 0.002% of the population each year (Langton Hewer, 1997; Warlow, 1998). About 130,000 stroke survivors live in the UK, with three-quarters having lasting disabilities (Cifu and Lorish 1994). Common problems include hemiplegia (paralysis), *apraxia* (movement planning problems, see glossary for terms in italics) and visual field deficits. People with right-hemisphere strokes often have additional visuospatial problems. They may not be able to draw, carry out visual tasks like jigsaws, find their way around or recognize people.

One particularly devastating consequence of stroke is aphasia, or a language disorder. This typically occurs after a left CVA, because, in the majority of people, language is processed by the left side of the brain. Aphasia affects all aspects of language. So hearing people with aphasia

* This work was funded by Wellcome Grant 053239.

have difficulties understanding and producing speech and problems in reading and writing (see Sarno, 1991; Parr, Byng and Gilpin, 1997). Figure 19.1 provides examples of aphasic speech.

MM (Marshall, Pring and Chiat, 1993)

Describing her weekend:

Mother's Day . . . er . . . Nicola . . . meals . . . flowers . . . er chocolates

Describing an episode of Home and Away:

er . . . house . . . dinner . . . nice . . . oh yes drinking . . . er man . . . er police . . . oh (gestures finger wagging) yes

RD (Ellis, Miller and Sin, 1983)

Describing a picture:

A bun bun (bull) is er churching (chasing) a boy or skirt (scout). A . . . boy skut (scout) is by a bone . . . poe (post) of pine . . . a . . . post . . . pone (post) with a er tone toe (line?) with washingt (washing) hanging on.

(presumed targets in parentheses)

Figure 19.1 Examples of aphasic speech.

Aphasia and sign language

Left hemisphere strokes can also cause aphasia in Deaf users of sign language (see, for example, Sarno, Swisher and Sarno, 1969; Chiarello, Knight and Mandel, 1982; Poizner, Klima and Bellugi, 1987; Corina et al., 1992; Hickok et al., 1995, Hickok et al., 1996, Hickok, Bellugi and Klima, 1996, Hickok, Love-Geffen and Klima, 2002 and see Corina 1998 for review). This is consistent with imaging studies showing that sign language, like spoken language, is left dominant (see, for example, Hickok, Bellugi and Klima, 1998; MacSweeney et al., 2002).

There are striking similarities between sign and speech aphasia. Many hearing aphasic people have agrammatism, or a loss of *syntax*. They can produce single words, but not sentences, and typically omit verbs and grammatical markers (see MM in Figure 19.1). Poizner, Klima and Bellugi (1987) identified a similar pattern in an aphasic user of American Sign Language (ASL) and we have replicated this finding in British Sign Language (BSL) (see Figure 19.2).

Not all aphasic people have problems with syntax: RD (see Figure 19.1) produces grammatically correct sentences, but makes numerous mistakes with words. These are mainly *phonological*, or involve sound

Gordon is describing a picture of a kitchen scene. In the picture a boy steals biscuits from a high shelf while balancing on a stool. His mother is doing the washing up and water runs out of the sink.

STEAL ... BISCUIT BISCUIT BISCUIT...BOY...CHILD...BOY...TAPS ...RUNNING (water)...h – o – t TAP...PAIN (points to boy in picture)... (mimes falling)

Figure 19.2 An example of agrammatic BSL.

substitutions. Phonological errors also occur in sign aphasia, for instance in the form of handshape, location or orientation substitutions (see Corina et al., 1992). Figure 19.3 illustrates a handshape error made by a Deaf participant in our project.

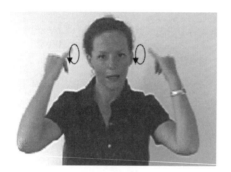
Target: SHEEP

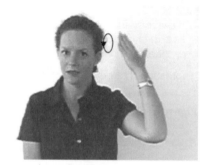
Error

Figure 19.3 Example of an Aphasic Phonological Error in BSL. The figure shows an unimpaired signer reproducing the error. Note that the error is produced with just the left hand, as the signer had a right hemiplegia.

Sign language aphasias are not only interesting because of the parallels they show with spoken language aphasias. They also enable us to explore aspects of language that are unique to sign, and so provide novel insights into how the brain processes language. One such aspect is the use of space. In sign languages, signing space can be used both topographically (for example, when describing the layout of a room), and syntactically. In the latter, sentence nouns are assigned consistent but arbitrary positions within the signing space, and verb signs move between these positions to indicate the subject and object of the action. Some studies suggest that these different uses of space dissociate following brain damage. So, people with right-hemisphere stroke who have visuospatial problems have shown impaired topographic but not syntactic space; while those with left-hemisphere strokes have shown the opposite dissociation (Poizner, Klima and Bellugi, 1987; Emmorey, Klima and Bellugi, 1995; Emmorey, 1996; Hickok et al., 1996). It seems that, although signing space is generally processed in the left hemisphere, the spatial skills of the right hemisphere may play a subtle role, particularly when tasks require the person to match a sign description to real world spatial relationships.

Most investigations of sign aphasia have been conducted with users of ASL, with few studies in other languages. We estimate that at least 100 Deaf people in Britain have strokes every year with perhaps a third of the survivors becoming aphasic. This largely hidden population poses a number of questions. What is the precise nature of their problems? What services are Deaf aphasic people offered and do these take account of their language and culture? The Deaf Stroke Project aimed to address these questions.

Test development

Investigating acquired sign language impairments is challenging. It may be difficult to determine the person's language abilities before the stroke, especially if there is no pre-morbid evidence (such as video recordings). Almost all hearing people acquire their first language from their parents, whereas Deaf users of sign language have various patterns of acquisition, which may affect competence even into adulthood (Emmorey et al., 1995; Morgan and Woll, 2002). Therefore, subtle difficulties observed after stroke may reflect a poor early language environment, or delayed acquisition.

Another difficulty is that BSL, like many sign languages, has a high degree of regional variation, particularly in the *lexicon* (Sutton Spence and Woll, 1999). Unimpaired Deaf people cope well with this. For example, we found that they can understand and produce different lexical variants in comprehension and naming tests. Deaf people following stroke may be less flexible. Therefore, an apparent failure on a test could arise from relative unfamiliarity with a regional sign, rather than a genuine language difficulty.

The third, and most obvious problem is the complete absence of appropriate language tests. One response might be to translate English aphasia tests into BSL. However, there are numerous reasons why this is not a good idea:

Control of variables

Language tests should be controlled for different variables, such as word frequency and age of acquisition. These factors affect processing in spoken language aphasia (Hirsh and Ellis, 1994; Jescheniak and Levelt, 1994) and are likely to be similarly influential in sign aphasia. However, we cannot assume that norms for English words apply to their translation equivalents in BSL, partly because of cultural differences and partly because many English words do not map directly onto BSL signs. There are also variables, like *iconicity*, which are relevant in BSL but less so in English.

Developing language-specific tests

Some assessments are similar across languages, such as tests of single word/sign comprehension. Grammatical assessments have to be more language centred. For example, English tests tend to focus on word order as this is the main carrier of sentence meanings, while the equivalent tests in BSL will focus on spatially specified syntax and verb modifications.

Selection of distractors

Tests of language comprehension often ask the person to point to a picture that matches a given word or a sentence. This picture is presented on a response card, together with carefully chosen distractors (or foils). For example, an English test might ask someone to point to a target picture (for example, 'cap') with distractors illustrating similar sounding words (for instance 'map' and 'tap'). This is testing whether the person can discriminate words. Sign discrimination may also be impaired in BSL aphasia. However, we cannot investigate this simply by translating the English text. Rather we need a novel task, involving signs with visually similar forms.

Cultural differences

Although British Deaf and hearing people share many cultural experiences, there are obvious differences. These lead to variations in concept and object familiarity, which should, in turn, influence test design. So a picture of a minicom is a more suitable test item than a radio for Deaf people; while the reverse is true for hearing people.

These are just some of the arguments against translating language tests. Our project, therefore, developed several new measures, which pay careful attention to the properties of BSL. The following section describes some of these and presents the results of testing with Deaf stroke survivors and Deaf controls. Controls were recruited from Deaf groups in the South of England. Most were elderly and none had neurological impairments. All used BSL as their preferred language.

The case history

A detailed case history (conducted in BSL) was obtained from each participant, often with a close friend or family member present. A family informant is particularly helpful when there is aphasia, which may prevent the person from responding fully to questions. The case history covers relevant background information (for example, family, work history, social contacts), the language history (for example, age of acquisition of BSL and pre-morbid use of English), the history of the stroke and problems since then. The case history will highlight changes in communication since the stroke. For example, the person may report sign-finding problems, or family members may comment that they have to sign more slowly to help a relative understand.

The sign-to-picture matching test

This explores comprehension of BSL nouns. The tester produces a single sign and the person has to point to the matching picture from a choice of five. The pictures show the target, a *semantic* distractor, which is related in meaning to the target, a phonological distractor, which has a similar sign form, a visual distractor and an unrelated distractor (see example in Figure 19.4). Visual distractors aim to identify people who use an *iconic* strategy in comprehension. So, in Figure 19.4, the visual distractor for dog (South-Eastern regional variation) is knife and fork, since the form of this sign could be interpreted as resembling cutlery. There are 40 items in the test. Twenty involve iconic signs and twenty involve non-iconic signs (iconicity was determined by ratings from Deaf signers and hearing non-signers). The test therefore enables us to explore whether understanding of signs after stroke is influenced by iconicity.

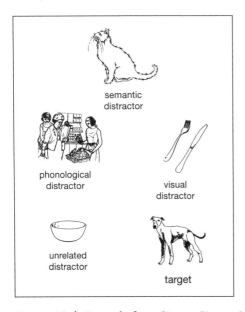

The target sign DOG is produced with two hands. In both hands, the index and middle finger are extended together and point downwards in front of the body. The sign for SHOP is very similar, although here all four fingers are extended together and point downwards.

Figure 19.4 Example from Sign to Picture Matching Test.

Controls and individuals with right hemisphere (RH) strokes scored close to ceiling on this test. The left hemisphere (LH) group made far more errors (mean correct score 79.5%, range 57.5% to 92.5%), the majority of which were semantic. Interestingly, there was no significant difference in their comprehension of iconic and non-iconic signs. There is already good evidence that iconicity does not affect the normal processing of sign language or its acquisition as a first language (see Petitto, 1987 and Emmorey, 2002 for reviews). The results of this test suggest that it is similarly uninfluential in aphasia.

Comprehension of verbs and sentences

Many aphasic people understand single nouns well but have problems with verbs and sentences (see Martin and Miller, 2002, for a review). To test for this possibility in BSL aphasia we developed the verb-and-sentence comprehension test. An individual watches a signed verb or sentence, which has to be matched to one of four pictures. Some sentences are simple, such as:

PICTURE WOMAN LOOK (the woman is looking at a picture)

while others are more complex, such as:

GIRL WOMAN (index to location a) BOOK SHOW (verb moves towards location a) (English gloss: 'a girl shows a book to a woman').

The distractors ensure that all aspects of the sentence have to be processed if the person is to succeed. So, in Figure 19.5, if the person misses one of the signs in the sentence, or fails to interpret the spatial syntax, he or she is likely to pick a distractor.

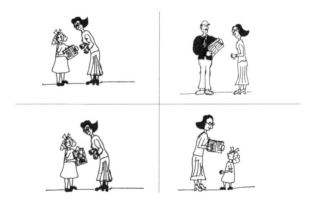

Figure 19.5 Example from the BSL Verb and Sentence Comprehension Test
GIRL WOMAN (index location a) BOOK SHOW (verb moves towards location a).

Again, the control and RH group were close to ceiling on this test, whereas the LH achieved a mean score of just 65% (range 30% to 82.5%). Many of their errors were reversals, so instead of pointing to the girl showing the book to the woman (target) they might point to the woman showing the book to the girl. This error pattern is also common in English aphasia (see, for example, Black, Nickels and Byng, 1992) and suggests that the person can understand the words in the sentence, but not the grammatical relationship between them. Interestingly, this parallel occurs despite the fact that, in English, the relationship is signalled by word order whereas in BSL it is signalled by spatial syntax.

Comprehension of locative sentences

Locative sentences, such as CHAIR BOX UNDER (The box is under the chair) express spatial relationships between objects. British Sign Language locatives can be specified in two ways: either lexically, using prepositional signs such as IN or UNDER, or by using *classifiers* to show the relationship between objects in topographical space. Signers fluent in BSL usually show a preference for classifier structures in their spontaneous production. We hypothesized that locatives may be difficult for BSL users following damage to either hemisphere, because they require intact processing by the left hemisphere language cortex and simultaneous spatial processing in the right hemisphere.

In this test a locative sentence has to be matched to one of four pictures. These show: the target; the reversal; a picture with the same objects in a different configuration; and a picture with different objects. So one target is BOX CUP ON (the cup is on the box), with distractors showing a box on a cup, a cup behind a box and a cup on a shelf. Sentences with lexical prepositions and classifiers are both tested.

As with the other language tests, this task posed no difficulties for controls, their mean score being 29/30. However, all stroke survivors were impaired, which supported our initial hypothesis. The LH group made mixed errors, whereas most errors of the RH group involved either picking the reversal, or the picture showing the objects in the wrong configuration. It seemed that different problems underpinned the performance of the stroke groups. Those with LH strokes had difficulty understanding all elements of the sentences, including the nouns. Those with RH strokes understood the nouns, but not their spatial configuration.

Production

A number of tests explored production. Nouns were tested by asking participants to name the targets used in the sign-to-picture matching test. We also asked people to describe the target pictures used in the verb and sentence comprehension test, to see whether production beyond the single word was affected. To elicit narratives, we asked each person to describe complex and sequenced pictures.

A novel computer task elicited locatives and classifiers. The person was shown a photograph of two objects in a particular spatial configuration (for example, a spoon next to a bowl). The picture then changed to show the same objects in a different configuration (for example, the spoon in the bowl) and the person was asked to describe the change. This picture sequence encouraged the use of classifiers, rather than lexical locative sentences, because classifier constructions are typically used to show changes in the spatial relationship between objects.

Most people with left-hemisphere strokes found these production tasks difficult. Some had virtually no output. Others could produce single nouns, but struggled when verbs or connected signs were required. The RH group generally fared better. However, some had extreme difficulties with locative classifiers, preferring to use lexical or signed English forms, with English word order, or even finger spelling to describe spatial relationships.

Summary of group performance

Like previous studies of lesioned signers, we found that people with left hemisphere damage were impaired on virtually all measures of BSL, whereas those with right damage were not. This is further evidence that sign language, like spoken language, is processed primarily in the left hemisphere.

Our RH group had difficulties with locative sentences, both in comprehension and production. Most of these people also had visuospatial problems – for instance, they could not copy pictures or reproduce patterns in a block design task (see Stanley pp. 301–2). Their problems with locatives were plausibly related to this, in that they could no longer use language to describe topographic space.

Some members of the RH group also had *pragmatic* problems, or difficulties in the use of language. So, although their signing was grammatically correct, it was often odd. They wandered off the topic in conversation, their story telling was incoherent and they missed out the punch line in jokes. Similar difficulties have been reported previously in both hearing and Deaf people with right hemisphere CVAs (Joanette, Goulet and Hannequin, 1990; Loew, Kegl and Poizner, 1997; Hickok et al., 1999).

Testing issues

We shall end this section with some general comments about testing Deaf people following stroke. Language assessment must be conducted by native signers or by Deaf investigators with highly fluent BSL. Only they have the required language expertise and knowledge of crucial issues, such as regional variation. Testing must also be flexible. For example, if a person has a visual field deficit or *neglect,* signs and pictures should be presented only on the unaffected side and in a vertical array. Testing must also take account of regional variation. The above measures use South East regional signs. When testing individuals from different parts of the country it is important to check whether these are known to the person, eg by using a family member as informant, and it may be necessary to replace some items with the person's own variant. Replacing target signs will result in the phonological distractor becoming invalid (since this item has a sign name which is similar in form to the target). Ideally, therefore, the phonological distractor should also be replaced. Of course, existing control data will no longer apply to a modified version of the test.

Finally, it is important to remember that individuals may have additional difficulties, over and above the effects of the stroke. One possibility is dementia, in which case relatives may report problems pre-dating the stroke, such as memory loss. There may also be co-occurring mental health problems or learning disabilities. Again, evidence for this may emerge from the case history and relatives' reports.

Individual case studies

The above tests were not only used to explore patterns of performance across groups, they also helped us to unravel the complex language difficulties of individuals after stroke. To illustrate this, we present two case studies, one of a person with left and the other with right hemisphere damage.

Maureen

Maureen was deafened at 18 months by meningitis. She attended Deaf school from the age of 5, was a lifelong user of BSL and active in the Deaf community. When Maureen was 70 she had a devastating left CVA, which caused a right-sided paralysis and severe communication difficulties.

When we met Maureen it was obvious that she retained excellent social skills. She smiled and waved in greeting and blew kisses when we left. As we signed our farewells, she reached for her calendar, in order to arrange the date for our next visit. Despite these skills Maureen had virtually no sign production. She could not answer questions, describe pictures or even repeat signs. We tried to cue her, by modelling signs and manipulating her good hand to help her achieve the handshape. Yet even with this degree of help, Maureen could produce nothing.

Maureen's hemiplegia might have restricted her signing. However, most people with hemiplegia sign well, albeit with only one hand.

Another explanation for her difficulties could be apraxia (Rothi and Heilman, 1997). All Maureen's planned actions were impaired. She could not gesture, beyond waving and pointing, and could not demonstrate the use of tools. One test for apraxia (Kimura, 1993; Sunderland and Sluman, 2000) involved imitating three actions in the correct order: pushing a button with the forefinger, grasping a handle and depressing a lever with the thumb. Maureen could not sequence these actions or formulate the correct hand posture for each one. The evidence pointed to severe apraxia.

We wondered whether Maureen still knew about signs, even though she could not produce them. To test this, we showed her pictures of various objects, together with icons representing three common BSL handshapes. Maureen had to think about the sign for each picture and point to its handshape (see example in Figure 19.6). Maureen scored no better than chance. It seemed that her mental representation of signs was impaired, which would be consistent with severe aphasia.

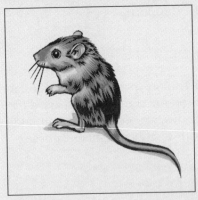

Task
Think of the sign for this picture, and point to the correct handshape

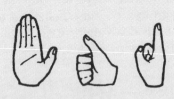

Figure 19.6 Example from the Handshape Judgement Test.

Further evidence for aphasia came from comprehension testing. On sign-to-picture matching she scored 25/40. Her understanding of verbs and sentences was even more impaired (12/40), as was her understanding of locatives (13/30). These comprehension difficulties were obvious in everyday interactions. So, to help her understand, we often used pictures, and signed slowly.

Although Maureen found it hard to understand BSL after her stroke, she understood gestures well. In one test we showed her pictures of four tools. We gestured the use of one, and she had to point to the corresponding picture. She scored 21/24, which was no different from elderly Deaf controls. This comprehension of gesture was useful, in that it opened up some rudimentary communication with the nursing home staff.

In summary, Maureen's stroke caused a severe aphasia, which impaired both her production and comprehension of BSL. She also had apraxia, which further restricted her sign production, and prevented her from using gesture. Although she could not produce gestures, she could understand them, which is evidence that gestures and signs are processed by different regions of the brain (see also Marshall et al., in press).

Stanley

Stanley was born deaf into a hearing family. He began to acquire BSL at the age of 5 when he attended a Deaf school and used it throughout his life as his preferred language.

When he was 56 Stanley had a severe right CVA, causing left hemiplegia and left neglect. As a result, Stanley might not notice people standing on his left side, and would ignore his paralysed arm, often leaving it dangling over the edge of his wheelchair. Fortunately, this problem improved over time.

Stanley had more general and long-lasting visuospatial problems. He found visual tasks, such as drawing and copying patterns, difficult. Faces were particularly problematic. For example, he could not recognize facial expressions of emotion (Ekman and Friesen, 1975), match pictures of the same face (Benton and Van Allen, 1973) or recall faces that he had seen shortly before (Warrington, 1984). Stanley reported everyday difficulties with faces. He had attended a day centre for people with disabilities for over a year yet could only recognize one member of staff there.

These problems might have a profound impact on Stanley's use of BSL, given that this is a visuospatial language. However, this was generally not the case. Stanley could still hold a conversation and coped well with a number of language tests, such as sign-to-picture matching, verb and sentence comprehension, and picture naming. Despite this, there were subtle communication difficulties. We noticed that Stanley's face lacked expression, even when he was signing about emotional events. His gaze tended to be fixed on the person he was addressing, with no changes to signal role shift or grammatical marking. It was often difficult to determine whether he was asking us a question, as his face lacked question markers. Stanley's appreciation of expression seemed equally poor. If we asked him a question using just facial markers he might simply stare at us, apparently unaware that a response was required. Stanley's social worker, who was a BSL user, confirmed that these problems were not present premorbidly.

It seemed that Stanley's visual problems had subtle effects on his signing, particularly with respect to facial processing. A test exploring comprehension of negation provided corroborating evidence. Stanley was shown two pictures, one of which was the negative of the other. For example, one pair showed a dog with and a dog without a bone. We signed either a positive or negative statement, which had to be matched to one of the pictures. Negatives were signed in two ways. In half the items the negative was marked purely facially (for example, with furrowed brows and a head shake). In the other half there was an additional lexical sign (NOTHING).

Controls and even most aphasic people found this test easy. Stanley, on the other hand, found it hard. His difficulties were not general, because he performed almost perfectly with positive items (15/16), and quite well with the lexically marked negatives (12/16). However, he consistently failed to detect negatives that were marked purely with face, and with these items his performance dropped below chance (5/16).

In summary, Stanley's visuospatial problems left many aspects of his sign language intact and he was not generally aphasic. There were, however, islands of difficulty, one of which involved processing sign language information on the face (see also Atkinson et al., 2004). To compensate for this, we never used grammatical facial markers in isolation when we were conversing with Stanley, but always added a lexical sign.

Access to services

Maureen and Stanley both received rehabilitation for their acquired disabilities. To what extent were they typical? Our project interviewed 48 Deaf stroke survivors. Accounts of rehabilitation varied greatly, partly because people could not remember what services they received, or were unclear about the roles of different professionals. With this in mind, about 70% of individuals recalled receiving physiotherapy and occupational therapy, whereas only 30% reported contact with a speech and language therapist (SLT). Those who had seen an SLT were mainly treated for swallowing problems, even if they had aphasia.

Experiences of services also varied. Some individuals reported positive encounters with creative and flexible staff, but there were also negative reports of attitudinal and communication problems. Lack of interpreting provision was a consistent theme in our interviews. Only four people reported that interpreters were provided by the hospital, and then only intermittently. In many cases, family members were called upon to provide communication support (see also Atkinson et al., 2002).

Survey of speech and language therapy providers (see also Marshall et al., 2002)

To find out more about rehabilitation we surveyed all SLT managers in Britain (N = 260). We asked whether their specialist stroke or neurology teams had received referrals of Deaf patients in the previous 5 years and, if so, what services were offered. We also asked if anyone in the team could sign, and whether they had access to interpreters.

Despite a reasonable response rate (60%), only 34 teams reported seeing Deaf stroke patients in the previous 5 years, with 39 people seen. Yet, using normal referral rates as a guide, we estimate that at least 220 Deaf people should have been referred in the same period. It seems that Deaf people with strokes are typically not being referred to SLT, possibly because medical staff (who are the main source of referrals) either cannot detect their acquired communication difficulties, or wrongly attribute these to their premorbid deafness.

The most common service offered to Deaf stroke patients was swallowing therapy, which reflected the dominant reason for referral. Fifty-four per cent of those referred were also given language assessment, but only 20% language therapy. Finally, we found that communication resources were far from ideal. Very few SLT teams working in the neurological field included skilled signers and 23% of respondents reported that they had no access to interpreters. Alarmingly, this was true of six of the services that actually treated Deaf patients.

Service recommendations

Meeting the needs of Deaf stroke patients is challenging, particularly when there are communication difficulties. These individuals represent a dispersed minority within the neurological caseload. Few rehabilitation specialists have signing skills and, until recently, there were no tools for assessing acquired BSL impairments. As we found in our survey, access to interpreters is not universal. Even if it were, working through interpreters is far from ideal. It is very difficult to interpret aphasic language accurately, particularly to a clinician who is not familiar with the unique properties of BSL. Rather, assessment should be conducted by clinicians fluent in BSL.

Despite these challenges, people from language minorities are entitled to equal access to services (Royal College of Speech and Language Therapists, 1996). One way of realizing this philosophy with respect to our population would be to establish a National Deaf Neurological Outreach Team. This would comprise rehabilitation specialists (for example, from clinical psychology, SLT and OT) who are skilled users of BSL and who could support/advise any neurological service throughout Britain faced with a Deaf referral. The team could continue to develop

BSL assessments and build upon existing knowledge about how neurological deficits affect sign language. Above all, they could help to ensure that Deaf people with strokes receive culturally and linguistically appropriate rehabilitation.

Conclusions

Our findings indicate that, as in all other language groups, sign-language impairments arise primarily from left-hemisphere damage. However, the signing skills of those with right CVAs were also affected. These individuals often had difficulty with language about spatial relationships and some, like Stanley, struggled with facially expressed elements. Our project also explored rehabilitation issues, particularly with respect to communication (an area neglected in previous research). We found that Deaf stroke survivors rarely received support for their acquired communication problems, and that SLT teams were not able to offer assessment or therapies that take account of the complex and often subtle nature of sign language breakdown. We argue that without specialist provision, eg in the form of a Deaf Neurological Outreach Team, Deaf people with acquired communication difficulties will continue to fall through the net.

Glossary

- *Apraxia.* Apraxia is a neurological deficit that impairs planned, purposeful movements, particularly those involving sequences. Apraxia is not due to paralysis, and spontaneous actions are unaffected – people will be unable to scratch their nose to request, but may do so automatically if it itches.
- *Classifiers.* Classifiers are a constrained set of handshapes used to denote categories of objects, which substitute for lexical signs in verbs of motion and location. So for example, flat objects (such as a piece of paper or a table) are represented by a flat handshape with the fingers extended and together, while long, thin objects (such as a pen or a person) are represented by an extended index finger. To express 'the pen is on the table', the hand representing the pen (extended index finger) is placed on top of the hand representing the table (flat hand, palm down).
- *Iconicity.* All sign languages include a number of iconic signs, where there is a relationship between the form of the sign and its meaning. For example, the BSL sign TREE employs a vertical forearm and extended and spread fingers that recall the trunk and branches of a tree.

Iconicity is not restricted to sign language, but is also observed in onomatopoeic spoken words, such as 'pop' and 'whisper'.

- *Lexicon.* The lexicon is the vocabulary of a language. The lexicon is constantly changing as new words are acquired and old ones fall out of use. The lexicon of BSL is productive, in the sense that new signs can be constructed, in a rule governed way, to express new or modified meanings (see Sutton Spence and Woll, 1999).
- *Neglect.* A person with unilateral spatial neglect fails to attend to stimuli or events occurring on one side of space. The neglected region is always on the opposite side of the CVA. So people with a right CVA may neglect stimuli occurring in their left visual field (neglect is more common in people with right than left CVAs). Possible signs of neglect include: failure to read words on one side of a newspaper, missing food on one side of the plate and only shaving one side of the face.
- *Phonology.* All languages have a phonology, which refers to the structure and formation of words through combinatorial units. For example, English words are composed from a constrained set of sounds, with rule governed combinations. The phonology of sign language is constructed from visual, rather than auditory, elements, including handshape, location and movement. Thus, BSL has a constrained set of handshapes with rules as to how they can be combined (see Sutton Spence and Woll, 1999).
- *Pragmatics.* Pragmatics refers to the use of language. In order to uncover the intention of a signer/speaker we need pragmatic skills. These go beyond the ability to decode the literal meanings of words or sentences. We also need to be alert to intonation and prosody (or the rhythm of the language), and be able to relate each sentence to the unfolding discourse and to our knowledge of the world.
- *Semantics.* Semantics refers to the meaning of language. When comprehending language we have to access the semantics of individual words/signs and of sentences. So, in the sentence: $DOG_{index\ a}\ CAT_{index\ b}\ BITE_{b\rightarrow a}$ (the cat bites the dog) we not only interpret the lexical meaning of CAT, but also its sentence meaning (as the agent or instigator of the verb). Strokes and other neurological disorders can impair the person's ability to access meaning from language. This may result in semantic errors, for example where the person calls a cat DOG, or points to a picture of a dog in response to the sign CAT.
- *Syntax.* Syntax refers to the organization of words or signs into sentences. Languages employ a number of devices to signal syntactic relations. For example, English uses word order and grammatical word endings (like -ed, -ing), while BSL employs spatial markers, such as indexing and directional inflection of verbs.

References

Atkinson J, Campbell R, Marshall J, Thacker A, Woll B (2004) Understanding 'not': neuropsychological dissociations between hand and head markers of negation in BSL. Neuropsychologia 42: 214–229.

Atkinson J, Marshall J, Thacker A and Woll B (2002) When sign language breaks down: deaf people's access to language therapy in the UK. Deaf Worlds 18: 9–21.

Benton AL, Van Allen MW (1973) Test of Face Recognition Manual. Neurosensory Center. Ames IA: Department of Neurology, University of Iowa.

Black M, Nickels L, Byng S (1992) Patterns of sentence processing deficit: processing simple sentences can be a complex matter. Journal of Neurolinguistics 6: 79–101.

Chiarello C, Knight R, Mandel M (1982) Aphasia in a prelingually deaf woman. Brain, 105: 29–51.

Cifu D, Lorish T (1994) Stroke rehabilitation: 5 stroke outcome. Archives of Physical Medicine and Rehabilitation 75(S): 56–60.

Corina DP (1998) Aphasia in users of signed languages. In Coppens P, Lebrun Y, Basso A (eds) Aphasia in Atypical Populations. Hillsdale NJ: Erlbaum, pp. 261–310.

Corina DP, Poizner H, Bellugi U, Feinberg T, Dowd D, O'Grady-Batch L (1992) Dissociation between linguistic and nonlinguistic gestural systems: a case for compositionality. Brain and Language 43: 414–47.

Ekman P, Friesen WV (1975) Unmasking the Face: A Guide to Recognizing Emotions from Facial Clues. Englewood Cliffs NJ: Prentice-Hall.

Ellis A, Miller D, Sin G (1983) Wernicke's aphasia and normal language processing: a case study in cognitive neuropsychology. Cognition 15: 111–44.

Emmorey K (1996) The confluence of spance and language in signed languages. In P Bloom, M Peterson, L Nadel, M Garrett (eds) Language and Space. Cambridge MA: MIT Press, pp. 171–209.

Emmorey K (2002) Language, Cognition and the Brain: Insights from Sign Language Research. Mahwah NJ: Erlbaum.

Emmorey K, Bellugi U, Friederici A, Horn P (1995) Effects of age of acquisition on grammatical sensitivity: Evidence from on-line and off-line tasks. Applied Psycholinguistics 16: 1–23.

Emmorey K, Corina D, Bellugi U (1995) Differential processing of topographic and referential functions of space. In Emmorey K, Reilly J (eds) Language, Gesture and Space. Mahwah NJ: Lawrence Erlbaum Associates, pp. 43–62.

Hickok G, Klima E, Kritchevsky M, Bellugi U (1995) A case of 'sign blindness' following left occipital damage in a deaf signer. Neuropsychologia 33: 1597–606.

Hickok G, Say K, Bellugi U, Klima E (1996) The basis of hemispheric asymmetries for language and spatial cognition – clues from focal brain damage in 2 deaf native signers, Aphasiology 10: 577–91.

Hickok G, Bellugi U, Klima E (1998) What's right about the neuroal organisation of sign language? A perspective on recent neuroimaging results. Trends in Cognitive Sciences 2: 465–8.

Hickok G, Wilson M, Clark K, Klima E, Kritchevsky M, Bellugi U (1999) Discourse deficits following right hemisphere damage in deaf signers. Brain and Language 66: 233–48.

Hickok G, Love-Geffen T, Klima ES (2002) Role of the left hemisphere in sign language comprehension. Brain and Language 82: 167–78.

Hirsh C, Ellis A (1994) Age of acquisition and lexical processing in aphasia. A case study. Cognitive Neuropsychology 6: 435–58.

Jescheniak J, Levelt W (1994) Word frequency effects in speech production: Retrieval of syntactic information and of phonological form. Journal of Experimental Psychology, Learning, Memory and Cognition 20: 824–43.

Joanette Y, Goulet P, Hannequin D (1990) Right Hemisphere and Verbal Communication. New York: Springer Verlag.

Kimura D (1993) Neuromotor Mechanisms in Human Communication. Oxford: Oxford University Press.

Langton Hewer R (1997) The epidemiology of disabling neurological disorders. In Greenwood R, Barnes M, McMillan T and Ward C (eds) Neurological Rehabilitation. Hove: Psychology Press.

Loew R, Kegl J, Poizner H (1997) Fractionation of the components of role play in a right-hemispheric lesioned signer. Aphasiology 11: 263–81.

MacSweeney M, Woll B, Campbell C, McGuire P, Calvert G, David A, Williams S, Brammer M (2002) Neural systems underlying British Sign Language sentence comprehension. Brain 125: 1583–93.

Marshall J, Pring T, Chiat S (1993) Sentence processing therapy: working at the level of the event. Aphasiology 7: 177–99.

Marshall J, Atkinson J, Smulovitch E, Thacker A, Woll B (In press) Aphasia in a user of British Sign Language: dissociation between sign and gesture. Cognitive Neuropsychology.

Marshall J, Atkinson J, Thacker A, Woll B (2002) Is speech and language therapy meeting the needs of language minorities: the case of Deaf people with neurological impairments. International Journal of Language and Communication Disorders 38: 85–94.

Martin R, Miller M (2002) Sentence comprehension deficits: independence and interaction of syntax, semantics and working memory. In A Hillis (ed) The Handbook of Adult Language Disorders. New York: Psychology Press.

Morgan G, Woll B (eds) (2002) Directions in Sign Language Acquisition Research. Amsterdam: John Benjamins.

Parr S, Byng S, Gilpin S (1997) Talking about Aphasia. Buckingham: Open University Press.

Petitto L (1987) On the autonomy of language and gesture: Evidence from the acquisition of personal pronouns in American Sign Language. Cognition 27: 1–52.

Poizner H, Klima ES, Bellugi U (1987) What the Hands Reveal about the Brain. Cambridge MA: MIT Press.

Rothi L, Heilman K (eds) (1997) Apraxia: the Neuropsychology of Action. Hove: Psychology Press.

Royal College of Speech and Language Therapists (1996) Communicating Quality. London: Royal College of Speech and Language Therapists.

Sarno J, Swisher L, Sarno M (1969) Aphasia in a congenitally deaf man. Cortex 5: 398–414.

Sarno M (1991) Acquired Aphasia. San Diego CA: Academic Press.

Sunderland A, Sluman S-M (2000) Ideomotor apraxia, visuomotor control and the explicit representation of posture. Neuropsychologia 38: 923–34.

Sutton Spence R, Woll B (1999) The Linguistics of British Sign Language. Cambridge: Cambridge University Press.

Warlow CP (1998) Epidemiology of stroke. The Lancet, 352(supplement III): 1–4.

Warrington EK (1984) Recognition Memory Test. Windsor: NFER Nelson.

CHAPTER 20

Non-organic hearing loss: detection, diagnosis and management

CATHERINE LYNCH AND SALLY AUSTEN

Introduction

Non-organic hearing loss (NOHL) is both clinically important and psychologically intriguing. Described as *responses to a hearing test indicating a greater deficit than can be explained by organic pathology*, explanations for this phenomenon have emerged from a variety of theoretical perspectives. This has resulted in a complex array of terms associated with the concept, including *functional deafness, feigned or simulated loss; psychogenic loss; pseudohypacusis; malingering; dissociative loss* and *conversion loss*. Methods for detecting NOHL and resolving true hearing levels will be discussed, together with diagnostic models and an outline of the basic principles of effective management.

The measurement of hearing: audiometry

Audiometry is the psychophysical measurement of hearing sensitivity, routinely employed from the cognitive age of 3 upwards. A behavioural response (such as pressing a button) is required whenever a test tone is heard.

When a positive response is forthcoming the test stimulus is made quieter; if a response is not apparent the intensity of the test stimulus is increased. The tester explores the region between response and no response, arriving at an estimation of threshold defined as the minimal level at which the subject responds two times out of three (British Society of Audiologists, 1981). This process is repeated for both ears separately at key frequencies across the normally audible range (250 Hz to 8 KHz).

A full test protocol necessitates approximately 140 responses. Around threshold, there is always some uncertainty, even for a well-motivated individual. Depending on attitudinal and/or personality factors

(Stephens, 1969; Aplin and Kane, 1985) there may be an inclination towards guessing or conversely an unwillingness to respond unless absolutely certain.

In spite of these artificial conditions, most audiometric tests are generally considered reliable with clinically acceptable test-retest differences. Where audiometric results are found *not* to reflect a true level of hearing, however, there can be several reasons. In the specific situation where the patient has influenced the outcome so as to appear less sensitive to sound than their true psychophysical threshold, the extra degree of recorded deficit constitutes an occurrence of NOHL.

Presenting features of NOHL

Jerger and Jerger (1981) estimate a prevalence of NOHL that is less than 2% in the general population: about 7% in children between 6 and 17 years and 10% to 50% in adults seeking compensation or in military-related audiology services. Put into context, even the 2% figure would imply several cases a month in a typical busy hospital setting.

The degree of NOHL can vary from a relatively small loss in one ear to an apparent complete loss of hearing bilaterally. In their series of 88 resolved NOHL cases, Gelfand and Silman (1993) found that 28% had non-organic components unilaterally and 72% bilaterally.

Many cases of NOHL present as an apparent superimposed deficit, augmenting an actual organic hearing loss (Gleason, 1958; Chailklin and Ventry, 1963; Coles and Priede, 1971; Gelfand and Silman, 1993). This non-organic overlay is the difference between the degree of hearing loss indicated by the patient and the actual underlying loss. A related phenomenon is the prior experience of organic hearing loss before onset of NOHL (Aplin and Rowson, 1986).

Attempts to profile psychological characteristics of persons presenting with NOHL have been made (Gleason, 1958; Trier and Levy, 1965; Aplin and Rowson, 1986). Greater degrees of emotional immaturity, social anxiety, instability and feelings of inferiority than the normal population have been suggested. Conclusions can be limited however by the specific nature of the populations under study (for example, a military setting).

Detecting NOHL

The detection of NOHL when it presents itself during audiometric evaluation is crucial for appropriate management. Failure to detect NOHL can lead to inappropriate intervention: the incorrect prescription of a powerful hearing aid or unnecessary surgery such as cochlear implantation. Furthermore, any missed psychological cause of NOHL could become entrenched, and ultimately less amenable to therapeutic input (Barr, 1963). Finally it may be considered socially inappropriate (even a criminal act) to divert funds intended to treat true disability.

Fortunately the ability to detect non-organic behaviour and determine true hearing levels is improving. Some cases of NOHL do still go unnoticed however. Studies by Spraggs, Burton and Graham (1994) and Lynch et al. (2001) indicate that significant numbers of NOHL cases were referred for tertiary level cochlear implant assessment, despite having passed through the hands of experienced clinicians.

Behavioural assessment

Often the nature of the referral (the medicolegal context, a teenager under stress, existing family deafness) will trigger an alert to possible NOHL. Individuals' attitude to their hearing loss can also provide clues. The patient may exaggerate some stereotypical characteristics of deafness such as cupping a hand to their ear or making exaggerated 'attempts' to lipread. Because they are somehow deriving benefit from the deaf role, they may exhibit an enhanced desire to discuss their hearing difficulties, contrasting with the typical embarrassment seen in cases of true hearing loss. This may culminate in the non-emotional state known as *la belle indifference* (Edgerton, 1994).

Where there is less overt intention to produce NOHL or a long-standing investment in the deaf or Deaf role, behaviour can be very congruent with that normally expected from a deaf person. Anecdotal reports include persons living in Deaf communities whose NOHL has gone unnoticed for years and even those who have adopted a deaf quality to their voice.

During initial contact, an alert clinician can take various opportunities to converse with the patient although manipulating a range of conditions, such as occasionally obscuring the possibility of lip-reading or continuing to converse while a supposed 'good' ear is blocked. This can help refine expectations of true underlying hearing levels prior to formal testing.

Audiometric assessment: specific techniques for quantifying NOHL

Once audiometry has commenced, an experienced clinician will be sensitive to any mismatch between apparent functional competence and emerging response levels.

Should it be suspected that standard audiometry is not yielding accurate results, there are several techniques that can be employed. Distinction is made between *subjective* tests that rely in part on the subject's active co-operation and cognitive effort versus *objective* tests that detect involuntary physiological activity.

Subjective tests

Studies simulating non-organic behaviour during audiometry suggest that a typical strategy for the patient is to adopt an internal loudness criterion or 'anchor' point, refusing to respond at levels quieter than this (Ventry, 1976; Gelfand and Silman, 1993; Gelfand, 1993). It is therefore useful for the tester to disrupt this criterion by refraining from the standard progression to higher intensity stimuli when no response is obtained. Longer than usual presentations are also useful, as the psychological effort needed to resist response increases with the length of the presentation tone. Similarly, leaving longer gaps between test stimuli encourages the patient to 'do something'. A key indicator of non-organic behaviour can be unwillingness to offer the normal amount of 'false positive' responses during such long gaps. A typical well-motivated patient will be tempted to make the odd false positive response, or ask for clarification and reassurance about the absence of stimuli (Chaiklin and Ventry, 1965).

Hosoi et al. (1999) recommend an approach designed for children whereby a non-functioning hearing aid is placed under the headphones, with the overt suggestion that this will enhance hearing. They report significant improvements in thresholds and speech recognition for NOHL cases, although the element of deception may not be acceptable to all. A simpler variant of this approach is deliberately to change the headphones to a larger circumaural pair, mentioning that the new ones work better, when in fact they are calibrated to perform the same measure. This will often have a positive effect on responses, particularly with children and less sophisticated adults. Other reframing techniques include asking the patient to say 'yes' when the stimulus is heard and 'no' when it is not. With less sophisticated NOHL patients the 'no' response can be reliably attached to the stimulus (Frank, 1976). This is unlikely to reveal NOHL in the determined adult, however.

When simple audiometric procedures (above) are ineffective in resolving the NOHL, tests exploiting various *non-intuitive psychophysical properties* of the hearing system can be useful. Only an unusually well-informed subject would be likely to second-guess the appropriate response. Examples include the fact that sound presented at high intensities through one headphone will at some stage be detected by the opposite cochlea as the pressure wave passes through the cranial structures. Assuming a functioning cochlea on the other side, presenting progressively louder sounds to a totally deaf ear should eventually elicit a response from the subject. Failure to obtain this 'shadow' response indicates deliberate suppression. A further non-intuitive property is that when two similar sounds are presented to both ears simultaneously, the origin of the sound is located to the ear with the more intense percept. The subject is often unaware that any sound at all has been presented to the other ear. The Stenger Test (Altschuler, 1970) exposes inconsistencies when a falsely 'denied' sound in the NOHL ear causes the sound that should otherwise be acknowledged by the opposite cochlea to seem inaudible. These techniques work best for unilateral NOHL.

Using speech (words) as test material is also often useful. Speech audiometry requires target words (or the constituent phonemes of target words) to be repeated. It is difficult to deny hearing words, especially if presentation levels are continually changing and the pace of presentation is quite fast. A person making a non-organic effort may choose to respond to every second or third word only then suddenly fail to respond at all, rather than show the typical slow degradation of accuracy with decreasing intensity. They may make errors within semantic category that indicate they had formed a mental image regardless of acoustical similarity (for example. responding with the word 'cat' for presentation of the target word "dog").

Objective tests

Objective tests benefit from bypassing the need for active cognition and co-operation on the part of the subject as they monitor the involuntary physiological response to sound. These techniques, while lacking the precision of a well-conducted subjective test, are usefully resistant to the effects of NOHL.

Neural activity evoked by the transmission of sound stimuli through the cochlea to the brain can be detected by appropriate recording equipment, usually incorporating electrodes placed either in the ear canal or the surface of the head. The threshold of the *evoked response* can then be statistically related to behavioural threshold.

There are several different techniques available, each focusing on different time periods after the onset of the stimulus, reflecting the different stages in neural transmission from ear to brain.

Performing the recordings can be lengthy, sedation may be required and analysis relies on skilful pattern recognition. Techniques proven useful for NOHL include auditory brainstem responses (ABR) and cortical evoked response audiometry (CERA), (Sohmer et al., 1977; Coles and Mason, 1984). The auditory steady state response, reviewed by Picton et al. (2003), also shows promise in this regard.

The array of tests described to explore NOHL as described above must be put in a practical context. With 15 minutes or less scheduled for audiometric testing per patient on a busy clinic, additional techniques will normally only be applied if the index of suspicion is sufficiently raised.

Diagnosing NOHL

The key requirement for efficient detection of NOHL is that clinicians stay alert to discrepancies that would indicate further testing. In settings where a poor rate of NOHL detection prevails, this may reflect the lack of a coherent model. A good model will aid diagnosis and prompt effective management strategies.

A review of the literature reveals serious conceptual problems relating to NOHL diagnosis, causes and significance. At one extreme NOHL can be seen as simply a pattern of inconsistent audiometric responses, signifying very little. At the other extreme, it may be viewed as a worrying sign of psychological dysfunction. The appreciation that all manifestations of non-organic behaviour do not spring from the same sources (Glorig, 1954; Williamson, 1974; Sohmer et al., 1977; Martin, 2002) is an important starting point for forming an effective understanding of the phenomenon.

Towards an improved model of NOHL

Previous descriptions of non-organic hearing loss have tended to create oversimplified dichotomies. Starkly contrasting concepts such as 'malingering' (which was considered conscious and in no way associated with psychological problems) and 'hysterical' or 'conversion' manifestations of NOHL (considered unconscious and indicative of psychological dysfunction) have been posited. Furthermore, the use of terminology reflected the lack of theoretical consistency. For example, Goldstein (1966) advocated that most NOHL was consciously simulated (malingering) rarely meeting the proper criteria for a psychogenic disorder. His view was that the patient was always aware of the pretence, though some would be unaware of their motivations. Other researchers felt that, in the absence of an admission from the patient, a clinician could never be sure of deliberate feigning and that most NOHL may well include a psychogenic factor (Hopkinson, 1967; 1973; Chaiklin and Ventry, 1963; Ventry, 1968).

Altschuler (1982) emphasized psychosocial precipitating factors such as gains afforded by employing the 'excuse' of disability to avoid challenging situations or explain failure. A prior experience of genuine hearing loss could seed the idea that there were benefits to be gained. The manifestation of a conversion disorder (the unconscious alteration of a physical condition due to underlying psychological conflict) is known to occur in other bodily systems, for example aphonia and paralysis. It is therefore plausible to expect that similar processes could affect the hearing system (Martin, 2002). Monsel and Herzon (1984) and Wolf et al. (1993) describe the psychodynamic origins of some cases of NOHL. Broad (1980) cites five paediatric cases. According to Beagley and Knight (1968), verified cases of fully unconscious hysterical or conversion deafness are quite rare, but do occur. Coles and Priede (1971) considered most cases to have a mixed aetiology, incorporating conscious and unconscious aspects to the NOHL.

Adding to the debate, Noble (1987) suggested that functional hearing loss in the context of a medicolegal assessment is, in fact, a legal rather than clinical entity. He warns against viewing criminal behaviour as pathological. The need to distinguish a person who is seriously pretending to be deaf in all aspects of life from those simply faking a loss for the purposes of testing is emphasized.

The Austen-Lynch model

Austen and Lynch (in press) attempt to bridge previous dissent by proposing a new model. Designed to align with the Diagnostic and Statistical manual of Mental Disorders – Fourth Edition (DSM-IV) (American Psychiatric Association, 2000), non-organic hearing loss is conceived as three categories arranged on a continuum. Specific diagnosis is dependent on two associated factors: 'degree of intention' (replacing 'consciousness' in previous schema) and 'type of gain': see Figure 20.1.

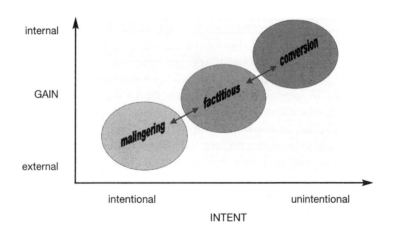

Figure 20.1 Categories on a continuum.

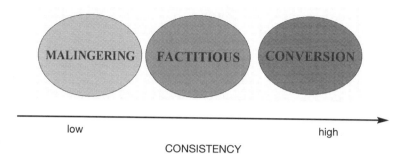

Figure 20.2 Consistency of response during testing

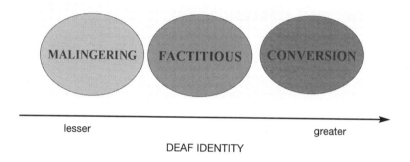

Figure 20.3 Deaf identity and lifestyle.

The Austen-Lynch model retains the *malingering* and *conversion* explanations for NOHL. Crucially, however, it suggests that many cases of NOHL fit the new intermediate category of *factitious hearing loss.* Here benefit from secondary gains is apparent, the gain having often become somewhat woven into the person's identity. Although the behaviour does have an intentional element, the gains of the 'factitious' group are predominantly psychosocial or emotional. This differentiates them from the 'malingering' group whose gains tend to be monetary or related to the acquisition of externally defined goals. It also differentiates them from the 'conversion' group which, although sharing to an extent the psychic gains, shows unintentional behaviour patterns.

Typical scenarios where factitious hearing loss may arise include teenagers under academic pressure, where the NOHL provides a less shameful reason for poor performance. It also includes persons attracted to deaf peer groups for the camaraderie and support, even if their membership is not audiologically appropriate. Austen and Lynch (in press) provide specific case examples.

This model also suggests that degree of deaf lifestyle is associated with degree of intention. Thus, patients at the malingering end of the continuum will tend to adopt the deaf posture only for purposes of testing, whereas patients at the conversion end will be likely to be conducting a more Deaf or deafened lifestyle. The factitious category is intermediate in this regard.

Movement through (and even in and out of) the classifications can evolve as individuals live out the effects of their particular NOHL over a period of time. A further important feature of the model is that it says in itself nothing about *the degree of distress*, which may be as acute for someone in the malingering category as in the factitious or conversion category, and therefore assessment must be made on an individual basis.

Managing and treating NOHL

Since opinions vary as to the significance of NOHL, it is unsurprising that management strategies also differ. Is the behaviour a simple expedient act without deeper psychological importance or is it relevant to become concerned about this individual? Some authors imply that a pragmatic approach consisting of attempts to obtain improved audiometric responses, followed by explanation and reassurance, can normally suffice to 'cure' the non-organicity without recourse to deeper analysis (Andaz, Heyworth and Rowe, 1995). The problem is therefore considered to disappear with the emergence of a normal audiogram. A deeper focus on the behaviour is considered risky as it could lead to labelling and consolidation of the problem, a possibility raised by Veniar and Salston (1983). Others imply a more psychological approach from the outset, viewing NOHL as a possible indicator of serious psychosocial dysfunction or even abuse (Klotz, Koch and Hackett, 1960; Broad, 1980; Altshuler, 1982; Brooks and Geoghegan, 1992; Riedner and Efros, 1995). This would imply a responsibility on the part of the clinician to uncover any adverse circumstances. Getting the balance right between over reacting and under reacting to the sign of NOHL in any particular case is therefore an ongoing challenge.

Recommendations for management of NOHL

Our approach is aligned with that of Silver (1996) whose guidance, although focusing on conversion disorder, is largely applicable for other manifestations of NOHL. The recommendations are:

- avoiding direct confrontation with the patient regarding the fact of NOHL;

- avoiding reinforcing or trivializing the symptoms;
- creating an expectation of recovery;
- providing a benign explanatory model.

If creatively and sensitively implemented, this opens a channel for graceful resolution of the NOHL whereby the patient does not need to feel stigmatized and can move forward appropriately. Gelfand (2001) advises that directly confronting patients with diagnostic labels such as 'malingering' may cause harm and that avoiding such psychiatric terminology is desirable.

Although any of the terms used within the Austen-Lynch model (malingering, factitious or conversion) could be perceived by the patient as pejorative, it is perhaps the term 'malingering' that could offend most, possibly because it is the one the patient is most likely to understand. One of the strengths of this model is its association with the theoretical and diagnostic consistency of DSM-IV and that it reduces the confusion previously caused by the rather subjective application of labels. However, the authors are aware that some of DSM-IV's terminology can be dated and, that as the Austen-Lynch model evolves, it will need to absorb the terminology of subsequent, updated versions of DSM-IV.

Although adherence to the present terminology of the Austen-Lynch model is recommended for diagnostic purposes with patients, clinicians should of course feel free to use the terms that they consider are in the best interest of the patient.

Additionally, we strongly recommend efforts to determine the precipitating causes of the NOHL, leading on to a diagnosis using the model described above. This may be a simple process with evidence easily forthcoming or may require specialist input from clinical psychology or psychiatry. Even in the latter case, some diagnoses may never be entirely clear. Most presentations, however, should meet the requirements for one of our three categories – see Figure 20.1. Optimal management options will then relate directly to the diagnosis.

For the malingering category, the aim is to help the patient identify and reduce as far as possible any external factors contributing to the NOHL. This may include counselling coupled with practical advice and support. In cases of medicolegal compensation, a clear explanation of the medical implication of the findings is warranted, together with a sympathetic but practical attitude to any true organic component that may underlie the NOHL. Reactions are difficult to predict, but a degree of hostility may arise in this category of patient. The degree of distress will play a role in any decision to refer for more specific psychological help.

For the factitious category, the need for emotional dependence on secondary gains can often be alleviated through sensitive reframing, psychological exploration and counselling. Withdrawing the emotional structure provided by the NOHL can be painful and even depressing for the patient. The treatment phase may be short and uncomplicated, accomplished within the course of an ordinary clinical consultation, or require more prolonged unravelling and intervention through several sessions. Patients who are intentionally feigning deafness in order to get a cochlear implant are likely also to fit the diagnostic criteria for what is commonly referred to as Munchausen syndrome.

Effectiveness of treatment for both the above categories is to be measured not only by the behavioural resolution of the NOHL but also by an indication from patients that they have found a better adaptation to their precipitating stresses. Follow-up will be necessary to ensure that the NOHL does not re-emerge and that the key issues have been addressed. Cases not responding to management within the routine setting should be referred to appropriate mental health services.

Importantly, all cases thought to be within the conversion category merit skilled psychiatric intervention to avoid any transference of the effects of internal conflict onto another modality. In this category, degree of distress will be hard to determine without the help of mental health professionals, and the treatment may or may not involve unveiling the NOHL depending on any likely consequences and balance of risks. In most settings, such cases will be extremely rare, although those involved with tertiary interventions such as cochlear implantation may expect a higher incidence (Lynch et al., 2001).

Managing NOHL in children

Although the overall approach to managing NOHL is similar to that described above, certain special factors apply to children. Riedner and Efros (1995) advocate that *any* manifestation of childhood NOHL merits investigation. The trend in recent years has been to move away from focusing the responsibility for NOHL on the child (Barr, 1963) towards incorporating the wider social dynamics including family and academic stresses and possible abuse (Veniar and Salston, 1983; Brooks and Geoghegan, 1992; Riedner and Efros, 1995).

Where the patient's family has been involved in extending secondary gains (for example, by offering extra attention or colluding with avoidance of responsibilities) careful preparation for the unveiling of NOHL is needed and the child's school may need to become involved in the management plan. Parents and others who have shown concern may feel deceived by the child and here the use of the factitious category can provide a useful basis for explaining the child's behaviour. A graceful resolution (as above) can be adapted and extended to members of the family, reducing the impact of negative feelings. It must be remembered that the behaviour of clinicians towards the child will act as a powerful model, and a dismissive attitude or crude 'exposure' of the NOHL could have damaging consequences.

The multidisciplinary team: who is responsible for NOHL management?

Who within the audiology team and beyond is competent to make the diagnosis and facilitate management?

Deeper motivations and degrees of distress are not always apparent without psychological or psychiatric assessment, therefore all cases of persistent NOHL would ideally have access to mental health services geared to the special needs of deafness. Although this may be theoretically appropriate, such consultations are not easily resourced by most health care settings outside of specialist hospitals. Furthermore it is likely that many patients would themselves elect to avoid what may be perceived as a stigmatising event, risking a focus on their 'shameful' behaviour. Lynch et al. (2001) reported low uptake of internal referral to psychological services in their group of NOHL patients.

Martin (2002) suggests that audiologists' responsibilities stop at measuring the extent of 'real' hearing loss, whereas Austen and Lynch (in press) suggest that a range of professionals can play a part in providing input for the purpose of diagnosis. The failure to recognize the contribution of the wider team is likely to result in a low enthusiasm for dealing with NOHL efficiently. Audiologists and others without training in psychological intervention, however, should not counsel the patient directly and the proper professional distance must certainly be observed. Martin's appeal that audiologists should avoid value judgements regarding their patients is certainly important.

The individual's GP can also be seen as a focal point for well-rounded management. The non-organic behaviour may have presented previously in another physical domain or, if not successfully treated, could reassert itself at a later stage. The GP may have valuable insights into additional motivational factors, serving as a useful resource to assist exploration of the cause and facilitate resolution of the NOHL.

Conclusion

Non-organic hearing loss is a clinically important subject from the point of view of the welfare of patients, some of whom will be very vulnerable. It is also an intriguing example of an attempted adaptive human response to challenging circumstances, be they external or intra-psychic. We contend that *degree of intention* and *type of gain* is a valid way of factoring out individual motivations, leading on to effective individual management strategies and treatment. There is scope to develop the understanding of NOHL further and a continuation of the creative debate is anticipated.

References

Altschuler MW (1970) The Stenger Phenomenon. Journal of Communicative Disorders, 3: 89–105.

Altschuler MW (1982) Qualitative indicators of non-organicity: informal observations and evaluation. In Kramer JD and Armbruster JM (eds) Forensic Audiology. Baltimore MD: University Park Press, pp. 50–68.

Andaz C, Heyworth T, Rowe S (1995) Nonorganic Hearing Loss in Children- a 2-year study. ORL 57: 33–5.

Aplin DY, Kane JM (1985) Personality and experimentally stimulated hearing loss. British Journal of Audiology 19: 251–5.

Aplin DY, Rowson VJ (1986) Personality and functional hearing loss in children. British Journal of Clinical Psychology 25(4): 313–14.

Austen S, Lynch C (in press) Non-organic hearing loss redefined: understanding, categorising and managing non-organic behaviour. International Journal of Audiology.

Barr B (1963) Psychogenic deafness in school children. Audiology 2: 125–8.

Beagley HA, Knight JJ (1968) The evaluation of suspected nonorganic hearing loss. Journal of Laryngology and Otology 82: 693–705.

British Society of Audiologists (1981) BSA recommended procedures for pure-tone audiometry using a manually-operated instrument. British Journal of Audiology 15: 213–16.

Broad RD (1980) Development and psychodynamic issues related to cases of childhood functional hearing loss. Child Psychiatry and Human Development 11(1): 49–58.

Brooks DN, Geoghegan PN (1992) Nonorganic hearing loss in young persons: transient episode or deep-seated difficulty? British Journal of Audiology 36: 347–50.

Chaiklin J, Ventry IM (1963) Functional hearing loss. In Jerger J (ed.) Modern Developments in Audiology. New York: Academic Press, pp. 76–125.

Chaiklin J, Ventry IM (1965) Patient errors during spondee and pure-tone threshold measurement. Journal of Audiological Research 5: 212–18.

Coles RRA, Mason SM (1984) The results of cortical electrical response audiometry in medicolegal investigations. British Journal of Audiology 18: 71–8.

Coles RRA, Priede VM (1971) Non-organic overlay in noise-induced hearing loss. Proceedings of the Royal Society of Medicine 64: 41–63.

American Psychiatric Association (2000) Diagnostic and Statistical Manual of Mental Disorders (DSM IV) Washington DC: APA.

Edgerton J (1994) American Psychiatric Glossary, 7 edn. Washington DC: American Psychiatric Press.

Frank T (1976) Yes-no test for nonorganic hearing loss. Archives of Otolaryngology 102: 162–5.

Gelfand SA (1993) Organic thresholds and functional components in experimentally simulated exaggerated hearing loss. British Journal of Audiology 27: 35–40.

Gelfand SA, Silman S (1993) Functional components and resolved thresholds in patients with unilateral nonorganic hearing loss. British Journal of Audiology 27: 29–34.

Gelfand SA (2001) Nonorganic Hearing Loss. In Gelfand SA (ed.) Essentials of Audiology. 2 edn. New York: Thieme Medical Publishers, pp. 421–42.

Gleason WJ (1958) Psychological Characteristics of the Audiologically Inconsistent Patient. AMA. Archives of Otolaryngology 68: 42–6.

Glorig A (1954) Malingering. Annals of Otology, Rhinology and Laryngology 65: 154–70.

Goldstein R (1966) Pseudohypacusis. Journal of Speech and Hearing Disorders 31: 341–52.

Hopkinson NT (1967) Comment on 'Pseudohypacusis'. Journal of Speech Hearing Disorders 32: 293–4.

Hopkinson NT (1973) Functional hearing loss. In Jerger J (ed.) Modern Developments in Audiology. 2 edn. New York: Academic Press, pp. 175–210.

Hosoi H, Yoshiaki T, Kiyotaka M and Levitt H (1999) Suggestion audiometry for non-organic hearing loss (pseudohypacusis) in children. International Journal of Paediatric Otorhinolarngology 47: 11–21.

Jerger S, Jerger J (1981) Functional hearing disorders. In Auditory Disorders. Boston MA: College Hill Press, pp. 51–8.

Klotz RE, Koch AW, Hackett TP (1960) Psychogenic hearing loss in children. Annals of Otology, Rhinology and Laryngology 65: 154–70.

Lynch CA, Stott EM, Wintersgill SW, Graham JM (2001) Non organic hearing loss in the Cochlear Implant Clinic. Oral Presentation at British Cochlear Implant Group Spring Meeting, Llandudno, Wales.

Martin FN (2002) Pseudohypacusis. In Katz J (ed.) Handbook of Clinical Audiology. 5 edn. Baltimore MD: Lippincott Williams & Wilkins, pp. 584–96.

Monsel EM, Herzon FS (1984) Functional hearing loss presenting as a sudden hearing loss: a case report. American Journal of Otology 5: 407–10.

Noble W (1987) The conceptual problem of 'functional hearing loss'. British Journal of Audiology 21: 1–3.

Picton TW, John SM, Dimitrijevic A, Purcell D (2003) Human Auditory Steady – State Responses. International Journal of Audiology 42: 177–219.

Riedner ED, Efros PL (1995) Nonorganic hearing loss and child abuse: beyond the sound booth. British Journal of Audiology 29: 195–7.

Silver FW (1996) Mangagement of conversion disorder. American Journal of Physical Medicine and Rehabilitation 75(2): 134–40.

Sohmer H, Feinmesser M, Bauberger-Tell L, Edelstein E (1977) Cochlear, brainstem and cortical evoked responses in non-organic hearing loss. Annals of Otology, Rhinology and Larygology 86: 227–34.

Spraggs PD, Burton MJ, Graham JM (1994) Nonorganic hearing loss in cochlear implant candidates. The American Journal of Otology 15(5): 652–7.

Stephens SDG (1969) Auditory threshold variance signal detection theory and personality. International Audiology 8: 131–7.

Trier TR, Levy R (1965) Social and psychological characteristics of veterans with functional hearing loss. Journal of Audiological Research 5: 241–56.

Veniar FA, Salston RS (1983) An approach to the treatment of pseudohypacusis in children. American Journal of Diseases of Childhood 137: 34–6.

Ventry IM (1968) A case for psychogenic hearing loss. Journal of Speech and Hearing Disorders 33: 89–92.

Ventry IM (1976) Comment on article by Martin and Monro. Journal of Speech and Hearing Disorders 40: 282–3.

Williamson D (1974) Functional hearing loss: a review. Maico Audiological Library Series 12: 33–4.

Wolf M, Birger M, Shoshan JB, Kronenberg J (1993) Conversion deafness. Annals of Otology, Rhinology and Laryngology 102: 349–52.

CHAPTER 21

Training deaf professionals

JIM CROMWELL

Introduction

> You cannot know what you are entering into. (Counselling Psychology Training Course Director)

> What are we entering into?! (Clinical Psychology Training Course Director)

The above are quotations from training staff who have had or who continue to have deaf trainees on their courses. While each appears at face value a little helpless, the spirit with which they were said in fact reflects the opposite. Although it is inevitably important to prepare as comprehensibly as possible for both the trainee's arrival and continued training, it is similarly vital to accept that complete preparation is a fantasy – to not fret about the challenges the deaf trainee might both face and present to the course, or about the technicalities of communication support, deaf awareness, equal access to resources – to not become so embroiled in the practical challenges that all space for reflection, learning, and indeed *training* are lost.

> It is *attitude* that counts, not getting it perfect. (Deaf trainee)

The information in this chapter is based upon available literature, interviews with deaf trainees, courses that have trained deaf psychologists, and personal experience as a qualified clinical psychologist working with deaf people and supervising deaf trainees. This chapter will endeavour to provide the reader with as much advice, anecdote and food for thought as is feasible, but two caveats exist: First, no two deaf people are the same and so no operational checklist for courses will cover all eventualities. Second, that two interpreters, a notetaker, a palantypist, deaf awareness training and devout adherence to the Disability Discrimination Act themselves do not make a qualified psychologist. Training courses should not deny one the space to reflect upon and to *enjoy* the issues that may arise while facilitating a deaf trainee's progression through the course.

> A centipede was happy quite,
> Until a toad in fun
> Said, 'Pray, which leg moves after which?'
> This raised her doubts to such a pitch,
> She fell exhausted in a ditch,
> Not knowing how to run. (Mrs Edmund Craster d. 1874)

Disability Discrimination Act

While this chapter will emphasize the positively challenging side of training deaf psychologists, there is nevertheless a stick that should not be forgotten: discrimination legislation. In the US this is the Americans With Disabilities Act 1990 (ADA) and in the UK the Disability Discrimination Act 1995 (DDA). Both the DDA and ADA require services such as training courses to make 'reasonable adjustment' to allow fair and equal access for people with disabilities. 'Reasonable' is determined by the size of the service or the size of that service's budget, and the ADA has defined budget as the *total* available funds of the academic institution and not of the department alone. There is, therefore, a legal obligation to be accessible and fair, and it is nearly *always* illegal to deny a request for, for example, interpreter services (Gutman and Pollard, 1999).

Effects on training

It has been argued (Gutman and Pollard, 1999) that training courses *benefit* from a richness and diversity among their students, across the placements offered, and across the perspectives presented by the student body to itself and to the course. Robert Pollard Jr (personal communication, 2002), has noted also that:

- deaf trainees are pursued for leadership positions in advance of their hearing colleagues;
- hearing colleagues of deaf trainees are often strongly and positively affected by the experience;
- that training programmes are able to demonstrate very visibly their commitment to multicultural initiatives.

It is likely also that deaf trainees will possess skills that will enhance the training experience for their peers; perhaps a significant sensitivity to body language and expression, strengths in communicating in difficult and compromised situations and overcoming isolating and minoritizing attitudes. Gutman and Pollard (1999) add that the presence of a deaf trainee, with accompanying communication support, also focuses attention on communication processes – vital when one considers the coalface of therapy: *communication.*

Selection

Processing and shortlisting applicants, arranging and conducting interviews and then reaching a decision about which applications ultimately succeed are all time consuming and are often timetabled with little room for manoeuvre. It is, however, at this time that the course is first faced with challenges that must be addressed in order to give the deaf applicant a fair opportunity for selection. These challenges take time to address properly, but it is also important not to allow delays that may occur to impact negatively on the applicant, for example, by expecting the applicant to be interviewed later than everyone else or by forcing a longer wait to hear the result than for the hearing applicants.

The interview and selection process

Preparation for the interview process mostly concerns communication support. For prelingually profoundly deaf applicants, sign language interpreters are the most likely support to be needed. At interview, as it would be throughout the training experience, it will be important to try to find interpreters with experience of mental health settings and related jargon. More important information regarding the use of interpreters may be found elsewhere in this book. It is important for those involved in selection to be fully aware of the related issues before interview in order that issues of logistics do not compromise the time available for the applicant to prove herself. Like any tool, one must learn how to use interpreter support effectively, rather than just assuming that it will cover all the issues.

At interview, supposing that all issues of communication and access are appropriately addressed, it is possible to proceed with the selection process as normal – that is, equally and fairly. At a face-to-face panel interview, or a presentation to the panel, it is probable that the presence of interpreters will quickly not be felt. However in any *group* task, the examiners should be aware of further issues:

- *Time lag.* No matter how promptly the interpreter interprets, the deaf applicants will always be momentarily behind the hearing group members in the flow of the discussion, and examiners can misunderstand this as failure to follow the discussion. How the applicant involves herself in the discussion will probably be noted as part of the appraisal, but this should be considered carefully in the context of the interpreting situation. For example, if she appears slightly aggressive by talking over somebody is this a function of being behind in the conversation and needing to claim 'air time'? If she appears reluctant to take part, is this instead a function of time lag and an effort to *not* interrupt, such that her own contribution arrives late and appears incongruous? Group members should be respectful of 'interpreter-time' – that is, to monitor their own discussion and to not respond to an utterance until it is clear that it has been interpreted; so dispensing with the iniquity of the time lag by all experiencing it together. A good chairperson ought to manage this. It is also advisable to schedule additional time for formal selection procedures to allow for the impact of these issues to not disadvantage the applicant.

- *Interruption.* Some interpreters tend to act as advocates for the deaf person with whom they are working. It might be appropriate for the examiners to discuss beforehand with the interpreters and the applicant which of them is responsible for asserting the right of the applicant to take part in the discussion, such that it is possible for the examiners to know if they are evaluating the applicant or the interpreter at the time.

The selection process should always focus on the applicant's clinical skills and qualifications, not her hearing loss. Questions regarding how she might work with different clinical groups, how she might introduce herself as a deaf clinician, how she might introduce the interpreter, or how to deal with challenges from clients unfamiliar with a deaf clinician are all reasonable. Making assumptions about her clinical limits, making challenging comments about the feasibility of pursuing this career, of treating hearing clients, or of funding for interpreter services would all be inappropriate.

Allowing the applicant's hearing loss, or the support that entails, to influence the decision of whether or not to select would be illegal.

The training experience

It is desirable for the deafness of our trainee to not take centre stage and to minimally impact on the training experience of all parties, but in order for this to happen as smoothly as possible it is necessary, paradoxically, to face up to it from the start. Throughout training, issues will arise that will bring the deafness to the forefront once again, so in order to limit the chances of this happening it is helpful to address as many issues as possible from the outset. It will be helpful to educate trainees and staff regarding use of interpreters. Deaf awareness training ought also to be offered, and can be purchased easily from deafness-related charities and organizations, introducing the idea of deaf people as a cultural and linguistic minority rather than as a disabled group. This shift in perspective provides a discussion point for trainees, which contributes positively to their training as well as presenting an important paradigm shift for relating to their deaf peers. Interestingly, whereas deaf awareness training is best offered by professional providers (as it is of a higher quality, and makes the focus Deaf people in general and not a particular person), trainees have found that on *placements* it is better conducted personally, with an interpreter, because then the placement is meeting the trainee in the context of the issues of deaf awareness and she is seen to be proactively helping them understand a situation that is likely to be new to them. Certain training course staff have even attended sign language courses in advance of their trainee's arrival. This should in no way be seen as an obligation but it demonstrates considerable commitment to the trainees, and it is surprising how much conversational sign language it is possible to learn in a relatively short time – reducing the sometimes exhausting need to rely on interpreter support for even the simplest conversation.

Preparation attenuates anxiety, and deaf trainees have pointed out that their *own* anxieties are considerably reduced by their courses having evidently prepared for, or at least considered, the various issues. A course that is quietly confident in its ability to offer a fair and equal training opportunity demonstrably puts the trainee at ease, whereas those that are manifestly agitated appear to their trainees to be seeing the deafness first and the trainee second. The trainee can experience course staff continually asking and checking about deafness-related issues to be unsupportive.

Teaching

As already mentioned regarding selection, communication support will need to be discussed with the trainee and booked in advance of the teaching modules. Sign language interpreters are in very limited supply and it will be necessary to book them well in advance and ideally use the same people for each lecture of a block of teaching. They most commonly work as single-handed freelance workers but ought ideally to be booked in pairs so that they may support each other and alternate the role of active interpreter. A single interpreter will need a 5–10 minute break every 40 minutes and should have a longer break after 2 hours. Without these breaks the amount of error in the translation reaches significant levels and the deaf trainee can no longer be said to have equal access to the taught material (Kyle and Woll, 1985). One course has pointed out the importance of remembering that two interpreters take up two seats! An extra two bodies can make what was an adequately sized classroom suddenly inadequate. Another course also mentioned that as soon as they had a deaf trainee, acoustic difficulties of certain rooms, hitherto unnoticed, became apparent. Sign language interpreters will make it their business to hear everything said in the room properly and will interrupt in order to seek clarification. Using a quiet room with good acoustics will limit the amount of interruption from the interpreters.

Lecturers, particularly those visiting from outside, will need to be

- informed that there is a deaf trainee on the course and to consider how that might (or might not) influence how they present their session.
- provided with information about interpreters and what to expect.
- told how to use interpreters and about the need for breaks.
- asked to provide copies of their notes and handouts to the interpreters at least the day before the lecture is to be delivered.
- given a little deaf awareness information such as advice not to talk while writing on a board, or cover the mouth, or talk while showing a slide unless they are simply reading the contents of that slide. If slides are to be used, they should not be used in a darkened room. Video footage presents special challenges to the interpreters, who would be helped by the opportunity to review the tape in advance of the session. Where the use of role play might seem onerous with interpreters, it has in fact been found to be quite straightforward, with fellow (hearing) trainees reporting that the interpreter is not a hindrance.

Appraisal

Trainee psychologists are usually appraised by written submissions (case reports and essays), process report (discussion and self-appraisal based upon an audiotape of a particular clinical session), and supervision on placement. The process report presents obvious difficulties due to the use of audiotape. With a deaf client the session could be videotaped, although it is hard to clearly record two people signing a conversation in a room. Even if the session were videotaped, while the trainees would be able to go through it and comment on the process, the staff appraising would be required to rely upon the interpreter for access to the recorded clinical work, and while not immediately prohibitive, a comprehensive discussion of the *process* of the session requires access to more of the session than just the *content*. Some courses expect trainees to transcribe the recording for the report. For deaf trainees this would require a process of translation as well as transcription and I would suggest that the former should be the responsibility of an interpreter. Appraisal more than anything else needs to be demonstrably *fair* for all concerned. The special nature of the process report indicates that the deaf trainees cannot be appraised in the same way as their hearing peers, and a modality-for-modality trade by way of using video instead of audio does not effectively address the issue. Those courses that have faced this already have found that it highlights the need for a system that judges trainees against equal standards but makes no stipulation about the means. It may be possible, for example, for a qualified psychologist with signing skills to observe a session and then to discuss process with the trainees and course staff.

Written work

It has been suggested (Conrad, 1979) that the median reading age of deaf school leavers is nine. While trainees will have a reading age commensurate with their academic record it is worth considering the context of this statistic.

Deaf signers converse in a language that cannot be written, which differs considerably in grammatical form from the dominant language locally, and that involves some concepts and linguistic structures that cannot easily be translated into English. Because signed languages cannot be written, the first *written* language of even a native signer will be that of the hearing society in which they live. Hearing people almost always speak and write the same language and so exposure to written words continues to shape their speech just as everyday exposure to speech shapes and refines their written skills. This mutually beneficial relationship between the verbal and written language is not available to deaf people.

When appraising the written work of a deaf trainees it is important to be clear about what is being appraised. While people's written English and the concepts they are conveying are, of course, significantly related (a concept must be clearly expressed for us to appraise it confidently), they are nevertheless distinguishable in certain ways – for example an intelligent exploration of 'scitzophrenia' is no less intelligent because of the dreadful spelling. For courses requiring a good first degree as an entry requirement this issue ought not to arise, but for those with different admissions criteria it may. For them it may be worth treating the deaf trainee as a student with English as a foreign language and to adhere to the guidelines and principles already established for that.

With a good interpreter, particularly if the same one is used for supervision as for the direct clinical work, the appraisal conducted by supervisors at the end of placements should be unproblematic.

Peer group

Most courses agree that peer support is an invaluable part of the training experience and, although it cannot be engineered or specifically timetabled, the early days of training are often deliberately moderately paced in order to allow the trainees time to get to know each other and to join as a group. In most cases there will be only one deaf trainee in a cohort and it is easy for that person to become marginalized – she is difficult to talk to, hard to understand, may confront others with their own inevitable misconceptions and politically sensitive attitudes, and is often accompanied by two interpreters. Courses can probably do no preparatory work in this regard, but it is worth being aware of the special effort *all* the trainees will have to be making in order for them to join effectively as a group. The deaf trainee will be all too familiar with this need but it remains a difficult though not insurmountable gap to bridge:

> I either had to be on the fringe and watch and understand nothing, or be proactive and get involved – ask what the conversation was etc . . . But then the focus shifted to me, i.e. I became dominant in the conversation. I hated not being able to just passively soak up conversation. (Deaf trainee)

The trainee will often also feel that she is the last to know everything and this may make her feel on the fringes of the group at best.

Where there is another signer on the course the benefits are probably obvious (although that person should *never* be used as a cheap alternative to a qualified interpreter). However, there is then a danger that the deaf trainee and fellow signer create their own microgroup talking only to each other, leaving a communication vacuum between them and the group. This can also happen with the deaf trainee and interpreters and the trainee would be well advised to prevent this from happening for fear of excluding herself from that important source of informal and moral support, her peers.

A few years of postgraduate vocational training, in which one is often expected to practise what has only just or is yet to be taught (while also attending taught modules) and to somehow produce a large and impressive-looking piece of research, is *stressful*. Those teaching courses will be familiar with the ways in which these stressors promote anxiety, which manifests in many ways. It is perhaps no surprise that the presence of a deaf trainee in the group can become the target for feelings *actually* related to the training experience. For example, hearing peers have been noted to become angry if their deaf peer understands a point or passes an assessment and they have not, and it seems clear that they feel threatened by this *disabled* trainee. Hearing peers may suspect that the deaf trainee reflects tokenism on the part of the course and sometimes these suspicions are aired in anger.

Deaf trainees will ultimately be able to share most stresses with the group as they will be course-related issues, such as difficult clients, looming deadlines and omnipotent ethics committees. There will, however, be additional stresses of working in two languages at once (as reading and lectured material will be presented in English and sign respectively), of meeting a client for the first time who has not met a deaf person or worked with an interpreter, and of interpreters not arriving when the family has arrived for therapy. It may be the case that such things can only be truly shared by talking to other deaf psychologists, but practically it may be prudent to allow for such discussions during meetings with the trainee's tutor or supervisor.

Placements/internships

Before the year begins, course staff should have considered whether to provide the deaf trainee exclusively with deaf clients, hearing clients or a mixture. Local constraints, of course, are the major determinant but, those aside, a broader discussion should take place about the competencies that would be expected to be derived from the placements, commensurate with the award at the end of the course, and whether or not they would be gained from only seeing deaf or hearing clients. Courses differ in the competencies they expect to be met in order to confer the particular award of that programme. A question may be raised of whether or not a trainee who sees only deaf people should be awarded a qualification that is restricted in terms of enabling the person to see only deaf clients. Ultimately it is incumbent on the course to provide equal and fair opportunity to the deaf trainee to achieve the same qualification as her hearing peers, a qualification that makes no distinction about the hearing status of potential clients. Indeed, hearing trainees who meet only hearing clients during their placements are never awarded qualifications that disallow them from seeing *deaf* clients. It would therefore be unreasonable to argue that the deaf trainee must see hearing clients on placement in order to then be qualified to meet them in the future.

Courses may consider that fair and equal placement experience would be gained from expecting the trainee to attend exclusively hearing placements, but this makes the error of assuming that equality of means yields equality of opportunity, because the experience of a deaf trainee in a hearing placement is not the same as that of a hearing trainee in the same placement. Long debates about equality of experience can be quickly dispensed with by focusing on equality of access to the competencies expected by the examination board. The question to be asked when a placement is to be offered is the same for all trainees, deaf or hearing:

> Given the placements in which this trainee has already worked, would the next one continue to provide fair opportunity to gain the competencies expected of this award?

The audiometric profile or cultural affinity of the client group is irrelevant. Certain courses raised concern that hearing people may not want to see a deaf therapist. However, none of the UK deaf trainees interviewed for this chapter reported that their hearing clients had refused to be seen by them, because of their deafness or for any other reason. One trainee made a point of asking, at the end of therapy, what sort of effect if any her deafness may have had:

> One client in particular said that she preferred talking through the interpreter. She had worked with a hearing therapist before and found it made her feel vulnerable and exposed, she clammed up and dropped out of therapy, whereas through the interpreter the conversation was more paced and measured, and as a result she felt safer. (Deaf trainee)

Robert Pollard Jr (2002) described similar experiences. Although hearing clients have universally responded positively to their deaf therapists, the question is nevertheless raised of whether or not a client has the right to decline to see a therapist on those grounds. The best working answer to this is probably that clients have a right to be informed that their therapist will be deaf but that they may not have the right to reject that therapist (should they wish to). Clients should be informed that their therapist is deaf and often works with an interpreter and this seems to be most sensitively achieved by stating it very simply at the bottom of the first piece of correspondence with an offer to discuss this should the client so wish.

It is helpful for courses to target supervisors who have a real interest in supervising a deaf trainee. However, time must be allowed for supervisors to take the idea back to their teams for discussion as the team provides the context for the placement experience. An ideal placement would also offer a range of options to the trainee rather than, for example, just a small routine schedule of outpatient clinics, and would have a supervisor who is well integrated into the wider team. Courses have also found it beneficial to highlight to teams that the aim of the placement is parity of *outcome* in terms of skills and competencies rather than parity of *process* through the placement. A degree of flexibility and creativity with regard to the process of the placement and the opportunities presented, will be necessary to ensure a fair outcome.

Supervision

Supervisors of course have different styles; some are almost parental in the protection of their charge while others monitor the trainee's work from some distance and can feel absent. Some may seem controlling, others disinterested. If the course feels nervous about their trainee it may be tempting to locate a placement with a more comforting and protective supervisor. However, while a supervisor who is relatively present and supportive is desirable, one who is overly cautious and protective may unintentionally undermine and de-skill the trainee by appearing to be doubtful of her competence. The trainee's confidence will remain at its initial low level for longer than is necessary. Likewise, one who appears unsupportive and dismissive may empower the trainee and boost confidence much quicker, but at the risk of expecting her to cope with so much that she drops out of the programme. This is not to say that deaf trainees are more vulnerable or sensitive than hearing ones, but that training is onerous for all trainees and never more so than at the first placement, and the deaf trainee has the additional concern of working psychologically through interpreters with hearing clients. At least one course has addressed this issue by allocating the first (core adult mental health) placement in a broad adult mental health service for deaf people, so that the trainee could face all the usual anxieties and doubts about seeing people clinically without being concerned about interpreter issues, communicating with the supervisor, or working with hearing clients. Where ordinary clinical concerns at least partly addressed, the trainee can then move on to a hearing placement with enough cognitive and emotional space to be able to address more clearly the other hearing–deaf concerns.

Notably, it appears that it is not just the deaf trainee who fears the first hearing placement. Courses that have not trained a deaf psychologist before feel it also, and just as the confidence of course staff is picked up by the trainee who then feels correspondingly more positive, so a confident supervisor and a positive placement experience reassures the course. Clinical placements feel like the acid test for all the preparatory work conducted by teaching staff by way of teaching and assignments, and as such the first placement visit or appraisal can be very beneficial, not just for the trainee but for the course. There will also inevitably be considerable learning on the part of the placement supervisor (and indeed the whole team), and it is important to ensure that there is a mechanism for these experiences and insights to be handed over to the next placement and back to the course.

Summary

For a variety of reasons few deaf people have trained as psychologists at this time and so few courses will have faced the issues inherent in training a deaf psychologist. These issues are myriad. This chapter has attempted to provide a starting-point for thinking about, and planning the training of, deaf psychologists and in so doing has highlighted a variety of issues, concerns, and perhaps philosophical challenges. It would be no excuse to flagrantly disregard these issues but it remains the case that the ultimate aim is the successful training of a psychologist, and to compromise this by focusing exclusively on the *deafness* would be disastrous.

There is room in this exercise for curiosity, enlightenment and enjoyment for the deaf trainee, for the hearing peers, and for the course.

References

Conrad, R (1979) The Deaf School Child. London: Harper and Row.

Disability Discrimination Act (1995) www.disability.gov.uk/dda

Gutman V, Pollard RQ (1999) Working with deaf interns and internship applicants. APPIC Newsletter (November), pp. 12–24.

Kyle J, Woll B (1985) Sign Language: The Study of Deaf People and their Language. Cambridge University Press: Cambridge.

Pollard Jr, RQ (2002) Program for Deaf Trainees: Ten Years of Experience. Personal Communication.

United States of America (1990). Americans with Disabilities Act Handbook. Washington DC: US Government Printing Office.

CHAPTER 22

Older adults who use sign language

SALLY AUSTEN

Introduction

'Older and growing', or 'growing old'? If our aim is that older adults, or seniors, receive services that maximize their social, mental and physical wellbeing, then this must include older adults who are Deaf. However, this is far from the case in practice. In most areas of the world older sign language users are an invisible group whose needs go unnoticed. This invisibility is reflected in the paucity of published literature in this area. Thus, where references are absent in this chapter, the stated opinions are based on my own clinical experience or experiences shared with me by colleagues.

In an ageing general population, the prevalence of profound prelingual deafness is 1:1000 and approximately one in seven people have some degree of hearing loss (Davis, 2001). The relatively large number of deafened people, particularly in the older populations, leads to the assumption that all older people are deafened rather than born deaf. Consequently, the older born deaf person who is a member of the Deaf community and uses sign language is often forgotten. The needs of older Deaf sign language users are very different to those of the older deafened population. It is this signing group on which this chapter will focus.

Life Experiences

It may be asked whether a specialism focusing on older adults who are Deaf is really necessary given that there is already a body of knowledge on both older adults (generally hearing) and Deaf people (generally less than 65 years). However, to enable equality of access of opportunity and services, this group must be regarded as having unique needs.

For centuries, philosophers have associated the ability to think with the ability to speak, therefore portraying Deaf people as incapable of thought. There is now a clearer distinction between language and thought and the conclusion seems to be that whereas certain types of thought, such as theory of mind, do require language, it does not matter whether that language is a sign or a spoken language. Born in the early part of the twentieth century, our present Deaf older adults would have been referred to as 'deaf and dumb'. Although the term 'dumb' meant without speech, it was soon associated with stupidity and the assumption that Deaf people were stupid was reinforced.

Historical overview

When, in 1880 the Milan conference on the education of Deaf people banned sign language in education in order to promote speech and lip-reading, hearing aids were in their infancy and health services were too expensive for most people, with the result that residual hearing was not utilized in the way it is today. Believing that sign would inhibit oral skills, most schools forbade the use of signing and had varying degrees of punishment for its use. Signing in public became something to be ashamed of. Despite the blanket ban, children learned to sign in secret, often from children of Deaf families. However, the legacy remains and many older Deaf people still do not feel comfortable signing in public, or find it shocking that young Deaf people sign so openly.

Deaf schools in this era were predominantly boarding. This was a mixed blessing as for many Deaf children it was their first chance to meet other Deaf people and to develop a cultural identity and sense of belonging. (Older Deaf people, introduced for the first time, often ask each other which school they went to and draw conclusions about each other's identity, experiences and allegiances.)

On the other hand, advising parents not to sign in the home meant that many Deaf children had no useful language before going to school, the result being that many 2- to 5-year-old Deaf children went to school, possibly alone on a train, with no understanding of what was happening to them and not knowing if they would ever see their parents again. The long-term effects on attachment and confidence can be speculated upon and disconnection from families was common. As with many other 'care' institutions, it is now becoming clear that such schools had high incidences of physical and sexual abuse of the children, both by other children and by professionals (Sullivan, Brookhouser and Scanlan, 2000).

As a result of the banning of sign language in the early years, many Deaf older people had poor language development and professionals had fairly low expectations of students who were therefore generally steered into the 'trades' rather than towards academia. Certain trades became commonly associated with Deaf people – for example tailoring or cobblering. As a result, Deaf people had lower incomes and higher unemployment than their hearing peers (Harris, Anderson and Novak, 1995).

Both Deaf and hearing people of this age group will have lived through at least one World War. Deaf people were rarely accepted for active duty, but many had responsible jobs such as air-raid wardens and stretcher-bearers, in the absence of large numbers of hearing men. As with women, in some ways the war emancipated Deaf people, who were recognized as able bodied and useful citizens. Some Deaf older adults report that the greatest risk to their health during wartime was the regular 'blackouts' and smog, which restricted their vision and left them vulnerable to being knocked over.

Sign language

Each country has its own native sign language(s) that, just as with spoken languages, has natural variations dependent on region, social group membership and social situation. Languages can also vary depending on age, particularly in sign language. There are many features within BSL that differentiate older and younger signers and some young Deaf people claim that they cannot understand the signing of older Deaf people. Older people tend to use more finger spelling (Sutton-Spence and Woll, 1993) and fewer clear English mouth patterns than younger Deaf people.

One of the reasons for this development in BSL may be that few Deaf people are born to Deaf parents, which results in large changes in sign language between the generations. Secondly, improvement in hearing aid technology has meant that Deaf people have used more of their residual hearing to listen to and learn English. Where sign was banned children learned to sign from other children in secret as opposed to in the classroom or from parents. Although the number of children learning sign from their parents has not changed, the number learning to sign from teachers and younger Deaf role models in schools has increased. Since the 1970s there has been an increase in the number of schools allowing signing in the classroom. At the same time however Deaf schools are being closed in favour of the integration of Deaf children into mainstream schooling. The result is that Deaf children will experience sign that is respected by the establishment but will not be exposed to a large signing community (Sutton-Spence and Woll, 1999).

Bayley (2002) looked at the grammatical structure of American Sign Language (ASL) in different age groups and found that the oldest group's language was often grammatically unorthodox, the middle-aged group was very correct in its grammar and the youngest group, similar to the oldest group, was more unorthodox. Her explanation for this was that, in the US, the oldest group had learned sign secretly at Deaf schools with little or no influence from educators. Consequently their grammar was somewhat unformed. The middle-aged group was the first to be allowed to sign in the US and hearing professionals instilled into them the importance of correct ASL grammar, which, being ambassadors for the newly accepted signing, they stuck to fairly rigidly. The younger group has benefited from the older group's persistence and the middle group's accuracy as it now has a language that has a sound grammatical basis but with which younger people have the confidence to experiment and adapt to their own cultural needs.

A third reason why older people's BSL varies is that some signs reflect the appearance of objects. For example, as technology has advanced the telephone has gone from a two handed device, to a dumb-bell shaped object and now to one with an aerial that is held in the palm of the hand. An older person may still use the sign of the two-piece phone whereas the younger will use the more modern sign. Signs also reflect the current culture. Younger Deaf people may not know the sign for 'pawn shop' whereas the sign for 'email' may not be known by some of the older generation (Sutton-Spence and Woll, 1999).

Deaf club: its importance and demise

For many older Deaf people the Deaf club has a great importance. The hub of the community, the Deaf club would be the place to pass on language, history and culture. It was the place for socializing, leisure activities and courting. Social workers for the Deaf would often do their work there; some clubs even had their church there. Bingo, storytelling and holidays were the stuff of Deaf clubs. Each geographical area had one and for leisure purposes, people often travelled only as far as the Deaf club or, on special occasions, to other Deaf clubs.

Times have changed, and younger Deaf people have spread their wings. The increased ease of transport and technology has meant that they can travel far and wide to meet Deaf people of their own age and do not frequent the Deaf club with the same dedication or enthusiasm. Deaf clubs are therefore becoming less influential in the Deaf community and some are closing down as their numbers dwindle. This may be perceived as a great loss to older adults who are not as able to embrace technology and travel in the same way as the younger generation. The Deaf club has possibly been replaced by the Internet as the place to find information; text phones, emails and pagers have become the way to communicate and pass on information. Finally, instead of the camaraderie among large numbers of the Deaf club, arising from members having been to the same Deaf school, the younger generation has wider educational options, attending a variety of schools, colleges and universities.

Social workers

Social workers for the Deaf have an unusual history. Initially the first social workers for the Deaf were all missionaries who, like their foreign travelling counterparts, had learned a language (sign) in order to minister to the community. Like other missionaries abroad they found that the tasks required of them exceeded that of spiritual welfare and that they were needed for many practical tasks including guidance and particularly for interpreting. In order to fulfil these goals, the social worker was often situated in the Deaf club and available at all hours to help Deaf people with almost any problem. As social and missionary work has developed professionally, it has become apparent that there is a fine line between helping a community and patronizing or controlling it (colonizing it).

Interpreting is now a profession in its own right and Deaf people are encouraged to book and instruct interpreters independently. Rather than being available at all times, social workers now tend to have separate offices and to take on specific pieces of casework for circumscribed lengths of time. For some older Deaf people, the degree of independence is not necessarily welcome.

The changing demographics of the Deaf community

Changes to the Deaf community can be attributed to a number of factors. First, inoculations being a relatively recent phenomenon, many of the older population would have been deafened via diseases such as rubella, scarlet fever, mumps or measles, which are generally decreasing in developed countries. Although inoculations against certain diseases are now commonly available, they are not taken up by all sections of the population equally. In the UK, white families started inoculating their children before black families, so the proportion of black to white Deaf people will have grown throughout the older person's lifetime. In immigrant and refugee populations where inoculation and medical intervention is limited, causes of deafness that are no longer seen in First World populations are relatively common. Furthermore, these Deaf immigrants have often received little formal educations so are arriving in the UK with little or no signed or spoken language skills.

Second, the survival rates of children who contracted diseases have changed. In our elderly cohort's youth, children who were multiply handicapped through rubella or meningitis may have died or would have been sent away to residential institutions leaving a population of Deaf people who tended not to have additional difficulties. Nowadays more multihandicapped people are surviving medical conditions such as rubella, meningitis and prematurity so the proportion of additional physical, mental and psychiatric difficulties of the population is changing.

Third, neonatal screening and cochlear implants have recently begun to impact on the Deaf community. Whereas, in the 1940s children would often have been of school age before their deafness was diagnosed, it is now relatively common to see small babies and toddlers with hearing aids or cochlear implants. With this new technology the emphasis may once more be on steering children towards oral, as opposed to signing, skills. Older Deaf people who have already seen their Deaf community dwindle as Deaf schools are closed in favour of mainstreaming and the Deaf clubs close as young people reject them, may also fear that their language and culture will be eradicated by these developments.

Deafness and service need

Although understanding the language, culture and history of older Deaf people can make for greater degrees of individual understanding, it is worth nothing if it does not affect service delivery.

With aging, so the need for services increases, in the domains of social, physical and mental wellbeing. Crucial to the accessing of all of these services is the recognition of sign language. Many older Deaf people can relate stories of decades of linguistic struggle, oppression and neglect and, as they approach their later years, it is understandable that they hope that the Deaf and hearing communities will share the effort of communication. However, instead of linguistic sanctuary the older Deaf person is more likely to find linguistic isolation.

Isolation

Changes in family structure have meant that older adults are included less in the extended family. Working women, and women who have children late, are less available to care for the older people in their family. Many people now move away from their hometowns leaving older people increasingly isolated and therefore potentially increasingly vulnerable.

A possible problem for all older adults, isolation affects the older Deaf person more acutely. All older people experience friends dying and families moving away but this may be more significant for the Deaf person, who probably had a restricted number of social contacts. Most Deaf people of this age group have married other Deaf people and it may be that the couple are each other's only regular exposure to sign. When one partner dies the surviving partner will then experience a linguistic and social void. Whereas younger people or hearing people who are housebound may be able to connect with others using the telephone or the Internet, these are unlikely solutions for the older Deaf person. The effect of isolation on mental and physical health is often dramatic.

Isolation is not just about being alone. As people get older they may need to access care or nursing homes. A service user reports, 'Deaf old people by themselves [in a nursing home] are in prison' (Smith, 2001). Many health and social care policies emphasize the patients' human right to receive services in their own first language and yet, in a mainstream (hearing) retirement or nursing home it is unlikely that staff will be able to sign or that there would be assistive devices such as flashing door bells or text phones. Some staff with good will and awareness may learn some sign but staff turnover in care settings is generally rapid. Dedicated facilities for Deaf elderly people are the obvious solution but, as with other services for Deaf people, the lack of a critical mass often prevents progress. The relatively small numbers of Deaf elderly people who require either a retirement home or a nursing home would mean that one home would have to service a wide geographical area, requiring residents to move far from their area of origin and any remaining friends or family. As with other provision for small populations the debate between integration and congregation continues.

Although there is very little provision for Deaf people in nursing or retirement homes, there is also very little provision for Deaf people who want to remain living independently. Service from home helps, nursing visits or care in the community are rarely provided in sign language and Deaf professionals are in short supply generally.

Frailties and illness

With old age comes an increase in physical health problems. Deaf people of all ages have difficulties accessing health care services and there is anecdotal evidence that, as a result, Deaf people have a reduced life expectancy and experience serious misdiagnosis or non-diagnosis of life threatening conditions (Fritschy, 2003). The chance of a health care professional signing is remote and it is often difficult to book, and sometimes not ideal to use, interpreters. Many conditions require immediate medical attention whereas interpreters generally require booking in advance. Some Deaf people do not bother to see the doctor, as they know the communication will be so unsatisfactory.

Deaf people already have a higher than average prevalence of ocular difficulties, so failing eyesight, which so often accompanies aging, is an additional burden. Fritschy (2000) found that 80% of his older Deaf residents had serious eye diseases and 20% needed immediate eye surgery. A lifelong fear for most Deaf people, deteriorating eyesight affects the ability to communicate freely and leads to a loss of independence. Failing eyesight in a hearing older person is also distressing but those with intact hearing can compensate somewhat for their poor vision. For all people, however, learning new ways of coping gets harder with age.

Unique to signing Deaf people, motoric conditions such as arthritis or Parkinson's disease will affect the ability to communicate. Likewise frailty due to poor health may make lifting the arms and hands compound the difficulty to communicate in a way that speaking when really frail does not.

Stroke is the third most common cause of death in the Western world after heart disease and cancer (Zorowitz, Gross and Polinski, 2002) and in the UK it is the most frequent cause of disability. The prevalence is such that it is likely that 100 BSL users will have strokes every year, with a third acquiring lasting disabilities. Stroke is most common in older people and can have effects in four areas: physical disability such as paralysis or hemiplegia, visual problems, cognitive impairments and language disorders. Each of these will have similar functional and psychosocial effects as with a hearing person but may also have a significant effect on the Deaf person's ability to communicate in sign language. Furthermore, the use of sign will restrict stroke patients' access to existing assessment and rehabilitation services.

Mental health services for elderly Deaf people

There is no service specifically for Deaf older adults with mental health problems in the UK. Services across Europe are variable and many countries having no services. Holland provides the most extensive services for Deaf older adults with and without mental health needs.

Whereas the most common reasons for older-adult admissions to psychiatric hospital include dementia, depression or psychosis (the prevalence of the range of mental health problems in the Deaf community is at least as high as in the general population), one of the most common reasons for staying in hospital is the lack of appropriate care homes or home care (Johnston et al., 1987).

Older people generally under-utilize mental health services despite having a higher than average prevalence of emotional problems. In the hearing services it is likely that bereavement issues, anxiety, depression and social difficulties, go untreated. This is at least as likely for the Deaf older adult.

The missing patients

In the absence of specialist mental health services for Deaf older adults it is not difficult to conclude that this client group is being poorly served. Some people who require services will be isolated by their linguistic status, meaning that no one is aware of their needs and that they are neither assessed nor treated. Some may be inappropriately placed in a service for hearing people where the chances of misdiagnosis and mistreatment increase with the staff's lack of deaf awareness and inability to sign, and at the very least they may be isolated and unhappy. They may be in a care home for Deaf people that provides for their linguistic and cultural needs but not for their mental health needs, resulting in unmanaged distress for both patient and staff. Finally, they may have been accepted into a psychiatric service for Deaf adults that cannot provide the expertise in gerontology and does not have provision for the patient to move into longer term accommodation once the assessment and initial treatment have been completed. In the absence of specialist services, each solution is a well meant compromise but actually gives the message that older Deaf people do not have the same rights as older hearing people. In this way they can be given a second-rate service by professionals who do not have the specific skills and experience for the task required of them. There is also pressure on staff expected to be experts in every niche of mental health provision but who often find themselves working outside of their competence.

Difficulties in differential diagnosis

Assessment and treatment of sign language users by non-signing health professionals is common but far from ideal. Access to interpreters is limited and both professional and interpreter will need a lot of experience before being able to offer anything like equity of service to the Deaf patient.

For example, the most common differential diagnosis in older adults is between depression and dementia. Depression often mimics dementia: memory problems, psychomotor retardation, and social withdrawal being symptoms of both disorders.

It is frequently missed by GPs in the older hearing population so it is likely to be missed even more in Deaf patients. Depression is often associated with lack of a confiding relationship and social difficulties, which may be more common in a Deaf elderly person. Protective factors include the presence of an intimate confidante (Evans and Katona, 1993) as well as the presence of necessary social skills – for example, assertiveness and communication skills – accessibility of day centres and counselling related to life events such as bereavement. The increased likelihood of linguistic and social isolation for the Deaf elderly person means that many of these psychological protective factors are not available to them.

To provide equity of service, the hearing professional will have to have knowledge of Deaf culture. Without this knowledge, clinical judgement is restricted and the professional may turn to standardized measurements such as cognitive assessments and symptom measurement question-naires. At this point professionals in both hearing services and Deaf services experience difficulty. Few psychometric tests or questionnaires have been validated or normed for use with Deaf people. Thus, baseline data are extremely hard to assess or predict, whether they concern the individual or the Deaf control group. Psychometric measures to predict the Deaf person's premorbid capabilities (used to assess whether there has been a deterioration) are worthless, as the Deaf person's education and English language skills may not be indicative of their intellectual capacity. Often testing Deaf people provides information, not on their cognitive abilities as intended, but on the amount of residual hearing they had or the signing skills of their teachers.

Education provision, particularly to older Deaf people, has not been comparable to that for hearing people. Even if psychometric assessment of the individual were possible, it is debatable whether comparison with a hearing group is useful or whether comparison should even be with other Deaf people. If the latter, then one is further handicapped by the lack of large sample research into the 'normal' Deaf brain and cognitive abilities. Furthermore, given the many different causes of deafness (some acquired at the same time as assaults on the brain, and some of genetic origin) and the different linguistic and educational opportunities, it is dif-ficult to group all Deaf people together for the sake of research. Little is known, for example, about how frontal lobe activity or memory present in the 'average' Deaf person. Likewise, little is known about emotional or psychiatric disorders in Deaf people. Thus, the risks of misdiagnosis and therefore of mistreatment by professionals, even if they use an interpreter, are raised for Deaf people. Even within specialist services for Deaf older adults, the lack of comprehensive literature or evidence base must reduce the chances of equity of service.

Behaviour problems

It is common for older people with additional needs to develop behav-iours that challenge the service. These can be explained by stress, separation anxiety, nocturnal confusion, attention seeking, loneliness, boredom, organic disorder, fear of the future and inability to cope, and sensory deprivation or overstimulation. In hearing older populations, problem behaviours are twice as common in those with cognitive impairment as in those without cognitive impairment (Cohen-Mansfield, Marx and Rosenthal, 1990).

Problem behaviours are generally three times more common in the Deaf population than in the hearing population (Meadow, 1981). Assessment of an older Deaf person with behaviour problems may therefore be complicated by their premorbid presentation, in which case sophisticated assessment is required. It may be that a psychosocial difficulty that is just manageable for a hearing person would be unmanageable given the additional strains of coping with deafness and communication difficulties.

Suicide

The importance of mental health provision for elderly people is exemplified by the very high rate of suicide among this group (Bennett and Collins, 2001). Older people who have a depressive background, and particularly when associated with insomnia, hypochondria, delusional guilt and illness, are a particular suicide risk. Older people are far more likely to die as a result of a suicide attempt than are their younger counterparts. Discussing suicidal ideation is a sensitive task and not one that is ideally conducted in one's second language or through an interpreter. Introducing interpreters to the possibility of this before a session will be necessary.

Developmental tasks

Brown and Pedder (1991) reported that the final task of development was to adjust to the running down of physical health, the possible loss of mental functioning, the death of friends/relatives and then eventually of ourselves. Erikson (1965) identified the task of old age as that of integration (a sense of completion or feeling of being part of a cycle of renewal) with failure to achieve this leading to despair and despondency. The final phase of life can therefore be a time of depression, regret and fear or an opportunity to gain a sense of completion and satisfaction. Others have described the developmental tasks of older age as being to review one's experiences, to reminisce, to process one's losses and put one's emotional baggage in order. There is so often an emphasis on physical care and organic explanations that the emotional work is often avoided in the hearing older population, so it is even less likely to be addressed if the older Deaf person does not have access to specialist services that can meet their needs.

Freud (1905) said that 'near or above the age of 50, the elasticity of mental processes, on which treatment depends, is as a rule lacking . . .'

While the hearing elderly are being treated in a more equitable way now (compared with hearing younger people) with counselling, family therapy, CBT and with psychodynamic therapies being explored with this age group, there is a total absence (in the UK) of such services for older Deaf people. It could be hypothesized that this lack of resources comes from a belief that Deaf people are less capable than hearing people of utilizing these therapies. Thus, while Freud's remark is no longer believed in relation to hearing older people, it is possibly still applied to Deaf older adults.

In addition to the overt level of interaction in therapy, there is the covert dimension, wherein the client and therapist react according to responses learned in the context of other relationships. One role of the therapist is to focus on what is happening during the therapy session and to use the transference to reflect the difficulties in relating the client's experiences in the broader world. The therapy session is therefore a microcosm of the client's broader relationships and environment. The lack of therapy for older Deaf people reflects the experience of the person in the broader world – one of isolation, of not being talked to, of not being asked questions, of being invisible.

Conclusion

Deaf elderly people share some experiences with their hearing peers but also have some unique experiences that have shaped their lives. They may be at greater risk of linguistic and social isolation than hearing elderly people and may therefore be at greater risk of mental health problems. The paucity of specialized services for Deaf elderly people may result in misdiagnosis and mistreatment of physical and mental health problems or may prevent the older Deaf adult from successfully addressing the existential tasks of aging. In most areas of the world Deaf older adults are not provided with services comparable to those provided to their hearing peers.

References

Bayley R (2002) Variation in ASL: the case of DEAF. Conference presentation to the Deafway III, Galludet University, Washington DC.

Bennett AT, Collins KA (2001) Elderly suicide: a 10-year retrospective study. American Journal of Forensic Medicine and Pathology 22(2): 169–72.

Brown D, Pedder J (1991) Introduction to Psychotherapy. 2 edn. London: Tavistock/Routledge.

Cohen-Mansfield J, Marx MS, Rosenthal AS (1990) Dementia and agitation in nursing home residents: how are they related? Psychology of Aging 5(1): 3–8.

Davis A (2001) The prevalence of deafness and hearing impairment. In Graham J, Martin M (eds) Ballantyne's Deafness, 6th Edition, pp. 10–25.

Erickson EH (1965) Childhood and Society. Harmondsworth: Penguin Books.

Evans S, Katona C (1993) Epidemiology of depressive symptoms in elderly primary care attenders. Dementia 4(6): 327–33.

Freud S (1905) 'On Psychotherapy' Standard ed VII. London: Hogarth Press.

Fritschy OBM (2000) Deaf seniors and mental health. Conference presentation to the European Society of Mental Health and Deafness, Copenhagen, 2000.

Fritschy OBM (2003) What's happening in Europe for the elderly deaf? Present situation of the services. Keynote presentation to the European Society of Mental Health and Deafness, Austria.

Harris JP, Anderson JP, Novak R (1995) An outcome study of cochlear implants in deaf patients. Archives of Otolaryngology, Head and Neck Surgery 121: 398–404.

Johnston M, Wakeling A, Graham N, Stokes F (1987) Cognitive impairment, emotional disorder and length of stay of elderly patients in a district general hospital. British Journal of Medical Psychology 60(2): 133–9.

Meadow KP (1981) Studies of behaviour problems of deaf children. In Stein L, Mindel E, Jabaley T (eds) Deafness and Mental Health. New York: Grune & Stratton, pp. 3–22.

Smith M (2001) The Housing Needs of Older Deaf People: the Leeds Experience. Leeds: Leeds City Council.

Sullivan P, Brookhouser P, Scanlon M (2000) Maltreatment of Deaf and hard of hearing children. In Hindley P, Kitson N (ed.) (2000) Mental Health and Deafness. London: Whurr, pp. 149–84.

Sutton-Spence R, Woll B (1993) The status and function of fingerspelling in BSL. In Marschark M, Clark M (eds) Psychological Perspectives on Deafness. Hillsdale NJ: Erlbaum, pp. 185–208.

Sutton-Spence R, Woll B (1999) The Linguistics of British Sign Language: an Introduction. Cambridge: Cambridge University Press.

Zorowitz RD, Gross E, Polinski DM (2002) The stroke survivor. Disability and Rehabilitation 24(13): 666–79.

CHAPTER 23

Working with survivors of
sexual abuse who are Deaf

SUE O'ROURKE AND NIGEL BEAIL

Introduction

Clinicians frequently have to face the issue of working with survivors of
child sexual abuse (CSA). Prevalence figures vary according to precise
methodology, but it is estimated that around 10% of the adult population
may have suffered some form of sexual abuse as children. Figures rise to
30%–33% of the female outpatient psychiatric population (Cahill,
Llewelyn and Pearson, 1991a). The literature on this subject is vast and it
is a challenge to distil the relevant research, evaluate the various treatment approaches and apply them to an individual. An attempt will be
made here to do this in order to apply the literature to work with Deaf
people. At first glance deafness may not appear to be a 'special case' and,
of course, Deaf people are not so different from hearing people. However,
the language and culture of deafness, the history – shared and individual
– of Deaf people in relation to the hearing majority, all impact on the
understanding of abuse and the way it is approached in therapy.

This chapter will examine the literature pertaining to the treatment of
survivors of CSA, focusing on literature with an empirical basis in examining efficacy of different treatment approaches. The aim is to then relate
these findings to work with Deaf survivors.

It is acknowledged that a history of CSA is associated with a variety of
psychological disorders in later life, including eating disorders, depression and borderline personality disorder (BPD) (Cahill, Llewelyn and
Pearson, 1991a; Brown, 1997; Pettigrew and Burcham, 1997). Most of the
literature pertains to women and no attempt will be made here to address
issues specific to men who have suffered CSA. The assumption that the
key issues are relevant to both men and women may not be entirely valid,
but it is beyond the scope of this review to discuss men as a subset of survivors, as well as Deaf people. For a review of the literature relating to
male survivors of abuse, see Boyd and Beail (1994).

Long-term effects of CSA: treatment approaches

Although the association between a history of CSA and adult psychological disorder is clear, it must be noted that the causality is merely inferred and there is a lack of evidence relating to the psychological processes involved, mediating between the experience of abuse as a child and difficulties in adulthood (Finkelhor, 1984; Cahill, Llewelyn and Pearson, 1991a).

Jehu (1988) suggests a range of interventions based on idiographic analysis of the particular needs of the patient (for example, assertiveness training, problem-solving skills and therapy for sexual dysfunction). This again reflects the fact that CSA is associated with a multiplicity of later difficulties. As for working with the abuse itself, Jehu (1988) in common with others, emphasizes the importance of an empathic, non-judgemental therapeutic style, enabling disclosure in the context of a safe therapeutic relationship. The importance attached to detailed disclosure depends on the theoretical stance taken. A behavioural approach suggests detailed and repeated discussion of the abuse can help desensitise the client to memories of abuse, which may have been avoided (Cahill, Llewelyn and Pearson, 1991b). Others emphasize exploring the meaning of the abuse for the client, rather than emphasizing the detail (Jehu, 1988).

Descriptions of guilt and shame felt by survivors of CSA are evident throughout the literature and the re-attribution of responsibility to the offender emerges as a goal of therapy. Other descriptions suggest the therapy process is akin to bereavement, as the client mourns lost innocence and lost childhood (Cahill, Llewelyn and Pearson, 1991b).

Despite slightly differing theoretical approaches, there is broad agreement about the goals and components of therapy. However, there is a lack of empirical work in this area and literature tends to be anecdotal and ideologically driven.

Case study : intervention

Ms E was a 32-year-old woman referred to mental health services with a history of depression and thoughts of self-harm. Recent angry outbursts and difficulties in her relationship with her children had led to concerns for their welfare. After several months of therapy aimed at coping with her anger, she disclosed she had been sexually abused from 11–17 by her uncle. Therapy focused on the abuse for some time, allowing her to vent her feelings which she had never done before. The uncle had now died and Ms E was adamant that no one else should know. She benefited from the experience of disclosing the abuse in a safe therapeutic relationship and being believed. Therapy involved discussing feelings of guilt and re-attributing blame wholly to the perpetrator. Links were made between past experiences and the current difficulties in relationships and managing her emotions.

Some rigour is in evidence when focusing on clients' beliefs or thoughts, related to 'self-image and esteem'. Cahill, Llewelyn and Pearson (1991b) report a study by Jehu, Klassen and Gazan (1986) in which clinically and statistically significant improvements in clients' beliefs and mood states were found following therapy involving:

• making clients aware of their beliefs;
• facilitating recognition of distortion in beliefs; and
• substituting more accurate beliefs.

Some of the literature pertaining to treatment of Post-Traumatic Stress Disorder (PTSD) is relevant to the treatment of survivors of CSA. A paper by Smucker and Niederee (1995) describes a treatment for incest-related PTSD using imaginal exposure and rescripting. The former involves exposing the individual to the traumatic event in their imagination, under the guidance of the therapist, with the aim that they gradually habituate to the trauma with it therefore becoming less anxiety inducing. Rescripting enables the victim to 'rewrite the script' of the event, again in their imagination, allowing a feeling of control and reducing the potency of the event.

The case example cited by Smucker and Niederee is useful in outlining the approach and reported improvements suggest the individual no longer met diagnostic criteria for PTSD after 8 sessions. Unfortunately, no empirical data are presented, nor is there any description of general level of functioning or longer term gain.

Cognitive behavioural treatment

A paper by Echeburua et al. (1997) is an example of treating survivors of CSA who meet the diagnostic criteria for PTSD. In this study 20 women who were victims of sexual aggression, meeting the criteria for PTSD, were treated by either gradual self-exposure and cognitive re-structuring or progressive relaxation, on a weekly basis for 6 weeks; the latter being an attention control. Assessment tools were administered before and after treatment and at 3, 6 and 12 months follow ups. Results suggest that self-exposure/cognitive restructuring was superior to the control intervention at the end of treatment and in all follow-up periods. Although such results appear impressive at first glance, and the authors conclude, 'that the cognitive behavioural treatment has been proven effective', there are a number of limitations to this study. The authors concede that generalization is difficult, due to the small sample size, but contend that the sample was 'homogenous' as all met the diagnostic criteria for PTSD. However, the group consisted of victims of CSA (n = 9), which usually occurred more than 10 years previously, and victims of adult rape (n = 11), which occurred more recently. To conclude that these groups are homogenous based on diagnostic criteria – a rather blunt instrument – would appear somewhat hasty. Developmental stage of the victim, relationship to the perpetrator, use of weapons and other details relating to the precise nature of the offence, might all be important.

The measures used include well researched psychometric instruments, such as the Beck Depression Inventory (BDI) and the State-Trait Anxiety Inventory (STAI) with reliability and validity reported. Also used was the 'Scale of Severity of Post-Traumatic Stress Disorder Symptoms' (Echeburua et al., 1997). The psychometric properties of this measure are not reported, presumably as it has not been standardized. The study, which uses this scale to assess the presence/absence and degree of PTSD, would clearly have been strengthened by the use of a standardized instrument. Similarly, the Scale of Adaptation (Echeburua et al., 1997), which purports to reflect the degree to which sexual aggression affects daily life, has no data to support its reliability and validity.

Despite these limitations, the strength of this study is in suggesting that a brief intervention may have long-term benefits for victims of sexual assault with heterogeneous histories, but possibly similar psychological profiles. It also follows up subjects for 12 months and, as such, was the first study to look at longer term outcome. Given the large numbers of individuals who have suffered CSA, future research involving a larger sample using similar methodology and with improved measures, would significantly add to the field.

Group work

Group work using a cognitive-behavioural approach is similarly lacking in empirical bases. The University of Manitoba project was evaluated using a client satisfaction questionnaire and results were favourable. This project conceptualized the treatment as consisting of two domains:

- the general therapeutic conditions; and
- specific treatments for particular difficulties (for example, mood disturbances).

What emerges from this and other studies using self-report, is increased self-esteem and that the most helpful aspect of therapy is meeting others who share the same experience. More functional measures show less consistent improvement (Cahill, Llewelyn and Pearson, 1991b).

A literature review by de Jong and Gorey (1996) aimed to compare short-term and long-term group therapy for survivors of abuse. They too found very few empirical studies, citing only seven in which data are presented, compared with many theoretical or anecdotal articles. Of these seven studies only one involved long-term work and several were criticized on methodological grounds. The authors conclude that any number of unreported factors may have accounted for changes in short-term groups, whereas the central question of the relative efficacy of short versus long-term group work is, as yet, unanswerable.

Child sexual abuse and deafness

Until recently, reports of CSA in the Deaf population have been largely anecdotal (for example, Vernon and Rich, 1997). Kennedy (1990) found that teachers suspect that a large number of Deaf children have suffered abuse. However, a recent study suggests that 40% of Deaf adults in a community population may have been abused as children (Ridgeway, 1997). In this study, 102 Deaf adults, aged 16–60, were interviewed by a Deaf psychologist, using British Sign Language (BSL). The investigation of CSA was part of a wider study looking at mental health problems in the Deaf community. Ridgeway states that 'a number of studies have indicated that Deaf people are at higher risk of abuse', but fails to reference this claim. In her study, the interviews included an assurance that anyone disclosing abuse would be offered counselling. While the ethical reasons behind this are self-evident, the effect of such a 'reward' for disclosure on a population with little access to services is indeterminate.

The published preliminary findings of this study give little detail of methodology, but Ridgeway (personal communication, 1999) confirms that CSA refers to rape or attempted rape as defined by the Law Society. This narrow definition of CSA makes the results all the more remarkable. Although the interviewer was a native BSL-user, it is unfortunate that exact transcripts of questions are not available, as this prevents examination of the rigour of the interview process. However, the author presents these as 'preliminary findings' and more detail may be available for scrutiny at a later date.

There is no empirical research literature pertaining to the treatment of Deaf adults who have been sexually abused as children. Papers by Schwarz (1994 and 1995) bemoan the lack of accessibility of services to Deaf people and the use of non-specialist therapists who enter into therapy with an interpreter, believing this to be sufficient. Psychological therapy by a signing Deaf specialist is recommended, but beyond this there are no specific treatment considerations. Other workers in the field discuss specific considerations in accessing services and therapy. These include the Deaf person's lack of awareness of the possibility of disclosure, fears of rejection by the small Deaf community and fears of trusting the 'all-knowing hearing therapist' (Doornkate and Zwart, 1998).

Treatment

With regard to actual treatment content, a paper by Sullivan et al. (1992) looks at a programme for treating Deaf adolescents who have been abused, which may be useful when considering Deaf adult treatment protocols. In this American study 72 Deaf children aged 12 to 16 had been abused at a residential school. All were offered psychotherapy services, free of charge, but parents of 37 declined the offer, providing a no-treatment control group. All the children were rated on the Child Behaviour Checklist (CBC) (Achenbach and Edelbrock, 1983) before and after treatment, and independent t-tests ruled out pre-existing differences between the groups. The model of therapy used was based on Sullivan and Scanlan's recommendations for use with handicapped children (Sullivan et al., 1992). Treatment goals included educational components such as basic information about normal human sexuality and interpersonal relationships and developing a vocabulary to label emotions and feelings.

Therapy was carried out by qualified counsellors with specific training in the psychology of deafness, who were fluent in sign. Post-treatment ratings were carried out by raters, who were described as unaware of which children were receiving therapy.

Analyses of variance showed a strong treatment effect for both boys and girls, which was maintained at one year. By the authors' own admission, findings relating to girls are tentative, owing to the small numbers (n = 21) and the use of parametric statistics is questionable in this case.

This study provides evidence for the effectiveness of some intervention in ameliorating problems in adolescents who have been abused. However, it fails to demonstrate the specific value of this intervention, as it lacks an appropriate attention-control group. It may be that empathic attention and other non-specific aspects of therapy are sufficient to bring about such results. In addition, the assertion that raters of behaviour were unaware of which group the adolescents were in is questionable. Since they were carers/house-parents, it is reasonable to assume that their charges might discuss matters with them.

The study, by its own admission, provides outcome data without addressing psychological process. Neither does it offer any methodology specific to Deaf people. Indeed, the conclusion might be that some therapeutic intervention is worthwhile for Deaf children, as for hearing children. Having said that, what distinguishes this package of treatment for young Deaf people from that offered to hearing adult survivors is a strong education component. Given the lack of access to information experienced by Deaf people, one cannot assume the same degree of knowledge about sexual, relationship or other matters. Thus, this approach is worth considering for Deaf adults where the presentation may indicate a lack of basic information about sex, sexuality and relationships.

The literature on CSA for hearing people recommends group work, reporting significant enhancement of self-esteem and benefits to affect (see, for example, de Jong and Gorey, 1996). However, the nature of the Deaf community, which is extremely small, may make it difficult for group members to avoid meeting each other socially. This raises questions about confidentiality and the appropriateness of group work for this client group, as 'safety' and 'trust' are deemed all important. Indeed, experience would suggest that recruitment might be difficult as a result of fears of confidentiality being broken within the Deaf community.

Theoretical issues

Thus far, the literature indicates an association between CSA and adult psychopathology in Deaf and hearing people alike, but says little about causality and mediating psychological processes. A consensus of clinical opinion suggests that some therapeutic intervention within the context of a safe therapeutic relationship is valuable, and a number of interventions may have beneficial effects on self-esteem and subjective measures of wellbeing (Cahill, Llewelyn and Pearson, 1991b).

The dual representation theory of Post-Traumatic Stress Disorder, as discussed by Brewin, Dalgleish and Joseph (1996), offers a cognitive theory of the psychological sequelae of trauma, including single occasion or repeated CSA. This theory, accounting for much experimental and clinical data, conceives of PTSD as unsuccessful and incomplete processing of emotional trauma. It proposes that there is more than one type of cognitive representation of trauma – there being verbally accessible memories (VAMs) which can be openly retrieved from autobiographical memory, and situational accessible memories (SAMs), which are non-verbal memories that may be triggered by, among other things, therapy. The theory proposes integration of traumatic memories into the sense of self as a satisfactory end point of processing emotional trauma. Conversely, incomplete integration is seen to lead to the clinical picture of PTSD.

The clinical task then becomes one of facilitating integration. One aspect of this is to detect and overcome inhibitory processes, which prevent the completion of the processing of the trauma, such as dissociation.

Although the dual representation theory stands up well, in terms of existing evidence, a specific treatment strategy and resulting outcome research are, as yet, not forthcoming. However, one related area is work that focuses on dissociative phenomena as a mediating factor between the experience of abuse and later psychological disorder.

Dissociation

The phenomenon of dissociation refers to mental states of absence of differing degrees, some of which may be functional – for example, the numbness after trauma allowing the individual to recover sufficiently before dealing with emotional pain. Mild dissociative states occur in, for example, day dreaming, while at the extreme end, dissociative disorders can cause considerable distress. These include dissociative amnesia (a loss of memory for traumatic events) and dissociative identity disorder.

With regard to trauma, dissociation may involve flashbacks: from a vague sense of familiarity linked to the abuse, to traumatic and intrusive memories triggered by a variety of everyday cues. Often a key aspect of diagnosis of post-traumatic stress disorder, flashbacks are a dissociative experience, involving a state of absence, derealisation and identity confusion (Kennerley, 1996).

The concept of dissociation as a mediator between sexual abuse and the manifestation of psychopathology gains credence on theoretical and empirical grounds. Dissociation, as a means of coping, can be conceived of as an automatic or volitional means of avoiding intolerable cognitions associated with abuse (Young, 1994). High scores on measures of dissociation are also associated with a variety of disorders that are, in turn, associated with a history of CSA, such as borderline personality disorder (BPD), PTSD and eating disorders (Ross-Gower et al, 1998).

A study by Ross-Gower et al. (1998) investigated the mediating role of dissociation in a population of 45 consecutive referrals of women to a clinical psychology department. Of the 45, 28 had experienced some form of abuse, and 17 no abuse. Measures of psychological symptoms (Delusions-Symptoms-Sates-Inventory, DSSI), borderline personality (Borderline Personality Syndrome Index, BSI) and the Dissociative Experiences Scale (DESII) were administered. Acceptable levels of reliability and validity were reported. Abuse versus no abuse groups were compared. Multiple regression analyses were used for testing the mediating role of dissociation between reported CSA and psychopathology – although to meet statistical criteria, the independent variable was abuse versus no abuse (i.e. dichotomous) rather than looking at levels of abuse. A stepwise regression approach suggested dissociation as a complete mediator between CSA and subsequent psychopathology, in the sense of presence/absence of difficulties. However, it was unable to explain degrees of disturbance associated with reduction in levels of dissociative processes. They suggest cognitive and behavioural techniques to increase awareness of cognitive and emotional states, leading to dissociation as a critical treatment goal. If dissociation is seen as extreme avoidance of disturbing cognitions, then a failure to deal with the process prior to actually making explicit unpleasant abuse-related cognitions in therapy, would predict an inability to engage. As yet, the efficacy of addressing dissociative phenomena as a precursor to other intervention is unclear. However, this study would appear to offer a theoretical framework to understand how the trauma of CSA may lead to a variety of difficulties in later life and also possibilities for the development of future therapies.

Use of cognitive-behavioural therapy

Kennerley (1996) also suggests that cognitive-behaviour therapy (CBT) can be brought to bear on dissociative symptoms. She outlines a process of assessment and therapy involving the identification of triggers for dissociation; managing the dissociation reaction by teaching skills of distraction and 'grounding'; cognitive restructuring and graded exposure to the affect and cognitions leading to dissociation. Evidence is cited that exposure to traumatic imagery in PTSD does not lead to habituation when clients depersonalize or dissociate and it is suggested that once the client has a repertoire of skills in order not to dissociate, other areas of trauma such as flashbacks and self-harm can be tackled (Kennerley, 1996).

Evidence for the efficacy of using CBT to treat dissociative phenomena is anecdotal – Kennerley (1996) gives 4 case examples to illustrate the approach – or indirect, as in the case of Vaughan and Tarrier (1992). There is a need for empirical work to investigate the efficacy of this treatment approach.

Psychological processes and deafness

There is no attempt to date to address psychological process when considering the effect of CSA on Deaf people in particular. However, research from the non-deaf literature indicates the role of self-denigrating thoughts and dysfunctional beliefs can be related to deafness.

The fact that, by virtue of numbers and relationships to adults in authority, most Deaf children who are victims of CSA will be abused by hearing adults, suggests that thoughts and beliefs relating to deafness and hearing may be important when discussing cognitions related to abuse. The complication of a hearing therapist working with a Deaf client raises additional issues of trust, which may be explored within a cognitive approach, looking at thoughts, beliefs and assumptions about deaf and hearing people.

Taking the dual representation theory of PTSD, the fact that Deaf young people are frequently disadvantaged and may have difficulty making sense of what is happening to them, suggests that they may be at particular risk of being unable to engage in emotional processing that would allow for the integration of the trauma. Brewin, Dalgleish and Joseph (1996) cite a number of other reasons preventing integration, including a lack of a confidante or unwillingness to confide. In the case of deafness, one might add being unable to communicate effectively with parents or other hearing adults, being unaware of being *able* to discuss such matters and not having the 'words' (signs) to do so, either in terms of communication to others or in understanding oneself.

The assessment of dissociation in Deaf people is difficult, as questionnaire measures are not reliable or valid for this group, even when an attempt is made to translate them into BSL (Cole, 1989). Behavioural characteristics indicating dissociation may present differently – for example, a glance away in a hearing person may be of little significance, but in a Deaf person means they are no longer 'listening' and are cutting themselves off. Thus, the investigation of dissociative phenomena in Deaf people would appear to be a worthwhile area for future research. Deaf people would appear to be at increased risk for problems in this area, having to negotiate their identity in a hearing world, where to be Deaf is often to be stigmatized and ostracized (Higgins, 1980).

Case study: deafness

Mr D was a 42-year-old Deaf man referred for a neuropsychological assessment. With a history of impulsive and aggressive behaviour, the possibility of an organic basis to his difficulties was raised, possibly linked to his cause of deafness and meningitis. Neuropsychological assessment took place over several weeks and a good rapport was established. During the final session, he disclosed he had been sexually abused at his residential Deaf school by a hearing 'carer' and asked for further appointments to discuss this. In the weeks and months that followed, he described how, at age 8, he was unable to tell his parents what was happening, as he did not have the language to explain and they could not sign. He also gave many examples of deafness-related thoughts connected to the abuse, such as 'If I wasn't deaf, this wouldn't have happened to me'; 'hearing people always abuse people'; 'I am useless because I'm deaf'; 'If I hadn't been so stupid (because I'm deaf), I could have stopped it happening.'

It became clear that at this young age the traumatic experience of being sexually abused by a hearing person had begun to shape his view of how deaf people are treated by hearing people in some position of authority over them. This had led to many hostile encounters with hearing people over the years, further reinforcing his view of how he could expect to be treated.

Conclusions

There is a plethora of literature on the effects of CSA on adults but a lack of empirical research. Similarly, there is consensus about general components of treatment, but little evidence on outcome and almost no work addressing psychological process. The dual representation theory of PTSD and the role of dissociation offer a theoretical understanding of the long-term sequelae of CSA and is possibly an important component in therapy. However, there is no outcome research to date.

As for working with Deaf people, there is some suggestion that rates of abuse may be particularly high (Ridgeway, 1997), but there has been little work on treatment specific to this population. Prior knowledge of deafness suggests that an increased educational component may be necessary, and Sullivan et al. (1992) provides some guidelines for this, based on a programme for Deaf adolescents. Lack of access to information, for example, relating to laws regarding underage sex, may be evident in assumptions and misunderstandings. Thus, reattribution of responsibility may involve a strong educational component.

The hearing literature suggests self-denigrating thoughts are a target for cognitive restructuring. In Deaf people, this would appear to necessitate an assessment of thoughts about deafness. For example, the notion of 'if I had been hearing this would not have happened' may be addressed in therapy. Avoidance of negative thoughts by means of dissociation is suggested as a barrier to engaging in therapy and the means by which the traumatic effects of abuse are maintained to adult life. This has not been considered in Deaf people, but the assessment of dissociation in this group would appear to be an important and interesting area for future research.

References

Achenbach TM, Edelbrock C (1983) Manual for the Child Behavior Checklist and Revised Child Behavior Profile. Burlington VT, University of Vermont, Dept of Psychiatry.

Brown L (1997) Child physical and sexual abuse and eating disorders: a review of the links and personal comments on the treatment process. Australia and New Zealand Journal of Psychology 31: 194–9.

Boyd J, Beaill N (1994) Gender issues in male sexual abuse. Clinical Psychology Forum 64: 35–8.

Brewin C, Dalgleish T, Joseph S (1996) A dual representation theory of post-traumatic stress disorder. Psychological Review 103(4): 670–86.

Cahill C, Llewelyn SP, Pearson C (1991a) Long-term effects of sexual abuse which occurred in childhood: a review. British Journal of Clinical Psychology 30: 117–30.

Cahill C, Llewelyn SP, Pearson C (1991b) Treatment of sexual abuse which occurred in childhood: a review. British Journal of Clinical Psychology 30: 1–13.

Cole SH (1989) Cultural Identity and Coping in Deafness: A study of Deaf Adolescents' Problems and Self-Perceptions. Unpublished thesis, University of Guildford.

de Jong TL, Gorey KM (1996) Short-term versus long-term group work with female survivors of child sexual abuse: a brief meta-analytic review. Social Work with Groups 19(1): 19–27.

Doornkate L, Zwart E (1998) Organisational and Therapeutic Issues. Paper presented at the British Society of Mental Health and Deafness.

Echeburua E, Corral P, Zubizarreta I, Sarasua B (1997) Psychological treatment of chronic post-traumatic stress disorder in victims of sexual aggression. Behaviour Modification 12(4): 433–56.

Finkelhor D (1984) Child Sexual Abuse: New Theory and Research. New York: The Free Press.

Higgins PC (1980) Outsiders in a Hearing World: A Sociology of Deafness. London: Sage Publications.

Jehu D (1988) Beyond Sexual Abuse: Therapy with Women who were Childhood Victims. Chichester: Wiley.

Jehu D, Klassen C, Gazan M (1986) Cognitive restructuring of distorted beliefs associated with childhood sexual abuse. Journal of Social Work and Human Sexuality 4: 49–69.

Kennedy M (1990) The Abused Deaf Child: The Role of the Social Worker with Deaf People. A Report on the Conference by the National Council of Social Workers and Deaf People and the NDCS keep Deaf Children Safe Project.

Kennerley H (1996) Cognitive therapy of dissociative symptoms associated with trauma. British Journal of Clinical Psychology 35: 325–40.

Pettrigrew J, Burcham J (1997) Characteristics of CSA and adult psychopathology in female psychiatric patients. Australia and New Zealand Journal of Psychology 31: 200–7.

Ridgeway S (1997) Deaf people and psychological health – some preliminary findings. Deaf Worlds 13(1): 9–18.

Ridgeway S (1999) Personal Communication.

Ross-Gower J, Waller G, Tyson M, Elliott P (1998) Reported sexual abuse and subsequent psychopathology among women attending psychology clinics: the mediating role of dissociation. British Journal of Clinical Psychology 37: 313–26.

Schwarz DB (1994) Techniques in treating survivors of CSA: problematic areas in their application to the Deaf population. Jadara 28: 39–45.

Schwarz DB (1995) Effective teaching in treating survivors of CSA: problematic areas in their application to the deaf population. Sexuality and Disability 13: 135–44.

Smucker MR, Niederee J (1995) Treating incest-related PTSD and pathogenic schemas through imaginal exposure and rescripting. Cognitive and Behavioural Practice 2: 63–93.

Sullivan PM, Scanlan JM, Brookhouser PE, Shulte LE, Knutsan JF (1992) The effects of psychotherapy on behaviour problems of sexually abused deaf children. Child Abuse and Neglect 16: 297–307.

Vaughan K, Tarrier N (1992) The use of image habituation training with post-traumatic stress disorders. British Journal of Psychiatry 161: 658–64.

Vernon M, Rich S (1997) Paedophilia and deafness. American Annals of the Deaf 142: 300–11.

Young J (1994) Cognitive Therapy for Personality Disorders: A Schema-Focused Approach. Sarasota: Professional Resource Press.

Index